Sinonasal Tumors

Sinonasal Tumors

Alexander G Chiu MD
Professor and Chief
Division of Otolaryngology-Head and Neck Surgery
Department of Surgery
University of Arizona
Tucson, AZ

Vijay R Ramakrishnan MD
Assistant Professor
Department of Otolaryngology-Head and Neck Surgery
University of Colorado
Aurora, CO

Jeffrey D Suh MD
Assistant Professor
Division of Otolaryngology-Head and Neck Surgery
University of California, Los Angeles
Los Angeles, CA

Foreword

Eugene N Myers
MD FACS FRCS Edin (Hon)

JAYPEE BROTHERS MEDICAL PUBLISHERS (P) LTD

New Delhi • Panama City • London

Jaypee Brothers Medical Publishers (P) Ltd

Headquarter

Jaypee Brothers Medical Publishers (P) Ltd
4838/24, Ansari Road, Daryaganj
New Delhi 110 002, India
Phone: +91-11-43574357
Fax: +91-11-43574314
Email: jaypee@jaypeebrothers.com

Overseas Offices

JP Medical Ltd,
83 Victoria Street London
SW1H 0HW (UK)
Phone: +44-2031708910
Fax: +02-03-0086180
Email: info@jpmedpub.com

Jaypee-Highlights Medical Publishers Inc
City of Knowledge, Bld 237, Clayton
Panama City, Panama
Phone: 507-317-0160
Fax: +50-73-010499
Email: cservice@jphmedical.com

Website: www.jaypeebrothers.com
Website: www.jaypeedigital.com

Inquiries for bulk sales may be solicited at: jaypee@jaypeebrothers.com

Publisher: Jitendar P Vij
Publishing Director: Tarun Duneja
Cover Design: Seema Dogra

Sinonasal Tumors

First Edition: **2012**

ISBN 978-93-5025-282-6

Printed at Ajanta Offset & Packagings Ltd., New Delhi

Dedicated to

This book is dedicated to my parents Paul and Elizabeth, my wife Michelle and children Nicolas and Aidan in whom words are never enough to recognize the support, sacrifice and inspiration they have given me throughout my life. I would also like to recognize my mentors Drs Vaughan and Kennedy for their lessons in medicine, humility and compassion, and my former partners Drs Palmer and Cohen for their advice, friendship and support.

Alexander G Chiu

This book would not exist without the tireless efforts of prior generations of surgeons and researchers, and their patients—who have provided the wealth of information inside. I must personally acknowledge the many professors whose time and patience have contributed to my professional development, and are too numerous to single out. Special thanks to my parents and brother, who have also sacrificed many things along the way, and to CMM who has always inspired me to do great things.

Vijay R Ramakrishnan

I would like to dedicate this work to my parents Hong Won and Kilja Suh and my brother Brian and thank them for their love and support throughout the years. To my wife Anne, thank you for being my inspiration and for your patience and understanding during the drafting of this book. I would also like to show my deepest appreciation to Drs Kennedy, Chiu, Palmer, Cohen, and Blackwell, and thank them for their outstanding teaching and invaluable mentorship.

Jeffrey D Suh

Contributors

Adappa, Nithin MD
Rhinology Fellow
Department of Otorhinolaryngology-
Head and Neck Surgery
University of Pennsylvania
Philadelphia, PA

Blackwell, Keith E MD
Professor
Division of Otolaryngology-
Head and Neck Surgery
University of California, Los Angeles
Los Angeles, CA

Bleier, Benjamin S MD
Clinical Instructor
Department of Otology and
Laryngology
Massachusetts Eye and Ear Infirmary
Harvard Medical School
Boston, Massachusetts

Borges, Thomas MD
Assistant Professor, Neuroradiology
Department of Radiology
University of Colorado
Department of Radiology
Academic Division
Aurora, CO

Chiu, Alexander G MD
Professor and Chief
Division of Otolaryngology-
Head and Neck Surgery
Department of Surgery
University of Arizona
Tucson, AZ

Costantino, Peter D MD FACS
Executive Director
New York Head and Neck Institute
(NYHNI)
Senior Vice-President
Head and Neck Surgery Service Line
The North Shore-LIJ Health System
Director
Center for Cranial Base Surgery
NYHNI at Lenox Hill
Hospital-Manhattan
Eye and Ear Infirmary

Desai, Kena MD
Resident Physician
Department of Medicine
University of Colorado
Aurora, CO

Geiger, Geoffrey A MD
Department of Radiation Oncology
University of Pennsylvania
Philadelphia, PA

Hou, Andrew MD
Neuroradiology Fellow
Department of Radiology
University of Colorado
Department of Radiology
Academic Division
Aurora, CO

Kane, Madeleine A MD PhD
Professor of Medicine
Division of Medical Oncology
University of Colorado
Aurora, CO

Kennedy, David W MD
Professor
Department of Otorhinolaryngology-
Head and Neck Surgery
University of Pennsylvania
Philadelphia, PA

Kokot, Niels MD
Assistant Professor
Department of Otolaryngology-
Head and Neck Surgery
Keck School of Medicine
University of Southern California
Los Angeles, CA

Lal, Devyani MD
Assistant Professor, Mayo College
of Medicine and Senior Associate
Consultant, Department of
Otorhinolaryngology, Mayo Clinic
Phoenix, Arizona

Lee, John MD FRCSC
Department of Otolaryngology-
Head and Neck Surgery
University of Toronto, St Michael's
Hospital, Toronto
Ontario, Canada

Lin, Alexander MD
Department of Radiation Oncology
Abramson Cancer Center
University of Pennsylvania
Philadelphia, PA

Lin, Derrick T MD FACS
Assistant Professor
Department of Otology and
Laryngology, Massachusetts Eye
and Ear Infirmary, Harvard Medical
School, Boston, Massachusetts

Perez-Mitchell, Carlos MD
Director, Center for Cranial Base, Head and Neck Surgery, Hima Health San Pablo Group–Caguas, Caguas, PR
Assistant Professor
University of Puerto Rico School Medicine, Department of Otolaryngology-Head and Neck Surgery, Medical Science Campus
Rio Piedras, PR

Morong, Sharon MD MSc
PGY-4 Resident
Department of Otolaryngology-Head and Neck Surgery
University of Toronto
Toronto, ON

Nayak, Jayakar V MD PhD
Assistant Professor
Department of Otolaryngology-Head and Neck Surgery
Stanford University
Palo Alto, CA

Palmer, James N MD
Associate Professor
Chief, Division of Rhinology
Department of Otorhinolaryngology-Head and Neck Surgery
University of Pennsylvania
Philadelphia, PA

Patel, Zara M MD
Clinical Instructor
Department of Otolaryngology-Head and Neck Surgery
Stanford Sinus Center
Stanford University
Palo Alto, CA

Quon, Harry MD MS
Associate Professor
Co-Director
Head and Neck Multidisciplinary Program, Department of Radiation Oncology and Molecular Radiation Sciences, Johns Hopkins Medicine
Baltimore, MD

Ramakrishnan, Vijay R MD
Assistant Professor
Division of Otolaryngology-Head and Neck Surgery
Univerisity of Colorado
Aurora, CO

Reder, Lindsay S MD
Department of Otolaryngology-Head and Neck Surgery
University of Southern California
Los Angeles, CA

Reed, Jeremy T MD MPH
Rhinology Fellow
Department of Otorhinolaryngology-Head and Neck Surgery
University of Pennsylvania
Philadelphia, PA

Stripp, Diana MD
Department of Radiation Oncology
Abramson Cancer Center
University of Pennsylvania
Philadelphia, PA

Suh, Jeffrey D MD
Assistant Professor
Division of Otolaryngology-Head and Neck Surgery
University of California, Los Angeles
Los Angeles, CA

Vescan, Allan MD FRCSC
Department of Otolaryngology-Head and Neck Surgery
University of Toronto
Mount Sinai Hospital
Toronto, Ontario, Canada

Vira, Darshni MD
Resident Surgeon
Division of Otolaryngology-Head and Neck Surgery
University of California, Los Angeles
Los Angeles, CA

Foreword

In 1933, Ringerts described the management of inverted papillomas of the nasal and paranasal sinuses. He pointed out that this tumor was characterized by a substantial rate of recurrence. However, a close reading of his paper suggests that he felt that this was not so much recurrence as persistent disease. In hindsight we can see why because these patients were treated the same as a patient with nasal polyps by removal of the lesion by a snare or by evulsion. During my residency in the decade of the 60s, the same techniques were used. Patients with multiple recurrences had a radioactive substance inserted into the nasal cavity. The recurrence rate was still substantial, again related to the lack of exposure by these surgical approaches.

In the 1970s, as the maturation of the ENT surgeon into a head and neck surgeon occurred, several others and I gained adequate exposure in this area using principles of cancer surgery, particularly the lateral rhinotomy. The recurrence rate described by Vrabek, Calcaterra, and Myers in their series had recurrence rates close to zero. However, this was at a cost to the patient of a midfacial scar and often deformity related to displacement of the medial central ligament. Technological advances have enabled us to improve the curability of both benign and malignant tumors when applied to the sinonasal area. This includes improvement in imaging techniques (CT scanning was not even available until the decade of the 1980s), the evolution of endoscopic equipment for endonasal surgery, microvascular reconstructive techniques, and more precise pathological diagnosis based upon improvements and new developments in special tests we are now able to perform on these tissues. While these technological advances certainly play a fundamental role in the changing treatment algorithms of these patients, still one cannot overlook the surgical training both in the external and intranasal approaches to these tumors. From the earliest days in residency training, otolaryngologists are taught to use the nasal endoscope in functional endoscopic sinus surgery for benign inflammatory diseases.

Later on, in their training come more advanced techniques for advanced conditions such as the recently introduced and highly successful techniques for endoscopic endonasal skull base surgery. However, not all the tumors that are encountered can be managed solely with endonasal techniques and it will evolve that some patients will need to be treated endoscopically, some by external procedures, and some by both. It is important to continue to train our Residents and Fellows both in the endoscopic and the open techniques for removal of sinonasal tumors.

In ***Sinonasal Tumors***, there are many chapters elaborating on some of the scientific advancements in diagnosis such as improved imaging techniques and pathological diagnosis, as well as ample space devoted to the operative technique and adjunctive treatment with radiation and/or chemotherapeutic techniques. We are able to offer a more personalized treatment program for the individual patient now that we have a better way of defining the parameters of involvement and have more precise diagnosis. The editors of this book have brought together a highly qualified group of specialists both in diagnosis and treatment to bring these new paradigms of treatment of sinonasal tumors into perspective.

Eugene N Myers MD FACS FRCS Edin (Hon)
Distinguished Professor and Emeritus Chair
Department of Otolaryngology
University of Pittsburgh School of Medicine
Pittsburgh, PA

Preface

Sinonasal tumors have traditionally been a difficult disease process to treat, let alone cure. Although fairly rare, this heterogeneous group of cancers often carry a guarded prognosis given their aggressive nature and close proximity to the brain and orbit. Traditional studies and techniques have focused on radical resections, but even these surgeries have often resulted in less than optimal disease-free rates.

Over the past decade, we have seen an evolution in the management of these tumors. Although radical surgeries are still needed for advanced cases, minimally invasive techniques using endoscopic equipment, computer-guided navigation, and specialty tools built for the sinuses and skull base have changed the way we often operate on these tumors. Combined with earlier detection methods, improved diagnostic imaging, tissue sparing radiation protocols, more effective chemotherapy and increased experience with endoscopic skull base and neurovascular techniques, we are seeing improved morbidity and mortality rates.

The purpose of this book is to present a modern way to treat *sinonasal tumors* with respect to traditional tumor extirpation principles and the need for radical excisions when the indications arise. As technology improves and our long-term follow-up grows, we expect further successes in the management of tumors long thought to be difficult to treat.

Alexander G Chiu MD
Vijay R Ramakrishnan MD
Jeffrey D Suh MD

Contents

1

Past, Present and Future of Sinonasal Tumor Management

Alexander G Chiu, MD

INTRODUCTION

For many years, the management philosophy of sinonasal malignancies has been consistent with traditional oncologic teachings. *En bloc* resections, wide tumor margins and resection of vital organs with tumor involvement were traditional textbook teachings designed to optimize patient survival rates. Despite large skin incisions and radical surgical resections, reported survival rates for sinonasal malignancies were poor and functional outcomes less than desirable. Adjuvant therapies left much to be desired, as radiation therapy in the sinonasal region proved threatening to a patient's vision and chemotherapy was largely ineffective.

With the advent of endoscopic tools, instruments and techniques, a new treatment paradigm has slowly evolved in the management of sinonasal cancer. In-office advancements such as CT scanners and nasal endoscopy are routinely performed for patients with nasal complaints. This has led to earlier detection of tumors with resultant surgical resections of smaller tumors isolated to the sinonasal cavity and without gross orbit or brain involvement. Prior criticisms of endoscopic techniques, including the inability to control bleeding and repair of skull base and dural defects with a "watertight seal," have been answered with the proven success of endoscopic techniques for epistaxis control and cerebrospinal fluid (CSF) leak repair. With the recently demonstrated success of endoscopic piecemeal resection of T4 laryngeal cancers, the traditional oncologic dogma of *en bloc* resection has come under question. Piecemeal resection of tumors has not been shown to alter patient survival in laryngeal cancer and as a result, the principle of piecemeal resection for sinonasal tumors has become more acceptable. Coupled with advancements in tissue-sparing radiation therapy and new chemotherapeutic regimens against tumors which were previously thought to be chemoresistant, the management of sinonasal cancer has evolved from an era of radical resections to minimally invasive approaches with outcomes that equal, if not surpass, traditional results (Figs 1.1A to D).

TRADITIONAL ONCOLOGIC TEACHINGS

En bloc resection of malignant tumors is a major principle in which head and neck oncology was founded upon. Giants of the field, such as Billroth, Crile, Hayes Martin, Ogura and Conley, formulated

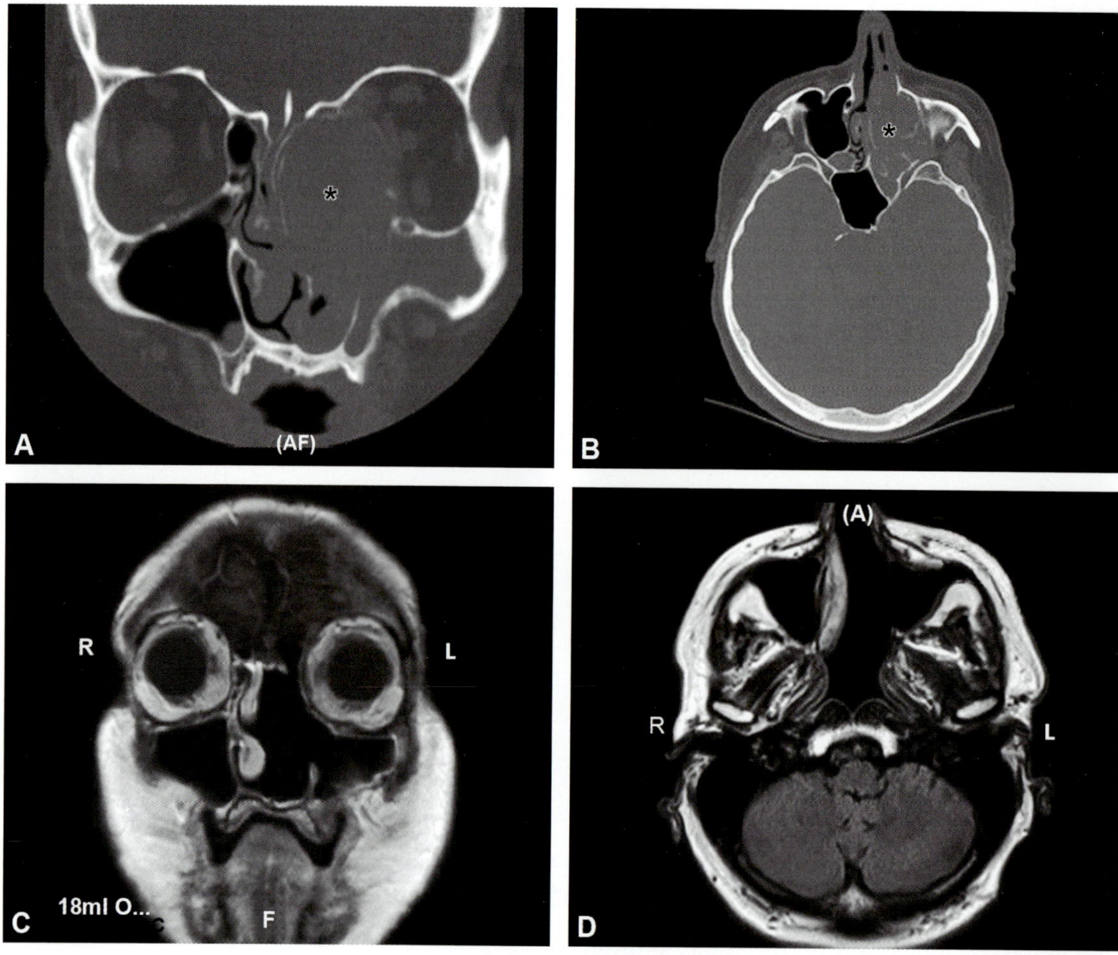

Figs 1.1A to D: (A and B) Preoperative coronal and axial CT scans of a patient with a left sided sinonasal mucosal melanoma.* (C and D) Coronal and axial T1-weighted MRI with gadolinium showing no disease 5 years following endoscopic surgery and radiation therapy.

their theories by the study of tumor spread, metastatic behavior, anatomical barriers and natural presentation of head and neck tumors.[1] Piecemeal resection of tumor was traditionally frowned upon as surgeons worried about tumor spill and resultant increase in regional or distal metastases.

Minimally invasive treatment of laryngeal cancers has been in application for quite some time and success in its practice has facilitated the acceptance of endoscopic sinus tumor management. Initial reports of transoral excision of laryngeal cancer date back to the late 1800s and by the early 1990s, case series of laser-assisted transoral excision of early glottic carcinomas were being reported.[2] Over the past 10 years, indications for minimally invasive approaches have expanded to include large tumors (T3 and T4) as well as recurrences after previous failed irradiation. With piecemeal resection and endoscopic transoral approaches, the minimally invasive technique has demonstrated oncologic safety and efficacy without increased incidence of metastatic spread.[3] Successful outcomes with large, bulky laryngeal cancers removed in piecemeal fashion have made it more acceptable to believe that sinonasal tumors could be removed in similar fashion and result.

The oncologic tenet of resecting tumor and obtaining clear margins still holds true for management of sinonasal tumors. It was once thought that traditional open craniofacial resection allowed for easier access to the margins, but with many of these tumors bordering the orbit, dura and cranial nerves, it is not easy to take a large margin without sacrificing a vital organ. In fact, the largest study looking at outcomes for open craniofacial resections was the International Collaborative Study published in 2005. Gathering 334 patients from 17 institutions, the positive margin rate was quoted at 30%.[4] As opposed to the naked eye, magnification using an endoscope gives the surgeon an advantage of accurate and detailed margins. This ability may make it possible to decrease the size of margin needed, thus sparing vital organs such as orbit and brain from being sacrificed solely for the purpose of taking a margin. The magnified view can also make tumor mapping more precise, especially in deep areas such as the pterygopalatine fossa and sphenoid sinus, where visualization and light illumination can be difficult in an open procedure.

RESULTS

Despite *en bloc* resections, radical facial incisions and wide tumor margins, results of traditional craniofacial resections have been disappointing. One case series published in 2006 presented 20 patients with mixed sinonasal histologies, with a 75% recurrence rate and a 65% 3-year survival rate.[5] The largest series to date, the International Collaborative Study Group, collected 334 patients from 17 institutions around the world, 32% of the tumors consisted of adenocarcinomas and 30% were squamous cell carcinoma (SCCA). As previously stated, their rate of positive margins was 30% and overall 5-year survival was 48.3%.[4] In 1999, Thaler and colleagues from the University of Pennsylvania described their results with endoscopic-assisted resection of sinonasal tumors. Performing the intranasal portion with an endoscope and the skull base component with a craniotomy, this report was one of the first to introduce the concept of endoscopic resection for malignant disease.[6] The following years saw the emergence of endoscopic-assisted and then purely endoscopic approaches, with esthesioneuroblastoma (ENB) being the most common malignancy removed solely with the endoscope. By the late 2000s, endoscopic resection of select malignancies has become an accepted practice in many of the leading cancer institutions around the world. Large skull base and sinonasal cancer centers located in London and Houston published case series of 49 and 93 patients respectively with 87–88% 5-year survival rates.[7,8] Although only after a 3-year follow-up, Chiu and Palmer demonstrated a 93.8% survival rate in 49 patients.[9] These results surpass those seen with open craniofacial resections. Although much of the success may be attributed to smaller staged tumors with a lower incidence of dural and soft tissue invasion, the fact remains that with earlier diagnosis and endoscopic techniques, improved survival rates and decreased complication rates can be achieved.

Adapting Lessons Learned from Inflammatory Disease and Benign Tumors and Applying to Malignancies

The results in the above endoscopic series are not only attributable to earlier tumor detection but also to improved surgical technique and increased endoscopic experience. Starting with techniques designed for the treatment of inflammatory disease, to gradual application to benign sinonasal tumors and followed by its use in combined neurosurgical cases of the skull base, i.e. pituitary tumors and anterior skull base meningiomas, endoscopic tumor surgeons have developed the skills and experience to safely and accurately resect sinonasal tumors while reconstructing dural defects to prevent major postoperative complications.

Functional endoscopic sinus surgery, first popularized in the early 1980s, paved the way for use of endoscopes in the sinonasal cavities.

Increased use and familiarity led to expansion of the endoscopic techniques beyond the sinuses to include the pituitary gland, orbits, anterior and middle cranial fossa. With this expansion came rapid technologic developments. Angled endoscopes, curved instruments, endoscopic bipolar forceps and clip appliers, endoscopic diamond drill bits, image guidance and now intraoperative computed tomography (CT) and magnetic resonance imaging (MRI) scanners are just some examples of the technology that has made minimally invasive surgery technically feasible for sinonasal malignancies.

One of the main criticisms of endoscopic techniques was the inability to control large blood vessels. Although management of the internal carotid artery remains a challenge endoscopically as it does with an open approach, control of the internal maxillary, anterior and posterior ethmoid arteries has long been a part of the endoscopic sinus surgeon's armamentarium. The use of bipolar forceps and endoscopic clips has made control of these arteries a core practice in the surgical management of epistaxis. These techniques can be applied to the management of tumors involving the cribiform plate, where the anterior ethmoid artery and posterior ethmoid arteries are often encountered. More posteriorly, experience with management of the internal maxillary artery for epistaxis and the surgical resection of juvenile angiofibromas, has given surgeons the experience and ability to control the posterior vasculature of sinonasal malignancies (Fig. 1.2).

Another traditional criticism of endoscopic techniques was the inability to create a "watertight seal" of the skull base after resection of tumors abutting skull base and dura. The need for the "watertight seal" often drove surgeons to perform a craniotomy for the sole purpose of reconstruction with a vascularized pericranial flap. This was thought to be the only method of reconstruction that would reliably prevent postoperative complications of a CSF leak, provide a barrier for tumor spread and withstand the effects of postoperative radiation

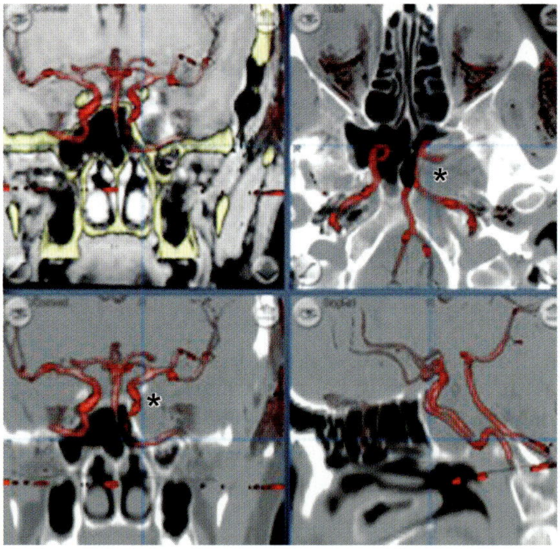

Fig. 1.2: CT/MRA fusion of a left middle fossa dermoid cyst bulging into the left sphenoid sinus.* This cyst was marsupialized into the sinus endoscopically. The image outlines the carotid artery in red.

therapy. From a technical standpoint, endoscopic sinus surgeons have been repairing skull base defects since the late 1980s. Cerebrospinal fluid rhinorrhea, meningoceles and encephaloceles have been shown to have a much higher rate of closure success with endoscopic techniques (95–98%) than open craniotomies (60%). The popularization of vascularized nasoseptal flaps for use in extended skull base procedures has improved the success of endoscopic reconstruction of large defects; there have been reports of decreased postoperative CSF leaks, and quicker healing, which has given greater comfort to surgeons that this type of repair could also withstand the effects of postoperative radiation (Figs 1.3A and B). The pericranial flap remains a great source of tissue for reconstruction, but now there are even reports of its use following endoscopic resection of tumors.[10]

Finally, recent experiences with combined neurosurgical endoscopic skull base cases have not only taught us lessons on skull base resection, but have also re-popularized the techniques of two-surgeon endoscopic resections (Figs 1.4A and B).

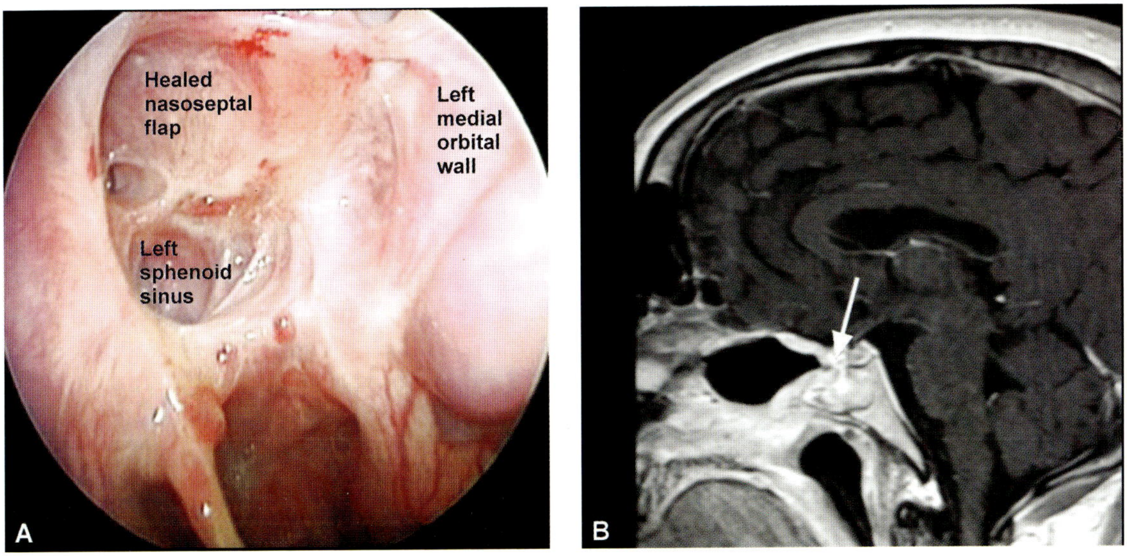

Figs 1.3A and B: (A) Endoscopic view; (B) sagittal T1 MRI view of a healed pedicled nasoseptal flap covering the ethmoid skull base (arrow).

In this technique the second surgeon is placed at the head of the bed or opposite to the primary surgeon. The extra hand(s) within the sinonasal cavity aids in retraction, excision and control of bleeding. In addition, techniques have been described that make more room in the nose for four instruments to be placed without restricting each other's movements. The septal slide technique and trans-septal approaches have been described so that one surgeon can work across the septum while the other manipulates the endoscope in the other nostril.[11,12]

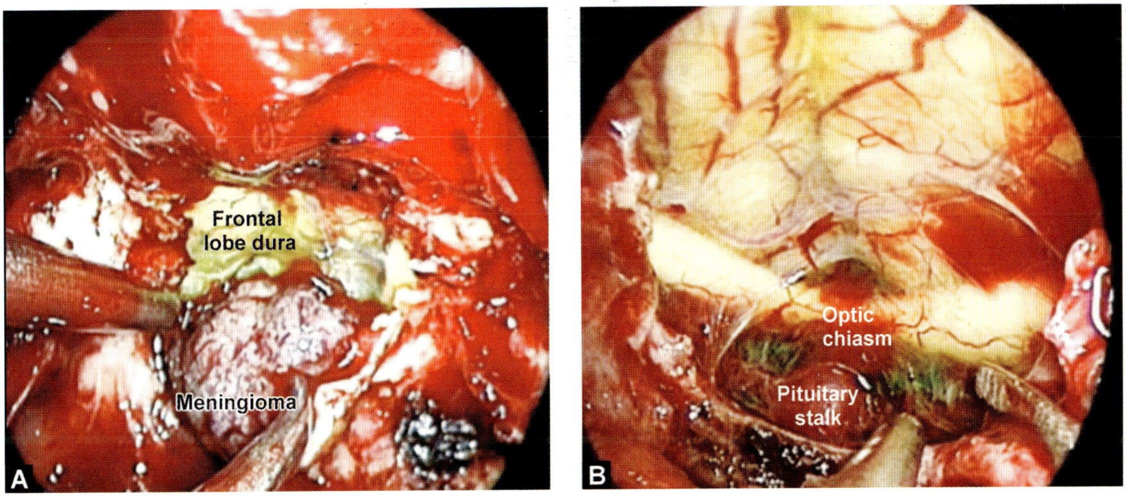

Figs 1.4A and B: (A) Endoscopic views of a 2-surgeon removal of a tuberculum sella meningioma (arrow); (B) Following resection, the optic chiasm and pituitary stalk are clearly seen.

SURGICAL PRINCIPLES FOR ENDOSCOPIC RESECTION OF MALIGNANCIES

In regards to sinonasal malignancies, many of the traditional oncologic principles have been replaced by new teachings. Some tenets remain true; the primary goal of surgical treatment remains the complete resection of tumor with negative margins, but *en bloc* resection remains impractical to the minimally invasive approach and piecemeal resection of tumor has become an accepted practice. Central to the concept of piecemeal resection is the identification of the tumor site of attachment. Originally a lesson learned from the treatment of benign sinonasal tumors such as an inverted papilloma, identification and *en bloc* resection of the site of tumor attachment allows for lower local recurrence rates.[13] While many sinonasal tumors have a broad base of attachment, thus requiring a wide resection of its base, there are select tumors such as adenocarcinomas and hemangiopericytomas that may be large, but are pedicled or have a small attachment to a non-essential structure (Figs 1.5A to D). Focusing on the resection of the site of

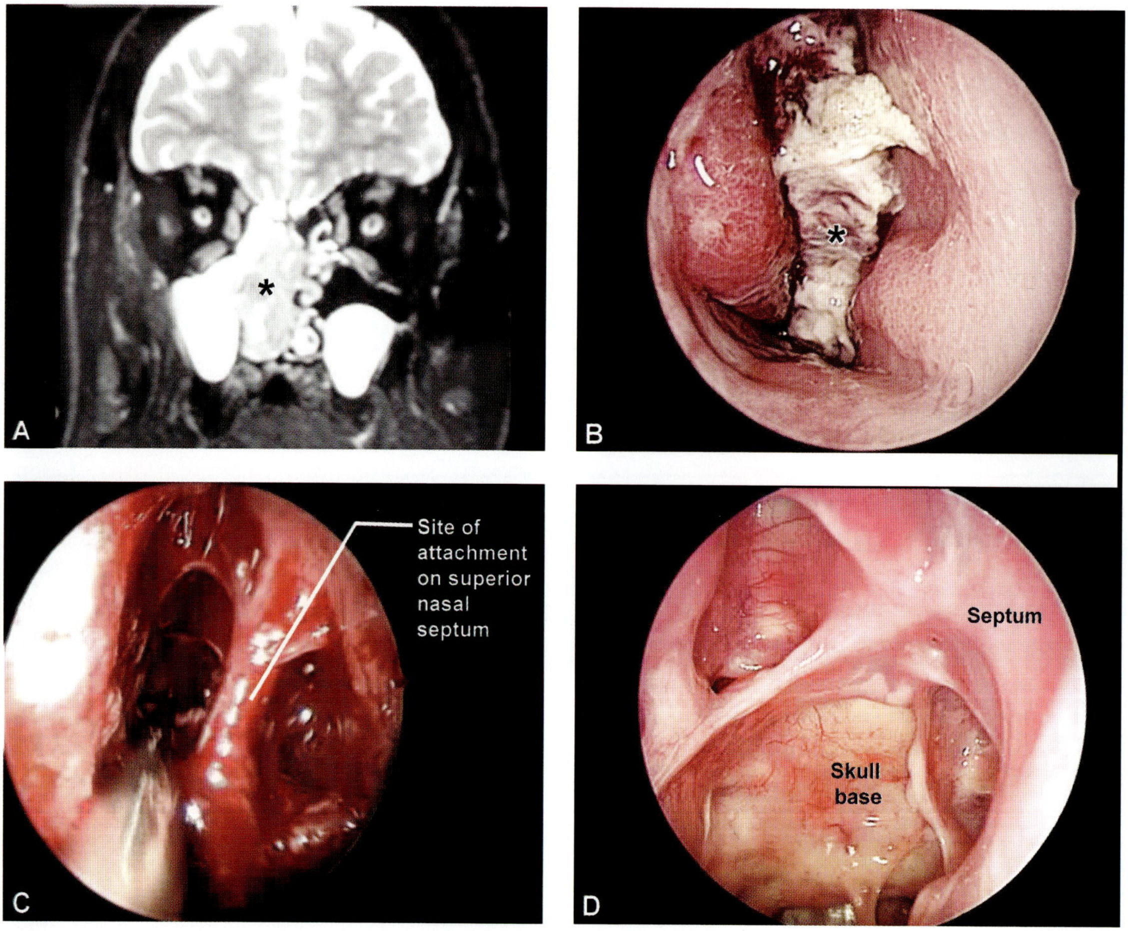

Figs 1.5A to D: (A) Coronal MRI scan of a sinonasal adenocarcinoma;* (B) The tumor filled much of the right nasal cavity;* but during endoscopic resection; (C) The tumor was pedicled on a narrow band of tissue attached to the nasal septum; (D) The portion of the septum housing the site of attachment was removed and the patient is disease-free 6 years after surgery alone.

attachment not only brings about a theoretically reduced chance for recurrence, but may also spare the patient a more morbid or invasive procedure.

FUTURE TRENDS

As technology improves, the management of sinonasal tumors will become increasingly less invasive. Robotic surgery, commonly employed for prostate and cardiovascular surgery, has taken a foothold in head and neck surgery with its treatment of base of tongue cancers. As robotic arms get smaller, there will be a time when an image-guided robot will be performing surgery in the sinuses and skull base. In addition to surgical techniques, improved radiation therapy such as proton beam radiation may also improve overall survival, especially for those tumors that have wide dural involvement or previously thought to be unresectable secondary to their proximity to the optic nerve or carotid artery. Chemotherapeutic regimens continue to improve, and its adjuvant use in select tumors such as sinonasal undifferentiated carcinomas, may allow for reduction of tumor burden and aid in preserving vital organs previously involved with tumor.

CONCLUSION

For the first time in many years, the management of sinonasal carcinoma has evolved with growing experience in endoscopic surgical techniques, technology and improved adjuvant therapies. Although, there are still some tumors that are better approached with an open surgical incision, i.e. those with wide dural or soft tissue involvement, endoscopic approaches have demonstrated a great potential to achieve results equivalent if not better than open approaches in select tumors. The main objective of this book is to highlight current management philosophies in the treatment of sinonasal tumors and to demonstrate modern techniques and advancements that have led to an evolution in management for this disease state.

REFERENCES

1. Wolf GT. Tradition, teamwork, and tailored treatment. Arch Otolaryngol Head Neck Surg. 2009;135(4):337-41.
2. Steiner W. Results of curative laser microsurgery of laryngeal carcinomas. Am J Otolaryngol. 1993;14:116-21.
3. Burns JA, Har El G, Shapshay S, et al. Endoscopic laser resection of laryngeal cancer: is it oncologically safe? Annals of Otology, Rhinology and Laryngology. 2009;118(6):399-404.
4. Ganly I, Patel SG, Singh B, et al. Craniofacial resection for malignant paranasal sinus tumors: report of an International Collaborative Study. Head Neck. 2005;27:575-84.
5. Granados-Garcia M, Celis-Lopez MA, Aguilar-Ponce JL, et al. Craniofacial resection for sinonasal tumors. Clin Transl Oncol 2006;8(2):119-23.
6. Thaler ER, Kotapka M, Lanza DC, et al. Endoscopically assited anterior cranial skull base resection of sinonasal tumors. Am J Rhinol 1999;13(4):303-10.
7. Howard DJ, Lund VJ, Wei WI. Craniofacial resection for tumors of the nasal cavity and paranasal sinuses: a 25-year experience. Head Neck 2006;28(10):867-73.
8. Hanna E, DeMonte F, Ibrahim S, et al. Endoscopic resection of sinonasal cancers with and without craniotomy: oncologic results. Arch Otolaryngol Head Neck Surg. 2009;135(12):1219-24.
9. Chiu AG, Suh J, Chi J, et al. "Endoscopic Resection of Sinonasal Malignancies". Presented at Spring Meeting of the American Rhinologic Society, Chicago; May 2011.
10. Zanation AM, Snyderman CH, Carrau RL, et al. Minimally invasive endoscopic pericranial flap: a new method for endonasal skull base reconstruction. Laryngoscope. 2009;119(1):13-8.
11. Ramakrishnan V, Chiu AG, Palmer JN. The septal slide technique for resection of lateral based sinonasal tumors. Am J Rhinol Allergy (in press).
12. Harvey RJ, Sheehan PO, Debnath NI, et al. Transseptal approach for extended endoscopic resections of the maxilla and infratemporal fossa. Am J Rhinol Allergy. 2009;23:426-32.
13. Woodworth BA, Bhargave GA, Palmer JN, et al. Clinical outcomes of endoscopic and endoscopic-assisted resection of inverted papillomas: a 15-year experience. Am J Rhinol. 2007;21:591-600.

2

Surgical and Radiological Anatomy of the Paranasal Sinuses

Jeremy T Reed, MD, MPH; Jeffrey D Suh, MD; Nithin Adappa, MD; James N Palmer, MD

OVERVIEW

Mastery of the anatomy of the paranasal sinuses is a prerequisite for any surgeon attempting to treat tumors in this area safely and effectively. The paranasal sinus region is complex, and varies greatly between individuals. Besides possessing clinical judgment and technical skills, a competent surgeon must also be a good anatomist. Surgical complications are often directly related to unfamiliarity with landmarks during dissection, or loss of orientation caused by pathology. This chapter will outline and summarize the basic anatomic concepts of the region, with an emphasis on relevant surgical anatomy.

EMBRYOLOGY OF LATERAL NASAL WALL

A series of five to six ridges first appear during the eighth week of development. Through regression and fusion of these ridges, known as ethmoturbinals, only three or four persist. After the regress of the first ethmoturbinal during development, its ascending portion forms the agger nasi and the inferior portion forms the uncinate process. The second ethmoturbinal forms the middle turbinate (MT). The third ethmoturbinal forms the superior turbinate. The fourth and fifth ethmoturbinals fuse to form the supreme turbinate (Fig. 2.1). These ethmoturbinals are ethmoid in origin, whereas the inferior turbinate (IT) arises from the maxilloturbinal which is not an ethmoid derivative.

BASIC ANATOMY

Nasal Cavity

Nasal Septum

The nasal septum is ordinarily a midline structure separating the left and right nasal cavities. It is composed of the vomer posteriorly, the perpendicular plate of the ethmoid bone superiorly, and the quadrangular cartilage anteriorly. At its superior margin the perpendicular plate of the ethmoid and nasal septum are continuous with the crista galli of the ethmoid bone. The crista galli is a midline, intracranial, bony extension of the ethmoid bone that provides an attachment for the falx cerebri. Posteriorly, the vomer is continuous with the sphenoid rostrum superiorly and the choanae inferiorly. The arch of the choana is a highly retained anatomic structure that the surgeon can reference for orientation when tumor growth has destroyed other anatomic landmarks. Inferiorly the vomer rests on the maxillary crest of the maxilla and palatine bones. Structural deviations of the septum affect

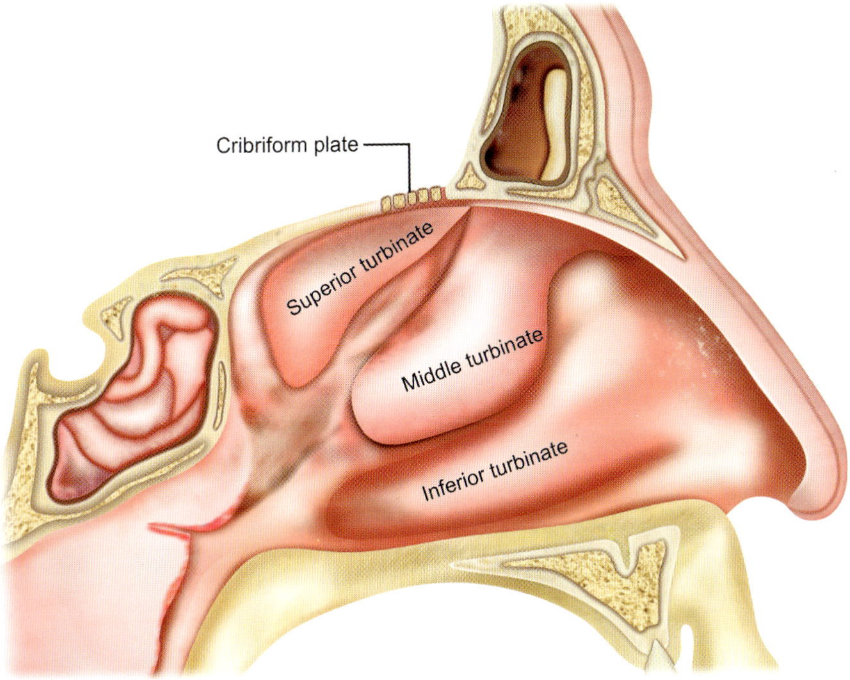

Fig. 2.1: View of lateral nasal wall.

nasal airway resistance. Deviation or deformity of the septum, producing asymmetry, is common, and was found in up to 79% of adults in one study.[1] Slowly progressive tumor growth within the nasal cavity will often create a septal deformity by pushing the septum to the opposite side without frankly invading into it. Another important concept in the nasal cavity is the nasal valve. The external nasal valve is formed by the columella, the nasal floor, and the nasal rim (or caudal border of the lower lateral cartilage). The internal nasal valve, which represents the narrowest part of the nose, is formed by the nasal septum, the caudal (lower edge) of the upper lateral cartilage, the anterior head of the IT, and the nasal floor.

Inferior Turbinate

The IT is largest of the nasal turbinates. It attaches anteriorly and laterally with the nasal surface of the maxilla and the perpendicular plate of the palatine bone posteriorly. The nasolacrimal duct empties into the inferior meatus at Hasner's valve near its anterior attachment to the maxilla. The turbinate plays important roles in protection of the lower airway and physiology of the nose. It functions in temperature regulation and humidification of inspired air, as well as filtration of foreign particles.[2] The vascular supply is the posterior lateral artery, a branch of the sphenopalatine artery (SPA) that enters the posterior aspect of the IT.[3] The artery then divides into two branches and run in a posterior-anterior direction. In some cases, an anastomosis with the facial artery may augment the blood supply at the anterior portion of IT.

Middle Turbinate

The MT forms the medial aspect of the middle meatus (Fig. 2.2). It serves as an important landmark in sinus surgery. The orientation of the MT runs along three different planes in its course from anterior to posterior. The anterior third of the MT runs in the

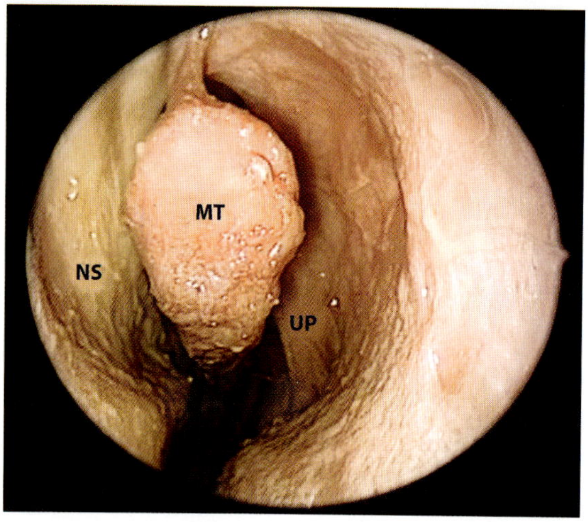

Fig. 2.2: Endoscopic view of left nasal cavity. Note the relationship between the uncinate process and MT in the middle meatus. NS: Nasal septum; MT: Middle turbinate; UP: Uncinate process.

sagittal plane, and is attached at the skull base to the cribriform plate.

Moving posteriorly, at the middle third, the turbinate reflects from a sagittal to a coronal orientation forming the basal lamella, or ground lamella. The basal lamella is attached to the lamina papyracea of the orbit laterally, and serves as a landmark to demarcate anterior from posterior ethmoid cells. Anterior to the basal lamella, the sinuses drain in the middle meatus. Posterior to the basal lamella, the cells drain through the superior meatus. The posterior third of the MT runs in an axial plane with its attachment continuing along the lateral nasal wall. The posterior end of the MT is adjacent to the sphenopalatine foramen. There are some distinct anatomic variations of the MT which will be discussed later in the chapter.

Superior Turbinate

The superior turbinate is found posterior and superior to the MT. It shares a common superior attachment with the MT, but is separated inferiorly by a meatus. The superior turbinate and septum both contain olfactory epithelium. The superior turbinate also serves as a reliable landmark when performing a sphenoidotomy as the natural ostium of the sphenoid sinus is generally located just medially and posteriorly to it. When the superior turbinate is small, a supreme turbinate may also be present.

Uncinate

The uncinate is a thin sickle shaped bone covering the natural maxillary ostium that helps direct sinus outflow posteriorly in the nose. Its anterior superior attachment is variable, possibly inserting onto the lamina papyracea, ethmoid roof, or MT (Figs 2.3A to C and 2.4). In one study, the uncinate process

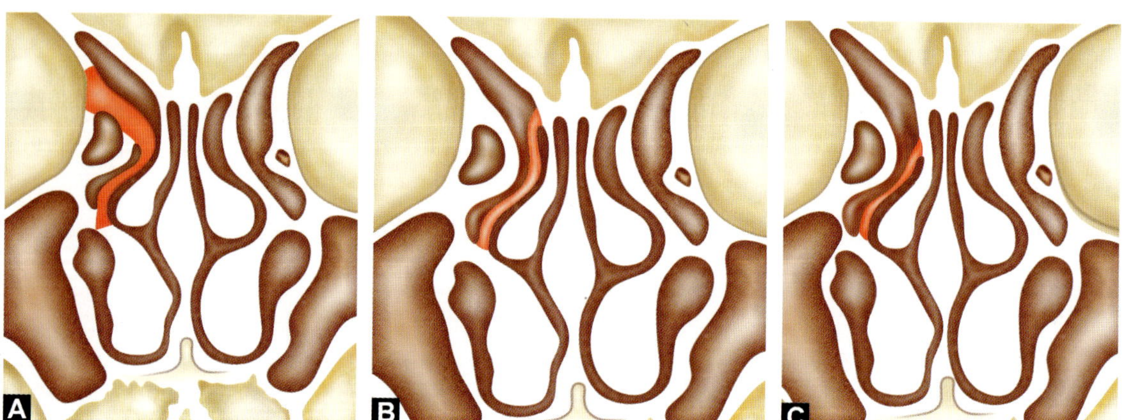

Figs 2.3A to C: (A) Uncinate attachment to lamina papyracea; (B) Uncinate attachment to skull base; (C) Uncinate attachment to middle turbinate.

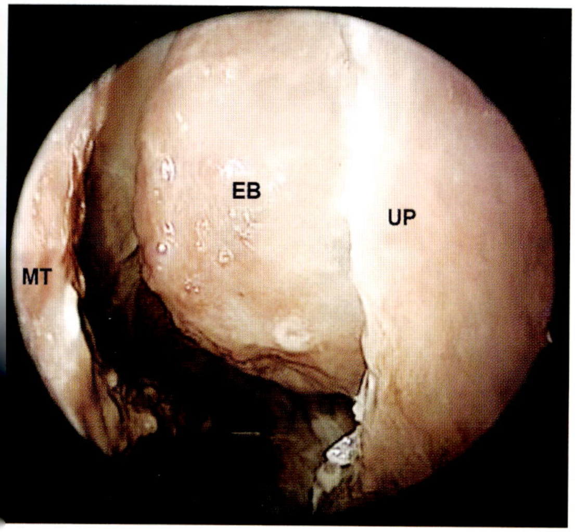

Fig. 2.4: After partial removal the uncinate process, the ethmoid bulla becomes visible in the middle meatus. EB: Ethmoid bulla; MT: Middle turbinate; UP: Uncinate process.

attached to the lamina in 54%, skull base in 24.5%, and MT in 21.5%.[4] However, these numbers can vary widely and there can be multiple attachments. The uncinate is ordinarily concave into the middle meatus, and parallels the anterior and inferior surfaces of the ethmoid bulla as it slopes inferior and posterior. However, a large nasal cavity tumor may displace a weakened uncinate laterally up against the lamina papyracea. Membranous dehiscences of the anterior and posterior fontanelles are separated by a bony projection inferiorly to the perpendicular plate of the palatine bone. The ethmoid infundibulum and natural ostium of the maxillary sinus are located lateral to the uncinate and are ordinarily not visualized on nasal endoscopy, when the uncinate process is present.

Orbit

The orbit supports and protects the eye. Seven bones compose the orbit: frontal, lacrimal, ethmoid, maxillary, sphenoid, zygoma, and palatine bones. The medial orbital wall consists of the frontal process of the maxilla, the lacrimal bone, the orbital plate of the ethmoid bone, and the lesser wing of the sphenoid. The orbital surface of the frontal bone and the lesser wing of the sphenoid compose the roof. The orbital surface of the maxilla meets the orbital plate of the zygoma and the orbital plate of the palatine bone to form the orbital floor. The lateral orbital wall is composed of the zygoma and the greater wing of the sphenoid.

Posteriorly, there are three openings into the orbit that provide blood supply, nervous innervation, and a potential route for tumor spread. The first, the optic canal, is encompassed in the bone of the lesser sphenoid wing and is located superior and medially at the orbital apex. The optic nerve and ophthalmic artery enter the orbit through this foramen. The second opening is the superior orbital fissure, where cranial nerves III, IV, VI, the lacrimal, frontal, and nasociliary branches of V1, and the superior ophthalmic and superior orbital veins pass. Inferior to the superior orbital fissure is the inferior orbital fissure through which the infraorbital nerve, artery, and vein transverse (Fig. 2.5).

Anteromedial in the orbit, where the frontal process of the maxilla meets the lacrimal bone, is the lacrimal fossa. The lacrimal fossa houses the lacrimal sac and is continuous with the nasolacrimal duct inferiorly. The nasolacrimal duct courses inferiorly and is encased in bone just anterior to the uncinate process. It opens into the inferior meatus

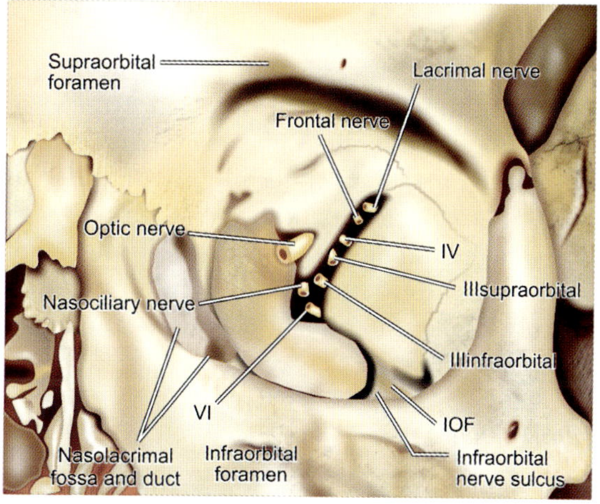

Fig. 2.5: Anterior view of a left orbital wall.

about 1-1.5 cm back from the anterior attachment of the IT to the maxilla.

Paranasal Sinuses

Maxillary Sinus

The maxillary sinus is the largest paranasal sinus. The adult volume can range from 8.5-15 ml, but it can also be hypoplastic or atelectatic. Agenesis of the maxillary sinus is found in up to 5-6% of adults.[5] The infraorbital branch courses along the roof of the maxillary fossa to exit at the infraorbital foramen. The floor of the maxillary sinus provides bone stock for the maxillary dentition. Occasionally the root of maxillary molars may be present in the antrum of the maxilla allowing periodontal disease and tumors to affect the sinus. The "true" maxillary sinus ostium is covered by the uncinate process, and leads into the infundibulum. Secondary openings, or accessory ostia, located posterior to the natural ostium have an incidence of at least 25%. Deep to the posterior wall of the maxillary sinus is the internal maxillary artery. The terminal branch of the maxillary artery, the SPA, enters the nasal cavity through the sphenopalatine foramen. The SPA frequently divides into multiple branches before leaving the sphenopalatine foramen, and in one study was found most commonly to divide into two major branches (76%), but may also divide into three branches (22%) or four branches (2%).[6] The sphenopalatine foramen and artery are located on the lateral nasal wall at the posterior limit of the maxillary sinus and just superior to the posterior attachment of the MT. The major branches of the SPA are the nasal septal artery (with branches to the MT and septum) and the posterior lateral nasal artery (with branches to the fontanelle and IT).

Ethmoid Sinuses

The ethmoid sinuses comprise the roof of the nasal cavity (Fig. 2.6). These sinuses are divided into anterior and posterior compartments by the basal lamella, the horizontal attachment of the MT to the lateral nasal wall (Fig. 2.7). The ethmoid bulla, an evolutionarily conserved landmark, is an anterior ethmoid cell that is laterally attached to the lamina papyracea. Opening the ethmoid bulla early in the dissection allows the surgeon to quickly and reliably establish the location of the medial orbit. Its anterior and inferior surfaces parallel the uncinate process from which it is separated from by the hiatus semilunaris. Dissection of the ethmoids is

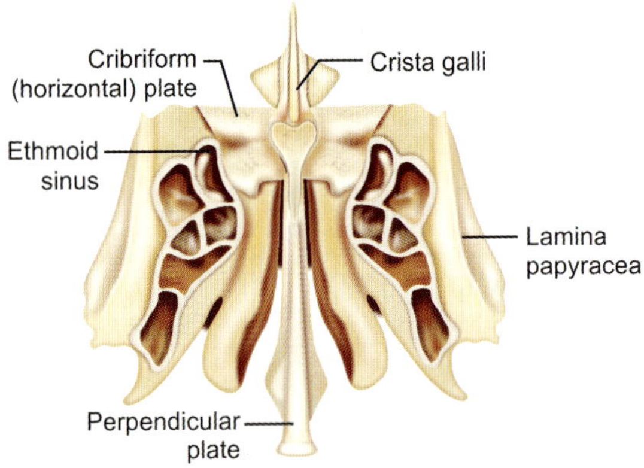

Fig. 2.6: Ethmoid bone.

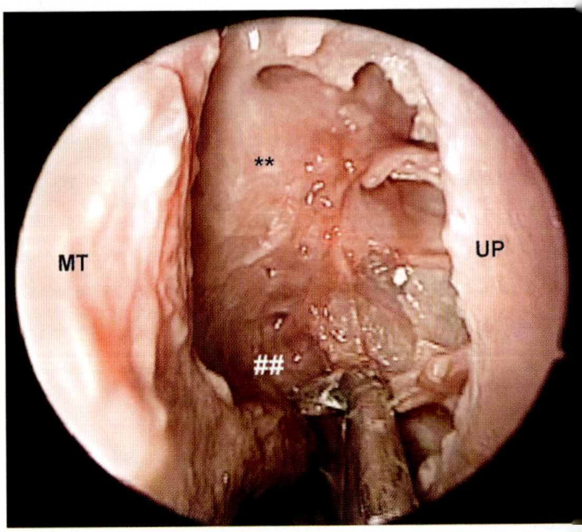

Fig. 2.7: Removal of the ethmoid bulla demonstrates the basal lamella: MT: Middle turbinate; UP: Uncinate process; **Vertical portion of basal lamella; ##Horizontal portion of basal lamella

easier to conceptualize with an understanding of the sinus lamella (Table 2.1). The 4 or 5 sinus lamellae are obliquely oriented and lie parallel to each other. With experience, these structures should be recognized during sinus surgery and are invaluable in maintaining orientation during dissection in the ethmoid cavity. The frontal, maxillary, and anterior ethmoid sinuses drain into the middle meatus. The posterior ethmoid cells drain into the superior meatus, while the sphenoid sinus drains into the sphenoethmoid recess.

Sphenoid Sinus

The sphenoid sinus is the most posteriorly located nasal sinus. Its roof is the planum sphenoidale which is the posterior limit of the anterior skull base. The optic nerve runs along the lateral roof of the sinus. The carotid artery runs vertically in its posterior-lateral wall. The intersinus septum separates the right and left sphenoid cavities. On occasion, the intersinus septum may track posteriorly to insert along the course of the internal carotid artery. It is important to make note of this preoperatively in order to avoid inadvertent internal carotid injury. It is also important to identify any bony dehiscences of the internal carotid and optic nerve in the sphenoid on CT imaging. Kennedy et al.[7] found dehiscence of the bony wall of the internal carotid artery in 25% of patients. In another study, protrusion of the internal carotid artery into the sphenoid sinus was identified in 30.3% of patients, and overt dehiscence in 5.3%.[8] Occasionally, a posterior ethmoid cell may pneumatize posterior and superior to the sphenoid sinus, creating an "Onodi cell." Onodi cells are important to recognize preoperatively on coronal and axial imaging because the optic nerve runs in the superior lateral roof of these cells (Fig. 2.8).

There are three patterns of sphenoid sinus pneumatization. The first type is the conchal (2.5%), in which the sinus pneumatization is minimal. The second type is presellar (10%) where the pneumatization extends to the anterior wall of the pituitary fossa. The third and most common type is sellar, where the pneumatization extends beyond the sella. This occurs in approximately 90% of adults (Fig. 2.9). Complete agenesis of the sphenoid sinus has an incidence of 1–1.5%.[5] Differentiating and recognizing these sphenoid variations is especially important when planning for transsphenoidal surgery.

Table 2.1 Ethmoid lamellae

1st lamella	Uncinate process
2nd lamella	Ethmoid bulla
3rd lamella	Middle turbinate
4th lamella	Superior turbinate
5th lamella	Supreme turbinate (when present)

Frontal Sinus

Frontal sinus anatomy is the most variable of the paranasal sinuses. Ten to twelve percent of the general population may have rudimentary frontal sinuses or completely lack frontal sinus pneumatization on one side. The average height of the frontal sinus is 24 mm, with a width of 29 mm, and depth of 20 mm. The posterior table of the frontal sinus is the boundary of the anterior cranial fossa. The frontal

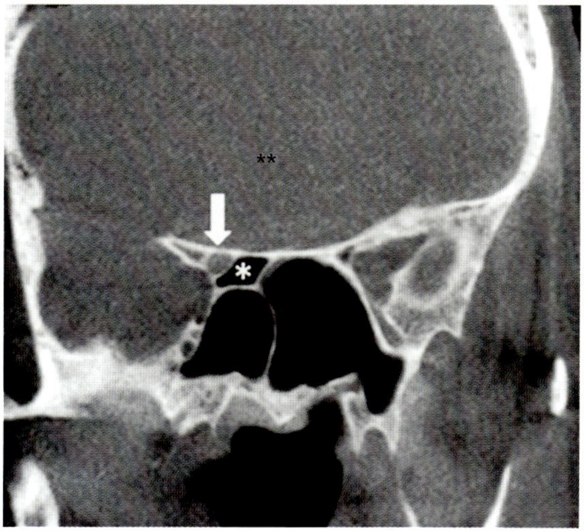

Fig. 2.8: Coronal CT scan. Note the relation of the Onodi cell to the optic nerve superiorly and laterally: (Arrow) Optic nerve; *Onodi cell.

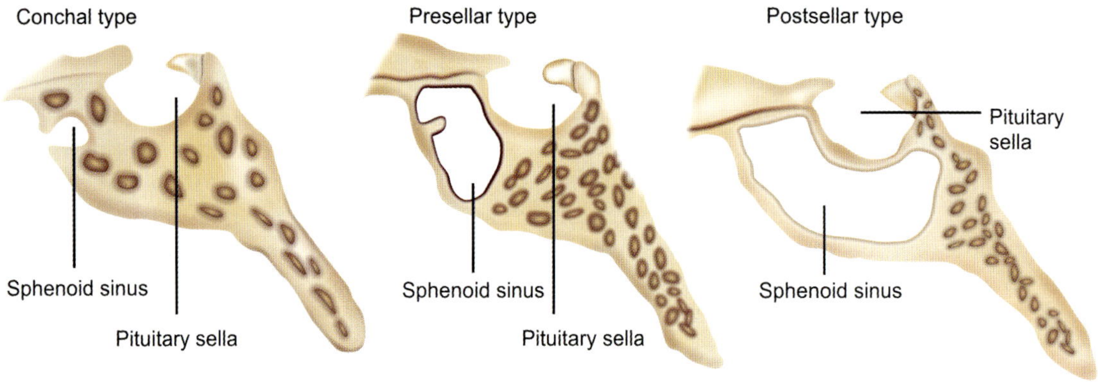

Fig. 2.9: Three different types of sphenoid pneumatization.

sinus ostium is located in the anterosuperior aspect of the middle meatus. Its location varies according to the site of attachment of the uncinate process. The frontal recess has four borders: the agger nasi cell anteriorly, the MT medially, the orbit laterally, and the supraorbital ethmoid cell and/or anterior aspect of the ethmoid bulla posteriorly. The variable anatomy of the sinus is best appreciated on sagittal CT imaging, including the anterior-posterior dimension of the frontal recess. A larger anterior-posterior dimension will facilitate dissection, especially if the frontal sinus needs to be opened widely. Kuhn described four types of frontal sinus cells, and this nomenclature is currently the most widely used[9] (Table 2.2 and Fig. 2.10). Two other types of cells are important to note preoperatively and intraoperatively: supraorbital ethmoid cells and intersinus septal cells. Supraorbital ethmoid cells are located posterior and lateral to the true frontal sinus and may be mistaken intraoperatively as the true frontal sinus.

Skull Base

The skull base forms the floor of the cranial cavity and separates the brain from the paranasal sinuses, orbit, and nasal cavity. Five bones make up the skull base. These are the paired frontal bones, paired parietal bones, ethmoid, sphenoid, and occipital bone. The skull base is divided into three regions: the anterior, middle, and posterior cranial fossa.

Table 2.2 Kuhn frontal cell types

Cell type	*Description*
I	One cell above the agger nasi
II	Two separate cells above the agger nasi
III	One large cell that pneumatizes into the frontal sinus
IV	Isolated cell within the frontal sinus

Cribriform Plate and Ethmoid Roof

The perpendicular plate of the ethmoid meets the cribriform plate to form the roof of the nasal cavity

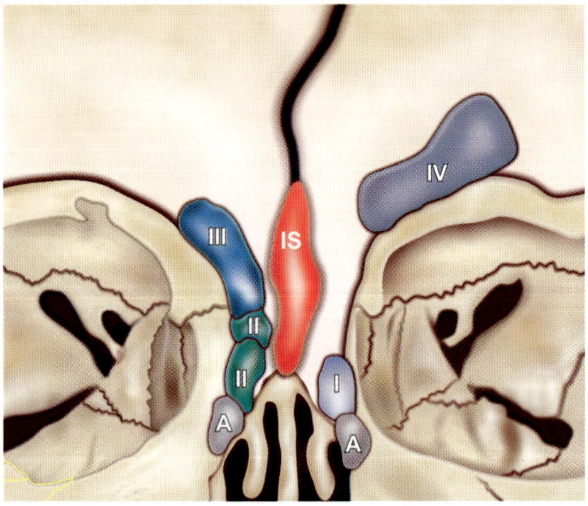

Fig. 2.10: Frontal sinus cells.

as well as the floor of the olfactory groove. The lateral lamellae of the cribriform plate are the vertically oriented lateral boundaries of the olfactory groove where the cribriform plate terminates. In one study, the lateral lamella was noted to be only 0.2 mm thick.[10] The height of the olfactory groove in relation to the ethmoid roof is important to note on coronal imaging preoperatively. Anatomic variations along the ethmoid roof are described by the Keros classification,[11] which measures the vertical height between the cribriform plate and the ethmoid roof. The lateral lamella of the cribriform plate represents the most common site of iatrogenic cerebrospinal fluid (CSF) leak in endoscopic sinus surgery, and can be more easily violated in Keros II and III cases. In this classification, the depth of the olfactory fossa is categorized as 1–3 mm (type I), 3–7 mm (type II), or 7–16 mm (type III). As the bone in this region is quite thin, increased vertical height lends itself to increased vulnerability. In Keros' original study of 450 cadavers, 12% were found to be Keros type I, 70% type II, and 18% type III.

Anterior, Middle, and Posterior Fossae

The anterior cranial fossa houses the frontal lobes. The anterior skull base is composed of three bones: the frontal, ethmoid, and sphenoid bones (Fig. 2.11). The anterior limit of the anterior skull base is the posterior wall of the frontal sinus. The roof of the sphenoid sinus, the planum sphenoidale, marks its posterior border. The anterior skull base slants inferiorly as one moves anterior to posterior through the nasal cavity. The frontal bone serves as the lateral border of the skull base and provides support for the frontal lobes superior to the orbits. The central skull base slopes medially, with the cribriform plate of the ethmoid bone as much as 1.5 cm lower than the roof of the ethmoid cavity.

In the midline, at the junction of the frontal bone with the ethmoid bone, is the foramen cecum (Fig. 2.12). The foramen cecum houses valveless emissary veins that drain into the sagittal sinus intracranially. The foramen cecum may also provide a route of extension for tumors and infection. Posterior to the frontal crest and foramen cecum is the crista galli. The crista galli is an interhemispheric bony extension of the ethmoid bone that provides attachment for the falx cerebri and sagittal sinus intracranially.

The central skull base includes the sphenoid body and the basal (clival) portion of the occipi-

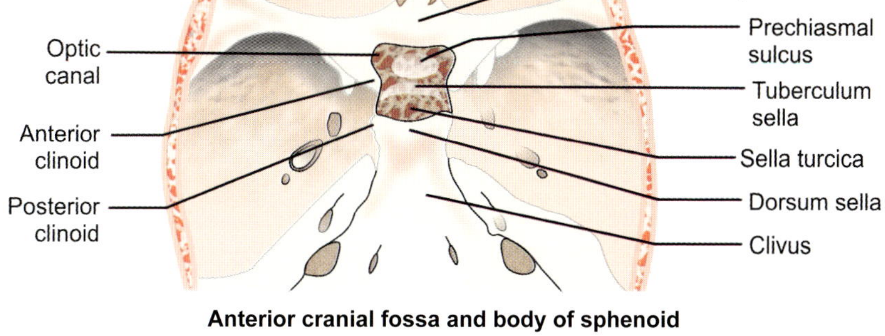

Fig. 2.11: Skull base with emphasis on anterior and middle fossa anatomy.

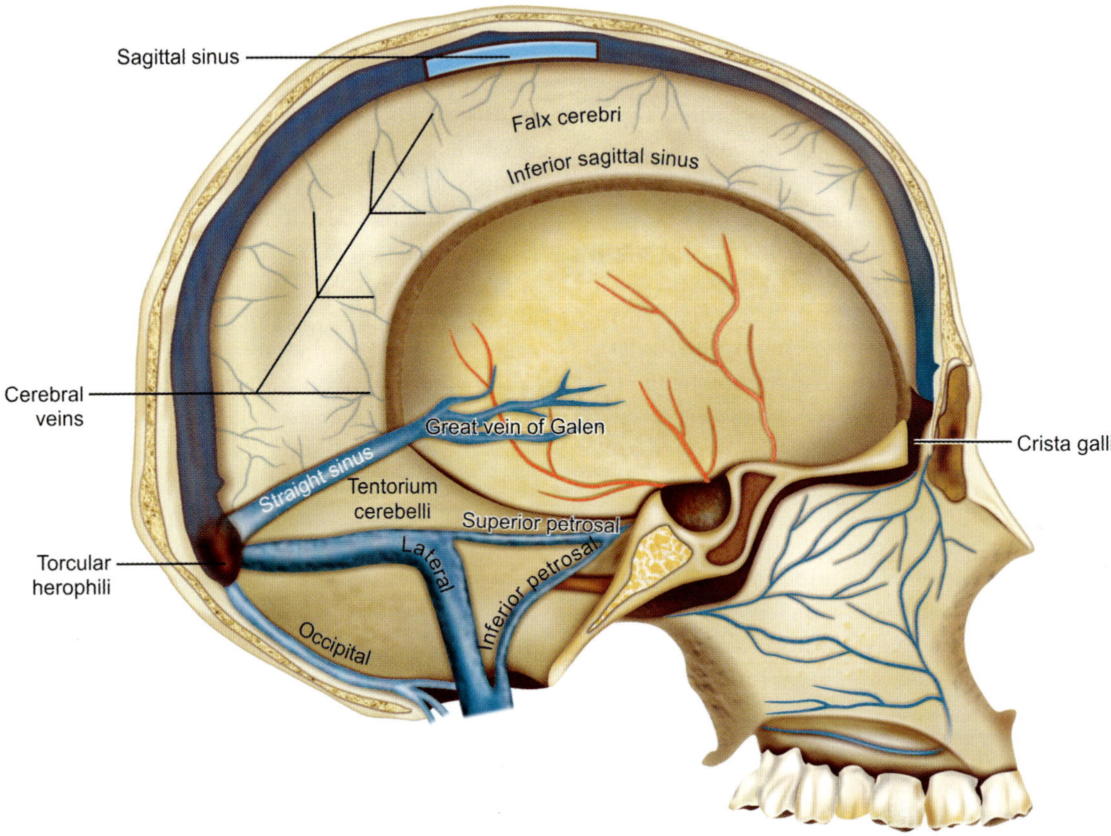

Fig. 2.12: Sagittal view of a midline skull depicting the sagittal sinus, the ethmoid bone, the foramen cecum and the frontal bone.

tal bone. The lateral aspect of the middle fossa is formed by the greater sphenoid wing, the temporal, zygomatic, maxillary, styloid, and palatine bones. The body of the sphenoid bone makes up the central portion of the middle fossa and houses the sella turcica. The sella turcica is a depression in the sphenoid roof that houses the pituitary gland. Just superior to the gland is the pituitary stalk and optic chiasm. The cavernous sinus lies lateral to the pituitary gland and the posterior sphenoid sinus. In addition to the internal carotid artery, the oculomotor (III), trochlear (IV), abducens (VI), ophthalmic (V1), and maxillary (V2) nerves run through the cavernous sinus (Fig. 2.13).

The posterior skull base is made up mostly by the occipital bone, with contributions from the sphenoid and temporal bones. Foramina include the internal auditory meatus/facial canal/stylomastoid foramen (CN-VII and VIII), the jugular foramen (CN-IX, X and XI), foramen magnum (CN-XI) and the hypoglossal canal (CN-XII).

Pterygopalatine and Infratemporal Fossae

The pterygopalatine fossa (PPF) is a small but important area as it contains numerous neurovascular structures. The boundaries of the PPF are as follows:

- Lateral: Infratemporal fossa via pterygomaxillary fissure
- Posteriorly: Pterygoid plates
- Anterior: Posterior surface of the maxilla

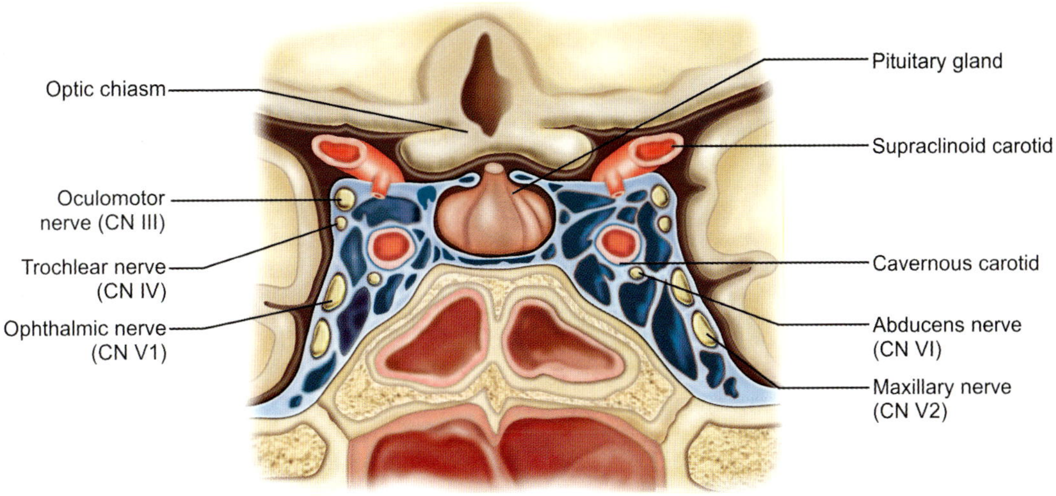

Fig. 2.13: Cavernous sinus anatomy.

- Inferiorly: Part of the floor is formed by the pyramidal process of the palatine bone.

There are numerous foramina in the PPF. Posteriorly is the foramen rotundum with the maxillary nerve (V2), vidian canal with the vidian nerve, palatovaginal canal, inferior orbital fissure, sphenopalatine foramen, pterygomaxillary fissure, and the palatine canal. Also within the PPF is the sphenopalatine ganglion, located posterior to the internal maxillary artery.

The infratemporal fossa (ITF) lies lateral to the PPF. Its boundaries are defined as follows:

- Anterior: Posterior surface of the maxilla
- Posterior: Styloid process, carotid sheath, and deep portions of the parotid gland
- Medial: Lateral pterygoid plate and superior pharyngeal constrictor
- Lateral: Ramus and zygomatic arch
- Inferior/Floor: None (continuous with neck spaces)
- Superior: Greater wing of the sphenoid.

Contained within the infratemporal fossa are the pterygoid muscles, the internal maxillary artery and its branches, the mandibular branch of the trigeminal nerve and its branches, the pterygoid venous plexus, and fat. Major foramina include the carotid canal, jugular foramen, foramen spinosum, ovale, and lacerum. The ITF continues medially to the PPF via the pterygomaxillary fissure.

Vascular Supply

The vascular supply to the skull base and paranasal sinuses is from both the internal and external carotid circulation. The internal maxillary artery is a branch of the external carotid artery that runs from lateral to medial, deep to the posterior wall of the maxillary sinus. In the infratemporal fossa, the maxillary artery provides supply to the temporalis muscle, and gives off the middle meningeal branch. As it passes through the pterygopalatine fossa, the maxillary artery branches into the superior alveolar, infraorbital, and greater palatine arteries before entering the nasal cavity as the SPA. After exiting the sphenopalatine foramen the artery splits into the posterior septal artery and into posterior lateral nasal arteries that parallel the superior, middle, and inferior turbinates. The posterior septal artery runs inferior to the natural sphenoid ostium and is often encountered when expanding a sphenoidotomy inferiorly. It is this artery that supplies posteriorly based septal flaps that are commonly used to reconstruct skull base defects.

The internal carotid artery may be divided into five segments: the cervical, the petrous, the intracavernous, the clinoid, and the supraclinoid segments. The cervical portion extends superior from the bifurcation of the common carotid to the carotid canal. The petrous portion of the internal carotid artery begins once this artery enters the carotid canal. After initial ascent within the carotid canal, the ICA turns anteromedially into the horizontal petrous segment. Just anterior to the horizontal segment of the ICA is the eustachian tube. After entrance into the foramen lacerum, the ICA runs under the petroclival ligament, turns superiorly, and transitions into the intracavernous segment. The artery ascends towards the posterior clinoid process and then turns anteriorly to enter the cavernous sinus. The ICA then runs anteriorly though the cavernous sinus towards the anterior sphenoid. Here at the anterior bend, it again turns superiorly and passes medial to the anterior clinoid process where it transitions into the clinoid segment. Finally, the ICA turns posteriorly and medially, running lateral to the optic nerve and medial to the anterior clinoid process as the supraclinoid segment. The intersection of the clinoid carotid with the optic nerve creates the opticocarotid recess, which is often evident endoscopically in the lateral superior wall of the sphenoid (Fig. 2.14).

The ophthalmic artery is the first branch of the ICA distal to the cavernous sinus. Once intraorbital, the ophthalmic artery branches into the posterior ethmoid, anterior ethmoid, supratrochlear, and supraorbital arteries. The anterior ethmoidal artery is located about 20 mm posterior to the lacrimal crest. The intranasal course of the artery is illustrated in Figure 2.15. This artery can either run along the skull base or below the skull base within a mesentery. The posterior ethmoidal artery lies about 10 mm posterior to the anterior ethmoidal artery within the orbit. Approximately 5 mm posterior to the posterior ethmoidal artery is the optic nerve.

ANATOMIC VARIATIONS

Certain anatomic variations are significant in that they may obstruct the infundibulum, or any part of the osteomeatal complex, interfering with the nasal air flow and mucociliary clearance of the frontal/

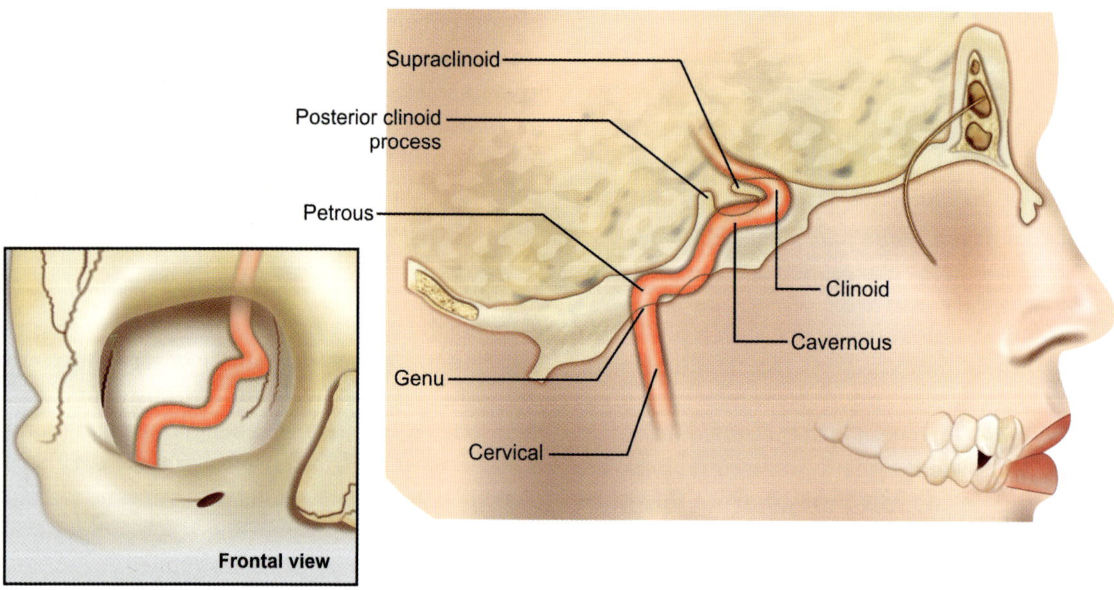

Fig. 2.14: Course of intracranial internal carotid artery.

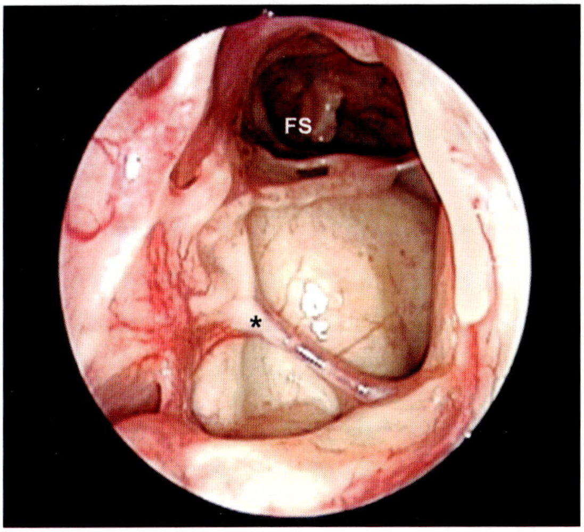

Fig. 2.15: Endoscopic view of left skull base after frontal sinusotomy: *Anterior ethmoid artery; FS: Frontal sinus.

maxillary, sphenoid, and/or ethmoid sinuses. Their presence should be identified clinically and radiographically, as their presence will influence the surgical procedure.[17] See Table 2.3 for relative frequencies of these anatomic variations. Another important variation is the Onodi cell, which is closely related to the optic nerve.

Concha Bullosa

Pneumatization of the middle turbinate (it may also occur in the superior and inferior turbinates, with far less frequency). Concha bullosa may be unilateral or bilateral.

Nasal Septal Deformity

Asymmetric nasal septum position that can displace turbinates laterally and narrow the middle meatus. Septal deviations can cause symptomatic nasal airway obstruction in some cases.

Paradoxical Middle Turbinate

The middle turbinate with its major curvature projected laterally, whereas in most patients it is toward the nasal septum. This may also narrow the middle meatus.

Haller Cell

Ethmoid air cell extending along the medial roof of the maxillary sinus. These cells contribute to narrowing of the infundibulum, and may restrict maxillary sinus drainage. In one study, a statistically significant increase in maxillary sinus mucosal disease was noted in patients with medium or large Haller cells (45.8%) versus those with small cells.[18]

Onodi Cell

The Onodi cell was first described by Adolf Onodi, a professor of laryngology, at the University of Budapest in Hungary in 1910. It is the most posterior ethmoid cell that pneumatizes laterally and superiorly to the sphenoid sinus and, due to its location, is intimately associated with the optic nerve. The presence of an Onodi cell can increase the risk of

Table 2.3 Anatomic variations

Study	*Concha bullosa*	*Septal deviation*	*Paradox MT*	*Haller cell*	*Onodi cell*
Zeinrich et al[12]	36%	21%	15%	10%	*
Mazza et al[13]	29%	*	11%	5%	9%
Kayalioglu et al[14]	28%	17%	10%	5%	*
Bolger et al[15]	53%	19%	26%	45%	*
Arslan et al[16]	30%	36%	3%	6%	12%

*Not evaluated

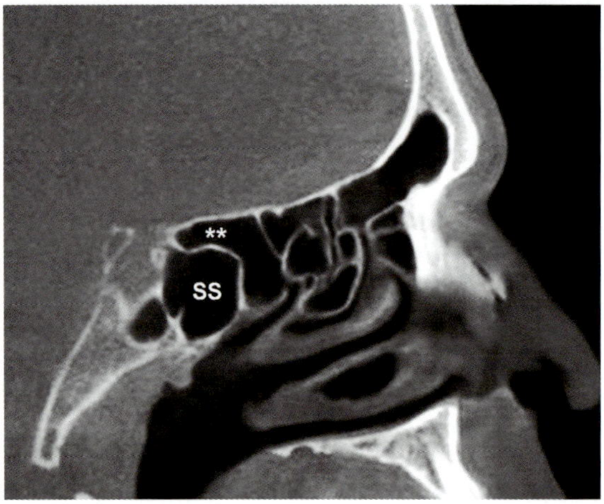

Fig. 2.16: Sagittal CT scan demonstration relationship between sphenoid sinus and Onodi cell: SS: Sphenoid sinus; **Onodi cell.

orbital complications during endoscopic sinus surgery (Fig. 2.16).

CONCLUSION

Technological advancements such as high resolution CT scans, intraoperative image guidance, and the availability of computer workstations for preoperative planning, has improved our understanding of surgical anatomy. However, even for experienced surgeons, the anatomy of the paranasal sinuses remains complex, and dissection challenging, due to its high variability. An intimate knowledge of the anatomic regions of the paranasal sinuses and skull base is essential for safe surgical management of all sinonasal pathology.

REFERENCES

1. Gray LP. Deviated nasal septum. Incidence and etiology. Ann Otol Rhinol Laryngol Suppl. 1978;87(3 Pt 3 Suppl 50):3-20.
2. Berger G, Balum-Azim M, Ophir D. The normal inferior turbinate: histomorphometric analysis and clinical implications. Laryngoscope. 2003;113(7):1192-8.
3. Padgham N, Vaughan-Jones R. Cadaver studies of the anatomy of arterial supply to the inferior turbinates. J R Soc Med. 1991;84(12):728-30.
4. Min, Y-G., Koh, et al. Clinical implications of the uncinate process in paranasal sinusitis: Radiologic evaluation. Am J Rhinology. 1995;9(3):131-5.
5. Orhan M, Govsa F, Saylam C. A quite rare condition: absence of sphenoidal sinuses. Surg Radiol Anat. 2010;32(6):551-3. Epub 2010 Jan 16.
6. Lee HY, Kim HU, Kim SS, et al. Surgical anatomy of the sphenopalatine artery in lateral nasal wall. Laryngoscope. 2002;112(10):1813-8.
7. Kennedy D, Zinrich H, Hassab M. The internal carotid artery as it relates to endoscopic shenoethmoidectomy. Am J Rhinol. 1990;4:7-12.
8. Birsen U, Gulsah B, Yasemin K, et al. Risky anatomic variations of sphenoid sinus for surgery. Surg Radil Anat. 2006;28:195-201.
9. Bent JP, Cuilty-Siller C, Kuhn FA. The frontal cell as a cause of frontal sinus obstruction. Am J Rhinol. 1994;8:185-91.
10. Kainz J, Stammberger H. The roof of the anterior ethmoid: a place of least resistance in the skull base. Am J Rhinol. 1989;3:191-9.
11. Keros P. On the practical value of difference in the level of the lamina cribrosa of the ethmoid. Z Laryngol Rhinol Otol. 1962;41:809-13.
12. Zinreich SJ, Abidin M, Kennedy DW. Cross sectional imaging of the nasal cavity and paranasal sinuses. Operative techniques in otolaryngology. Head and Neck Surg. 1990;2:94-8.
13. Mazza D, Bontempi E, Guerrisi A, et al. Paranasal sinuses anatomic variants: 64-slice CT evaluation. Minerva Stomatol. 2007;56(6):311-8.
14. Kayalioglu G, Oyar O, Govsa F. Nasal cavity and paranasal sinus bony variations: a computed tomographic study. Rhinology. 2000;38(3):108-13.
15. Bolger WE, Butzin CA, Parsons DS. Paranasal sinus bony anatomic variations and mucosal abnormalities: CT analysis for endoscopic sinus surgery. Laryngoscope. 1991;101:56-64.
16. Arslan H, Aydinlioglu A, Bozkurt M, et al. Anatomic variations of the paranasal sinuses: CT examination for endoscopic sinus surgery. Auris Nasus Larynx. 1999;26(1):39-48.
17. Kantarci M, Karasen RM, Alper F, et al. Remarkable anatomic variations in paranasal sinus region and their clinical importance. Eur J Radiol. 2004;50(3):296-302.
18. Stackpole SA, Edelstein DR. The anatomic relevance of the Haller cell in sinusitis. Am J Rhinol. 1997;11(3):219-23.

3

Imaging of Sinonasal Tumors

Andrew Hou, MD; Thomas Borges, MD

INTRODUCTION

The major goals of imaging sinonasal tumors are to identify the primary abnormality, determine its degree of aggression, delineate local extent of a tumor's margins, characterize perineural spread (PNS) and orbital invasion, and evaluate the skull base and lymph node involvement. Due to the complexity of these tumors, an imaging workup should include a combination of computed tomography (CT) and magnetic resonance imaging (MRI). CT is essential for evaluating bone involvement or destruction. MRI further characterizes soft tissue involvement and can better distinguish benign from malignant findings.

On CT, evaluating bone changes can be challenging as the radiographic appearance may not always be a proper reflection of a tumor (Figs. 3.1A and B). As a general rule, an aggressive process will cause irregular destruction with ill-defined margins of infiltration. Changes are often described as "osteolytic" and squamous cell carcinoma (SCC) most commonly exhibits this finding. However, this can also occur with metastatic disease, aggressive sarcomas and sinonasal undifferentiated carcinoma.[1]

Bone scalloping and remodeling often occur from a more long-standing benign process such as inflammation and polyps (Figs 3.2A and B); however, melanoma can also have this appearance.[2] Some aggressive tumors may remodel the bone, examples include malignant minor salivary gland tumors, large cell lymphomas, melanomas and olfactory neuroblastomas.[1]

Bone along the skull base has a limited ability to remodel and may deossify secondary to pressure, giving an aggressive and infiltrative appearance. When bone margins are sclerotic, a chronic relapsing process such as obstruction and/or infection should be considered. Sinus inflammation and infection, as seen in allergic fungal rhinosinusitis, can also cause extensive bone destruction. Aggressive bone changes involving the orbit, cribriform plate or posterior lateral maxillary sinus wall may indicate spread beyond the nasal cavity and paranasal sinuses. Contrast is most helpful for evaluating tumor along the meninges and orbit, along with characterizing post-obstructive sinusitis[3] and necrosis, which are typically nonenhancing. Lesion density on CT can also be quite variable as hypercellular neoplasms have similar Hounsfield measurements compared to chronic secretions, fungal infections or blood products.[2]

Magnetic resonance imaging provides the greatest detailed soft tissue evaluation without

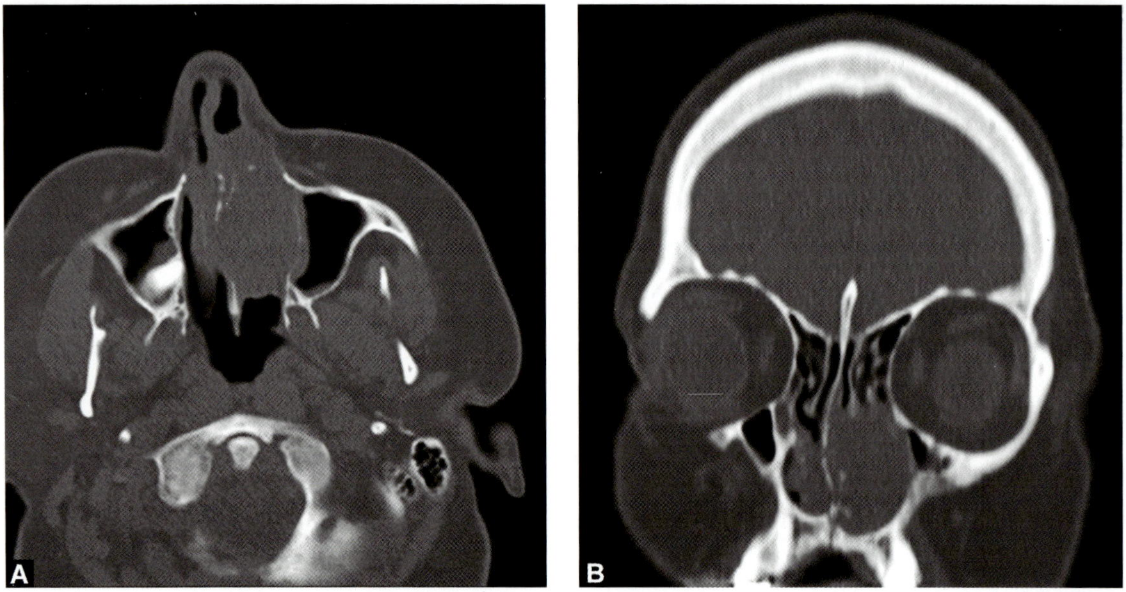

Figs 3.1A and B: (A) Axial; (B) coronal CT images in bone windows with a chondrosarcoma lacking matrix and deceptively benign appearing thinned bone.

ionizing radiation. Delineation of tumor from surrounding soft tissue inflammation depends on the signal differences of each. Often, tumors have a hypo-to-isointense signal on both T1 and T2-weighted MRI sequences when compared to brain and muscle. Tumors such as pleomorphic

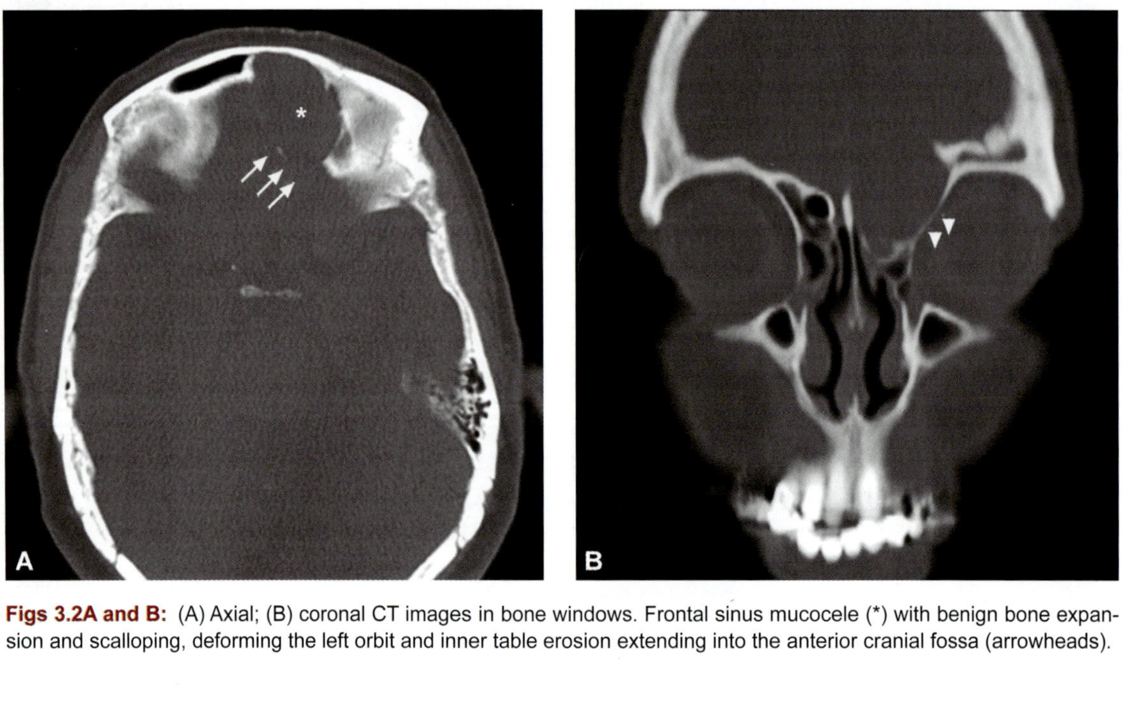

Figs 3.2A and B: (A) Axial; (B) coronal CT images in bone windows. Frontal sinus mucocele (*) with benign bone expansion and scalloping, deforming the left orbit and inner table erosion extending into the anterior cranial fossa (arrowheads).

adenomas, nerve sheath neoplasms, hemangiomas and inverted papillomas tend to be bright on T2-weighted MR images. Signal characteristics can overlap with benign secretions as protein and water content vary. As protein content increases to near 30% and water content decreases, signal will increase on T1-weighted and decrease on T2-weighted MRI sequences. Near or above 30%, the protein signal on both T1 and T2-weighted MRI sequences will drop and can appear as a void, similar to air. Tumors avidly enhance after contrast administration while retained secretions will not and only peripheral enhancement along the inflamed mucosa is apparent.[4]

With new and developing CT scanners, finding an ideal balance between radiation dose and image quality remains a challenge. CT protocols with 1 mm axial non-contrast images can provide isometric reformations on separate workstations and selected images can be captured to highlight specific details. Other protocols utilize 2–3 mm thick sections obtained in the coronal plane with the patient prone and the neck hyper-extended. In either protocol, 3 mm coronal reformatted images usually provide the necessary details in most cases and allow for easy viewing of the anatomic landmarks for sinus surgery, as well as the horizontally directed foramen rotundum and vidian canal.

Standard MRI protocols include non-contrast axial and coronal 3 mm T1 and T2-weighted images centered on the paranasal sinuses, while including the anterior and middle cranial fossa. Fat suppression on post-contrast MRI is especially helpful while examining the skull base as normal bright fat signal can hide subtle involvement. A complete evaluation characterizes abnormal tissue along the fat planes of the subcutaneous cheek, parapharyngeal space, pterygopalatine fossa (PPF), retroantral fat pad and masticator space.

PERINEURAL SPREAD

Approximately 2.5–5% of head and neck cancers exhibit PNS. Amongst sinonasal malignancies, the most common tumors are SCC (Figs 3.3A and B) and minor salivary gland tumors such as adenoid

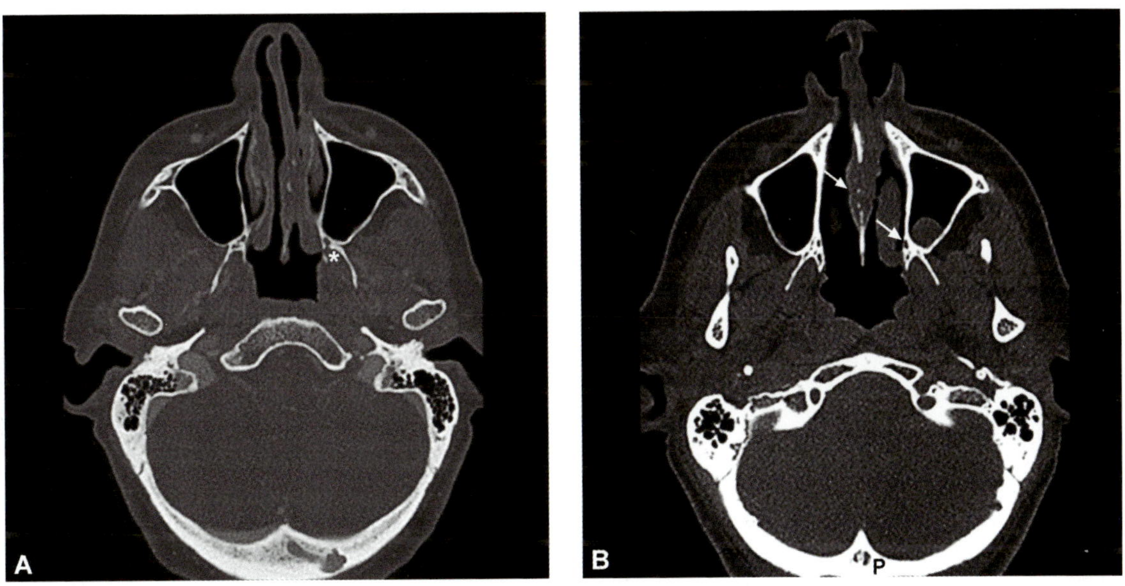

Figs 3.3A and B: Axial noncontrast CT images. (A) Bone; (B) Soft tissue windows. Subtle erosion of the left medial pterygoid plate (*) and widening of the left pterygopalatine canal (arrow). Permeative and lytic changes involve the nasal septum (arrowhead). Squamous cell carcinoma with perineural spread.

cystic carcinoma. For aggressive sinonasal tumors, the V2 division of the trigeminal nerve is the most common conduit for perineural tumor spread. Spread along the nerves is more often towards the central nervous system, although spread outward has been observed. Skip lesions can occur, making it imperative to evaluate the entire course of a nerve to fully characterize the extent of involvement.

The route of spread along V2 can begin via the infraorbital division in the roof of the maxillary sinus, or by infiltration of tumor into the PPF. This may continue through the foramen rotundum, into the cavernous sinus, through Meckel's cave and to the main trigeminal trunk[5] (Figs 3.4 to 3.6).

On CT, nerve involvement manifests as widening and erosion of fissures, foramina, and canals, as well as bone remodeling[6] (Figs 3.7A to C). Obliteration of the normal fat planes at the skull base foramina may precede bone changes as an early sign of nerve involvement.[7] On MRI, pre-contrast T1-weighted images are important to evaluate for replacement of the normal hyperintense fat within the PPF and along the basal foramina[5] (Fig. 3.5A). While contrast-enhanced CT rarely shows enhancement of tumor along nerves, post-contrast T1-weighted fat-suppression MR images allow the best visualization of abnormally-enhancing nerves[8] (Figs 3.4A and 3.5B).

Studies have shown an association between PNS and an enhanced risk of subsequent locoregional recurrence with decreased survival.[9] Therefore, it is crucial for perineural extension to be identified prior to treatment planning for appropriate and optimal therapy.

Orbital Involvement

Distinguishing between orbital invasion of tumor versus tumor in a periorbital location is often difficult, but of tremendous clinical importance, as the former portends a worse prognosis and may require a more aggressive and debilitating surgery. The line of demarcation is essentially formed by the periorbita. This is comprised of the periosteum from the seven bones forming the orbit and is continuous with the dura mater at the optic foramen and superior orbital fissure. Unfortunately, the periorbita is poorly delineated on imaging; CT has little discriminating capability between soft tissues and the periorbita.[10] On MRI, bone and periorbita are both hypointense on T1-weighted and T2-

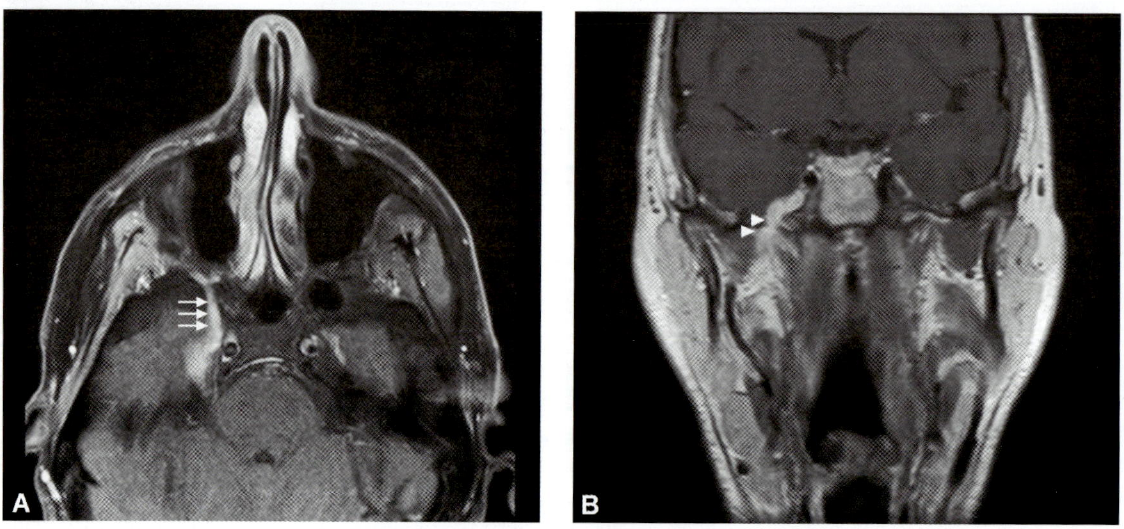

Figs 3.4A and B: (A) Post-contrast T1-weighted fat-suppressed axial; (B) Post-contrast T1-weighted coronal MR image. Perineural spread along the right trigemial nerve V2 (arrows) and V3 (arrowheads) segments.

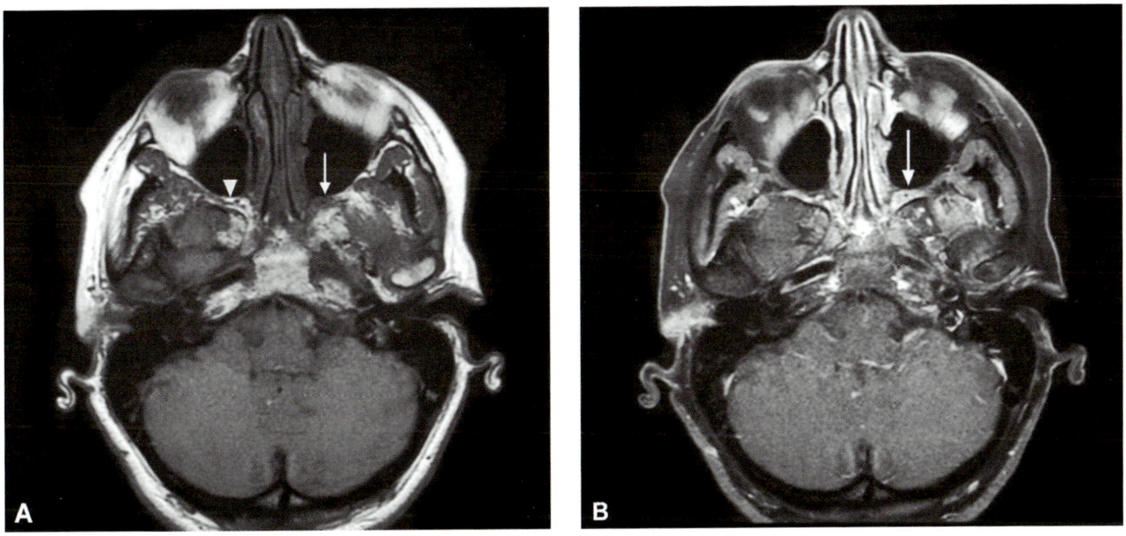

Figs 3.5A and B: (A) Pre-contrast T1-weighted; (B) Post-contrast T1-weighted fat-suppressed axial MR images. Left pterygopalatine fossa spread with obliteration (short arrow) of the normal fat (arrowhead) and enhancement (long arrow). Adenoid cystic carcinoma primary.

weighted images. Therefore, lack of this low signal continuity is relied upon to indicate a breach of the periorbita (Figs 3.8B and 3.9A).

Kim et al.[10] found tumors of the paranasal sinuses to be of slightly greater signal intensity than the bone and periorbita on T2-weighted images. Orbital fat invasion was better demonstrated on MRI, as CT poorly differentiated between tumor invading the orbital fat and tumor still limited to the periorbita.

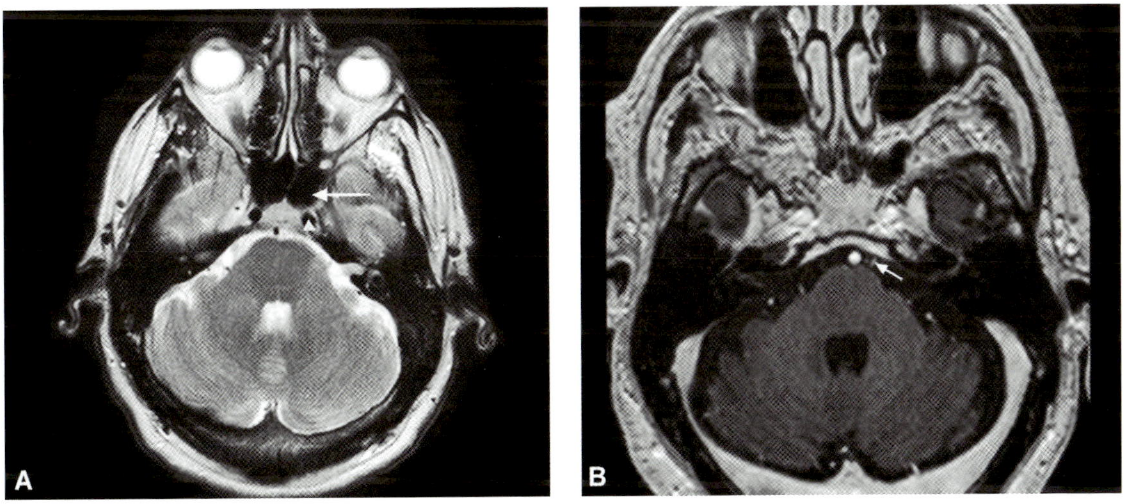

Figs 3.6A and B: (A) Pre-contrast T2-weighted; (B) Post-contrast T1-weighted axial MR images. Perineural spread along V2 with low signal intensity is along the left foramen rotundum (large arrow) as well as loss of normal fluid intensity within Meckel's cave (^). Note normal T2 hyperintensity within the right Meckel's cave (*). Enhancement within the cisternal portion of left cranial nerve V (small arrow) indicates spread to a more proximal location.

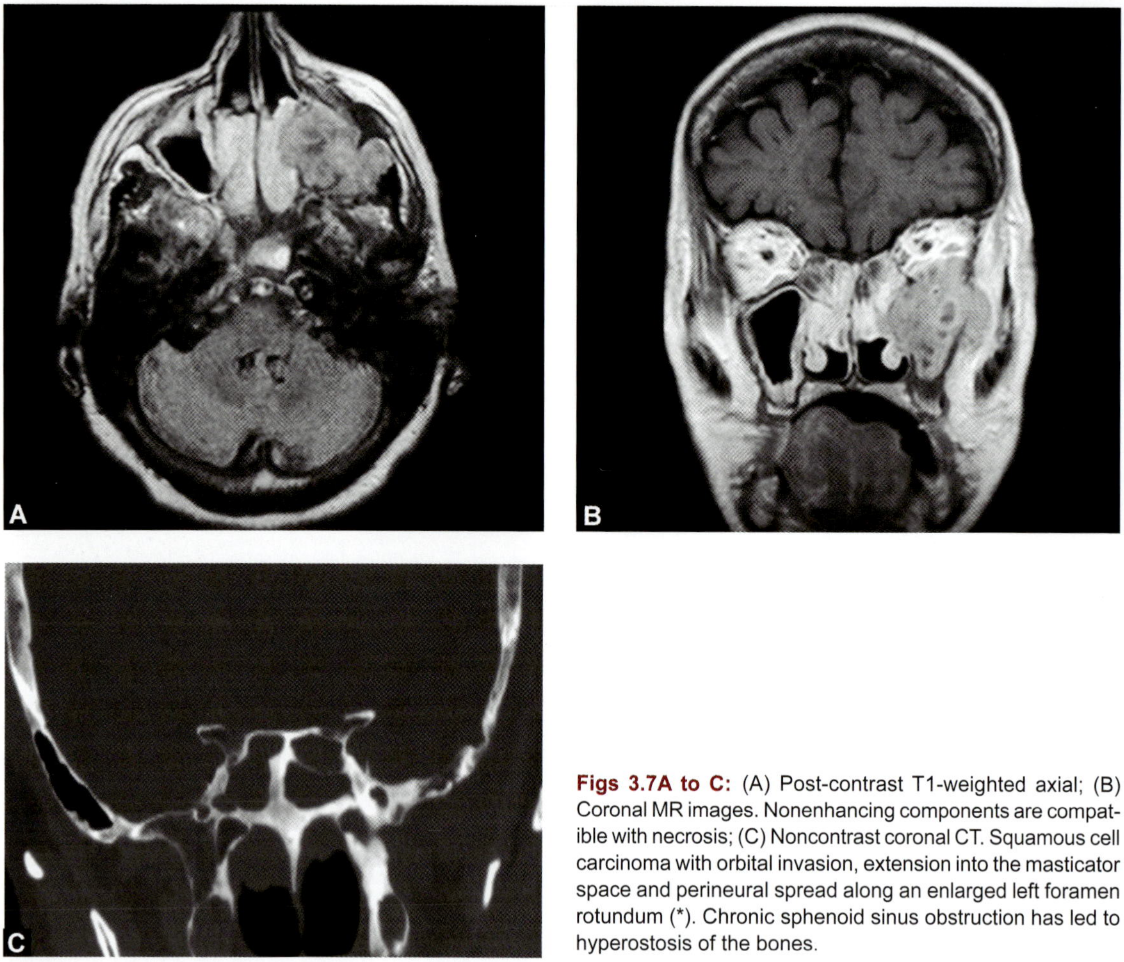

Figs 3.7A to C: (A) Post-contrast T1-weighted axial; (B) Coronal MR images. Nonenhancing components are compatible with necrosis; (C) Noncontrast coronal CT. Squamous cell carcinoma with orbital invasion, extension into the masticator space and perineural spread along an enlarged left foramen rotundum (*). Chronic sphenoid sinus obstruction has led to hyperostosis of the bones.

In a study by Eisen et al.[11] the presence of tumor adjacent to the periorbita was shown as the most sensitive imaging criteria to predict orbital invasion. Extraocular muscle enlargement or signal abnormality and infiltration of the orbital fat were the criteria with the highest positive predictive values.

Dural Involvement

Dural infiltration by tumor is an essential precursor to brain parenchymal invasion and is important to recognize preoperatively, as surgical resection and reconstruction becomes significantly more complicated. Post-contrast T1-weighted imaging is the key MRI sequence to evaluate for dural abnormalities. The pattern of enhancement is more important than just the presence.[1] Dural involvement is most likely when there is nodular enhancement as opposed to the linear reactive change seen in hyperemia and inflammation (Figs 3.10 to 3.12). Imaging findings, which have been shown to accurately predict tumor involvement of the dura, include the presence of pial enhancement, nodular dural enhancement and dural enhancement greater than 5 mm in thickness[12] (Figs 3.13B and 3.14B).

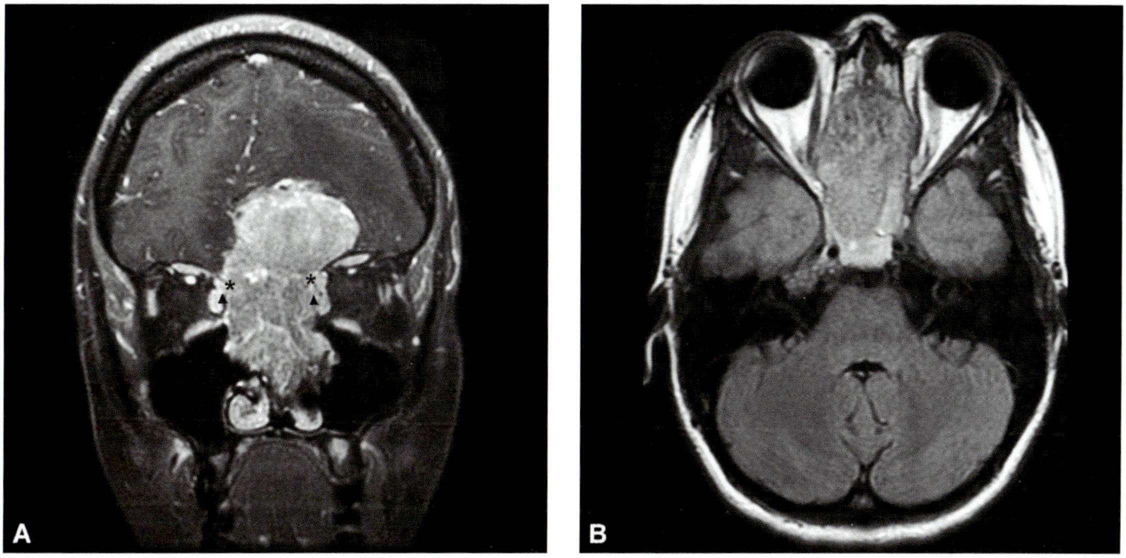

Figs 3.8A and B: (A) Post-contrast T1-weighted fat-suppressed coronal MRI, (B) Pre-contrast T2 FLAIR axial MR image. Sinonasal undifferentiated carcinoma eroding through the skull base and into both orbits along the medial rectus (^) and superior oblique(*) muscles, left greater than right. Medial orbital wall invasion on a T2 FLAIR sequence is displayed in (B).

Skull base invasion can manifest as infiltration of the marrow and lack of the normal bright signal on T1-weighted images. This tends to be non-specific however, since many processes such as anemia, HIV, lymphoma and osteomalacia can have similar findings.

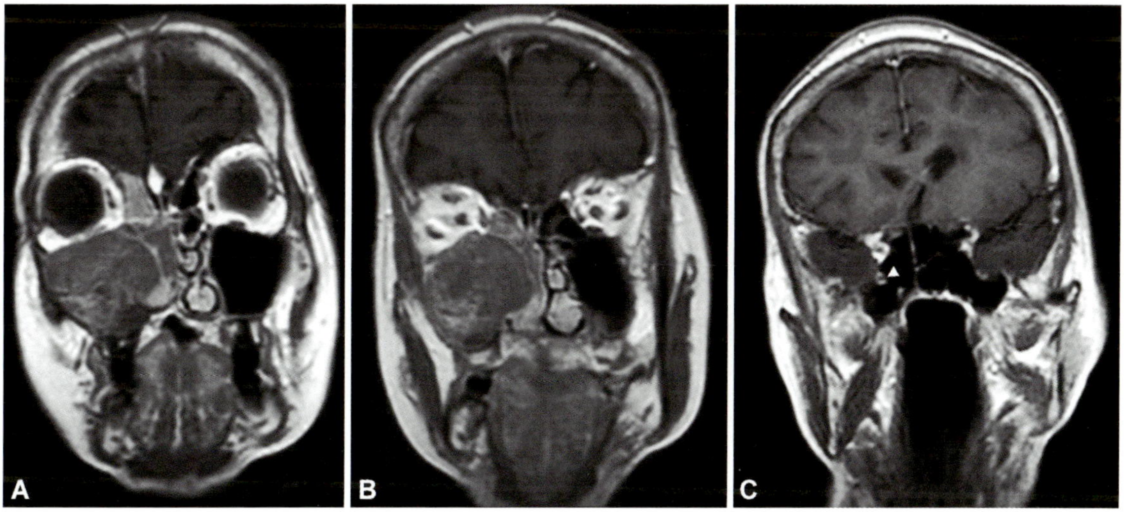

Figs 3.9A to C: (A) Pos-tcontrast T1-weighted coronal MR images. (A and B) Melanoma invading the right orbit, filling the entire right maxillary sinus and obstructing the right frontal sinus; (C) Perineural spread is along the enlarged right foramen rotundum (arrowhead).

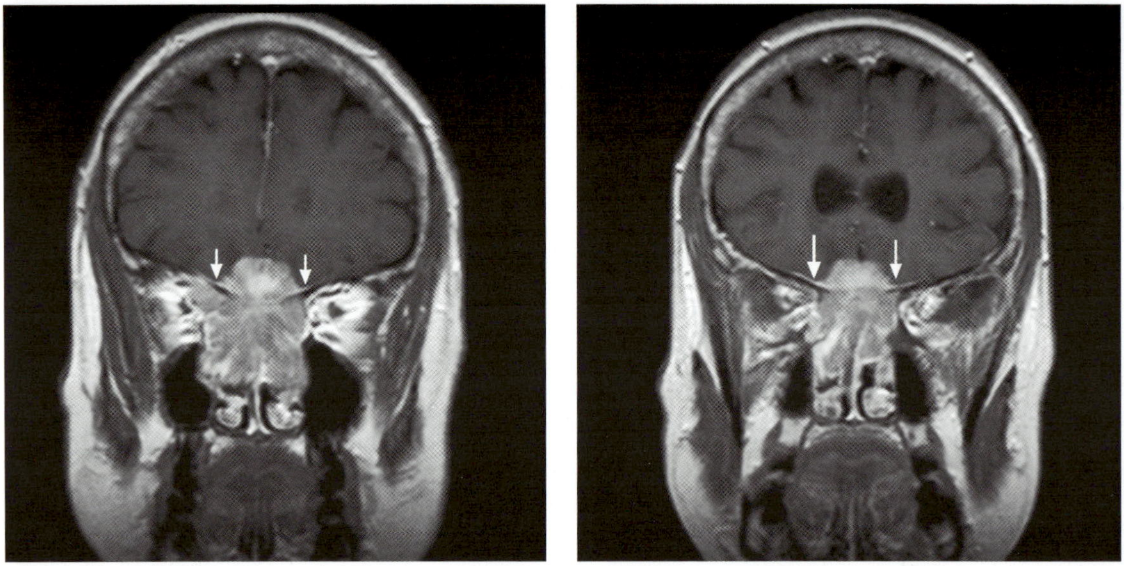

Figs 3.10A and B: (A and B) Post-contrast T1-weighted coronal MR images. Enhancing mass centered at the cribriform plate with portions extending into the anterior cranial fossa and upper nasal cavity. While the description is fitting for an esthesioneuroblastoma, the thickened dural enhancement (arrows) along the lateral margins of the mass is not typical for ENB. In fact, the enhancement is a classic appearance for a "dural tail" and this was a case of nasal meningioma.

Nodal and Distant Metastases

In addition to CT and MRI of the head and neck for characterization of the primary tumor and detection of locoregional spread, CT of the chest, abdomen, and pelvis is not uncommonly performed to assess for distant metastases. Unfortunately, these exams are limited as they provide anatomic information but are incapable of detailing biological activity. 18F-FDG-PET imaging can detect metabolic activity from neoplasm within lymph nodes or distant metastases and has been shown to affect patient management and prognosis.[13] Combined PET/CT has improved diagnostic accuracy with fewer equivocal findings in comparison to standard PET images in these patients.[14]

The role of follow-up with 18F-Fluorodeoxyglucose-positron emission tomography (18F-FDG-PET) continues to develop. Overlapping findings from resection, radiation and edema, as well as intracranial tumors near adjacent hypermetabolic brain pose a challenge. A review by Liu et al.[15] found an average sensitivity of 95% for residual or recurrent disease using 18F-FDG-PET, more than CT (76%) and MRI (78%). In certain instances, 201TL SPECT can be helpful in distinguishing tumor from radiation necrosis as only viable tumor will utilize intracellular transport for this K+ analog. Yet this modality can miss tumors below 1.5 cm in size. Yen et al.[16] compared SPECT/CT with 18F-FDG-PET and found overall sensitivity and specificity at 66.7%/100% and 86.7%/75% respectively.

SQUAMOUS CELL CARCINOMA

Squamous cell carcinoma is the most common sinonasal malignancy, accounting for up to 80% of cases. This occurs more often in men (2:1 male-to-female ratio) and has been associated with occupational exposures, such as nickel, wood dust, chromium and isopropyl alcohol. Sinonasal involvement is distributed amongst the maxillary sinus (25–60%), nasal cavity (30%), and ethmoid air cells (10%). Origin within the

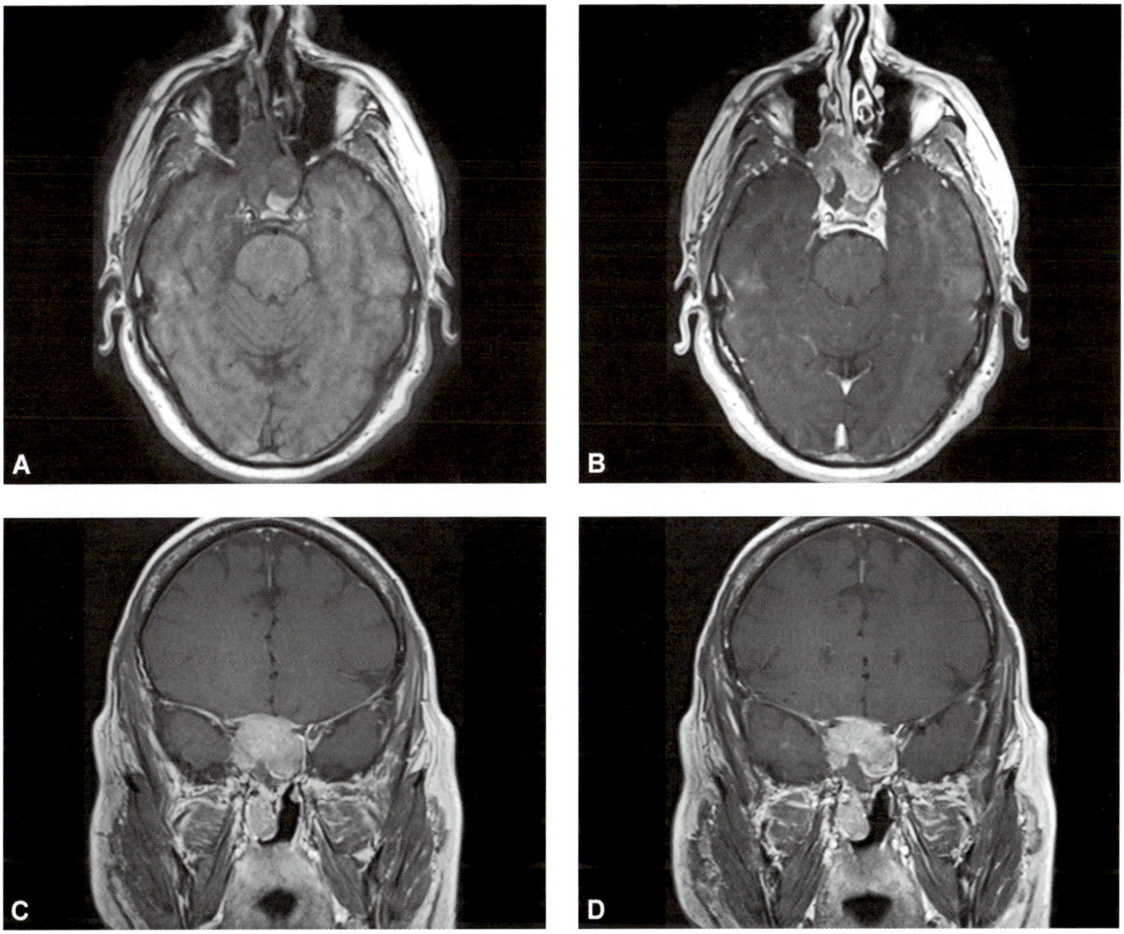

Figs 3.11A to D: (A and B) Pre- and post-contrast T1-weighted axial; (C and D) Post-contrast coronal MR images. Sinonasal undifferentiated carcinoma which is T1 hypointense and demonstrates heterogeneous enhancement following contrast administration. There is extension into the anterior cranial fossa along the thickened dura and the brain parenchyma is displaced, but not invaded.

frontal or sphenoid sinuses occurs in less than 2% of the cases.[17]

On CT, SCC appears as a soft-tissue density mass with heterogeneous enhancement. Bone destruction often has an aggressive appearance.

On MRI, SCC is typically isointense on T1-weighted imaging and isointense to hyperintense on T2-weighted imaging. Higher cellularity results in more hypointense signal than other sinonasal tumors. Enhancement is often heterogeneous with areas of nonenhancing necrosis (Fig. 3.7B).

ADENOCARCINOMA

Adenocarcinoma accounts for about 4% of primary sinonasal malignant neoplasms. These are more commonly found in workers of the hardwood and shoe industries as exposure to wood dust imparts a 900-fold increased relative risk of developing adenocarcinoma. These patients are typically men and the tumors have predilection for the ethmoid sinuses. A second subgroup is comprised of sporadic tumors, more often in women, which more

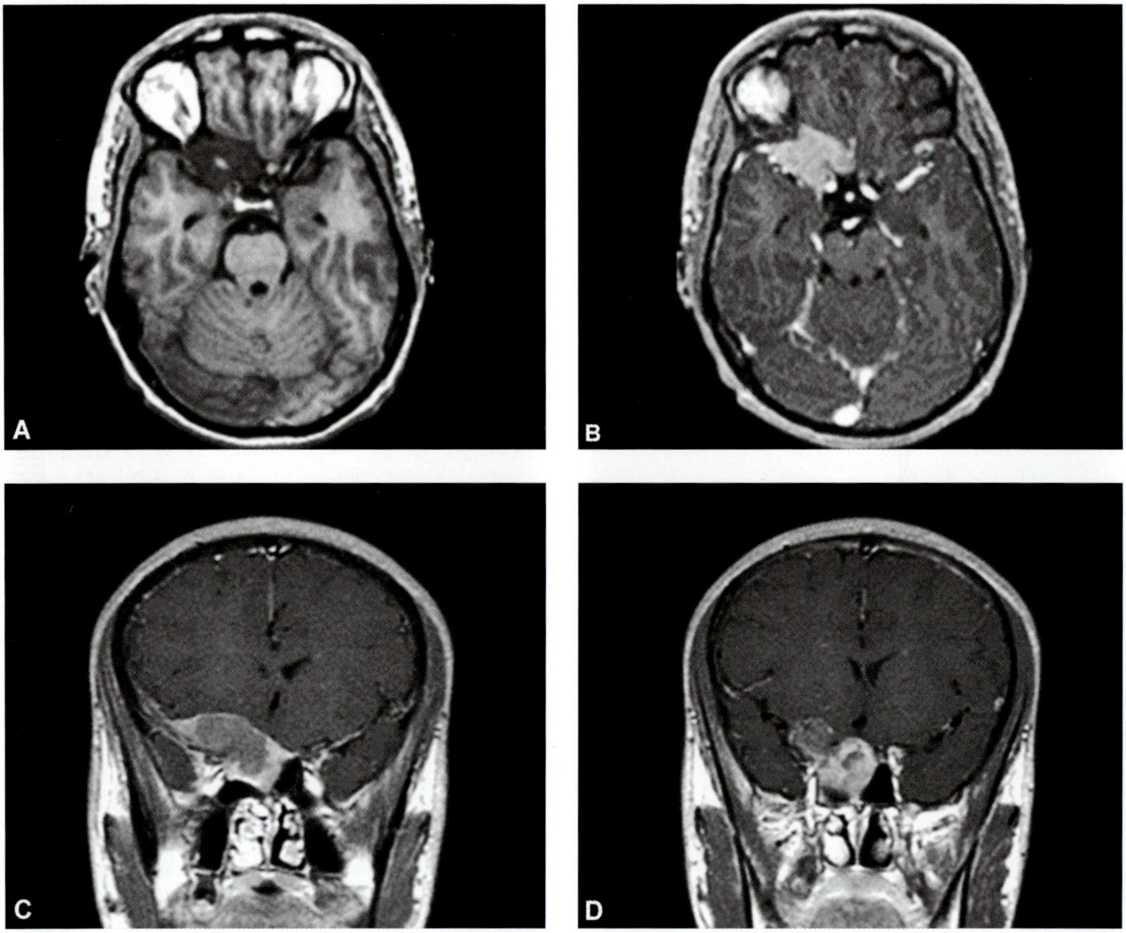

Figs 3.12A to D: (A) Pre-contrast T1-weighted; (B) Post-contrast T1-weighted fat-suppressed axial; (C and D) Coronal MR images. Expansile T1 hypointense mass involving the sphenoid sinuses extends along the anterior cranial fossa and sella, and has heterogeneous enhancement following contrast administration. The brain parenchyma is displaced, but not invaded. Findings are similar to those encountered in Figures 3.11A to D.

frequently arise within the maxillary sinuses. Nasal cavity and ethmoid sinus tumors usually become symptomatic prior to invasion of local structures while those of maxillary sinus origin often remain asymptomatic until an advanced stage.[18]

Tumors are typically hypointense on T1-weighted and hypointense on T2-weighted MR images. Enhancement patterns are variable.

Adenoid Cystic Carcinoma

Sinonasal adenoid cystic carcinomas usually arise from minor salivary glands, most commonly within the maxillary sinuses and followed by the nasal cavity (Figs 3.15 and 3.16). Direct extension from the palate may also occur, but is less common.[19] They comprise 5–15% of all sinonasal malignancies. These tumors are slow-growing, exhibit multiple local recurrences and have a protracted clinical course.[20] Perineural tumor invasion is characteristic and since skip lesions along nerves can occur, negative surgical margins are of equivocal significance.[21]

These tumors have a locally aggressive appearance, commonly presenting with a combination of bone erosions and sclerosis. Higher grade tumors

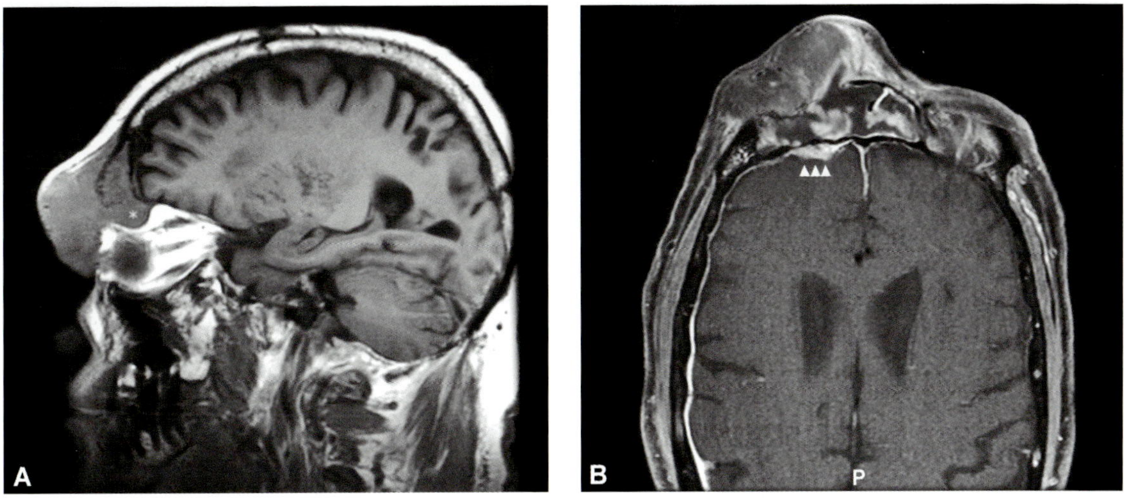

Figs 3.13A and B: (A) Pre-contrast T1-weighted sagittal; (B) Post-contrast T1-weighted fat-suppressed axial MR images. Large frontal sinus follicular cell carcinoma with orbital (*) and dural (^) invasion.

are intermediate intensity on T2-weighted imaging and are more frequent than lower grade tumors which can be T2 hyperintense.

Inverted Papilloma

Inverted papilloma (IP) is a benign sinonasal tumor which has been reported to develop into carcinoma or have concurrent carcinoma in 3–24% of cases.[21] These constitute 0.5–4% of nasal cavity tumors, commonly arising from the lateral wall and may extend into the maxillary or ethmoid sinuses. Extension into the frontal and sphenoid sinuses may also occur, but is less frequent. Larger IP tumors are associated with

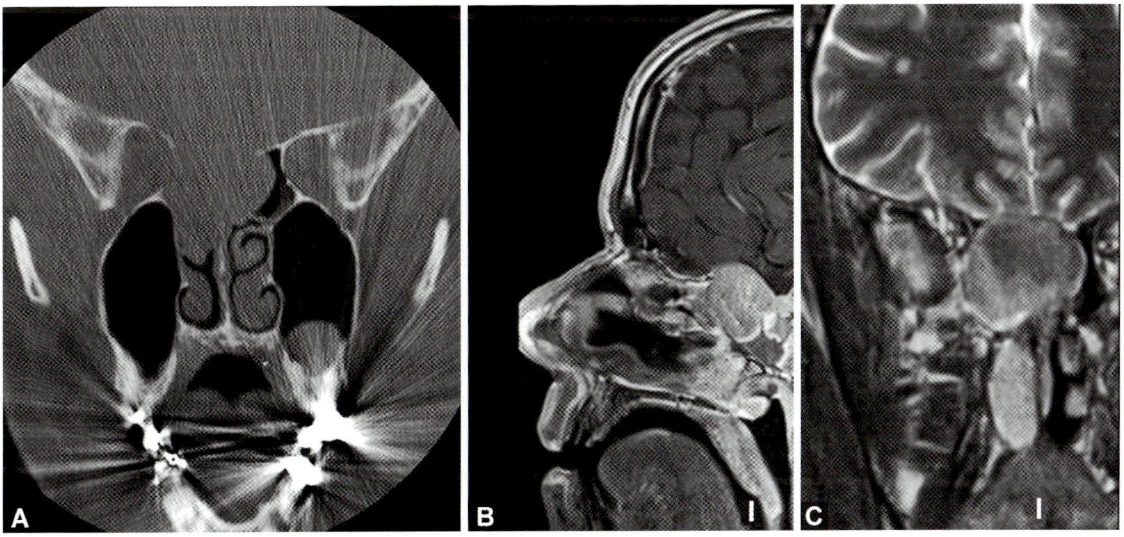

Figs 3.14A to C: (A) Noncontrast coronal CT; (B) Post-contrast T1-weighted fat-suppressed sagittal; (C) Pre-contrast T2-weighted coronal MR images. SNUC invading the skull base. Intracranial involvement is confined to the dura as there are normal signal returns from the adjacent gyrus rectus.

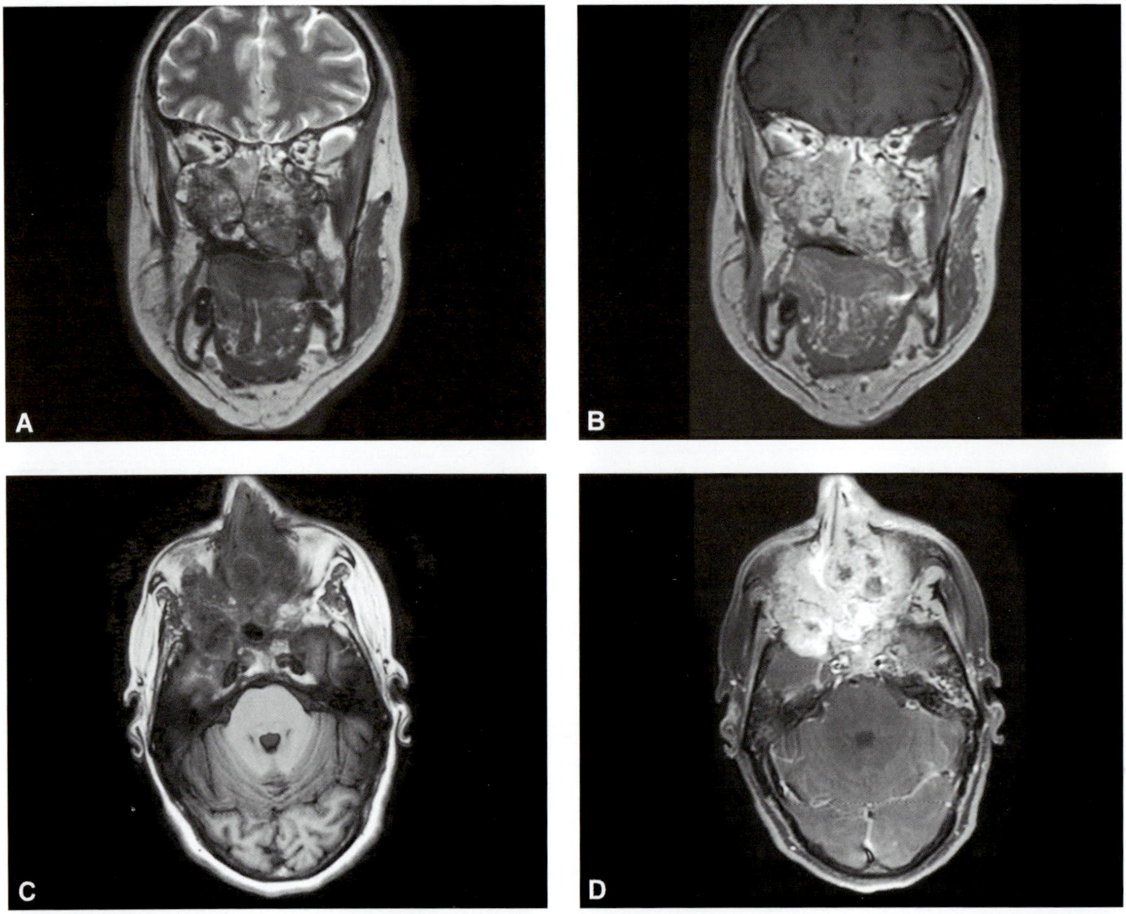

Figs 3.15A to D: (A) Pre-contrast T2-weighted; (B) Post-contrast T1-weighted coronal MR images showing a large mass occupying the entire nasal vault as well as filling the maxillary sinuses and involving the ethmoid air cells; (C) Pre-contrast T1-weighted; (D) Post-contrast T1-weighted fat-suppressed axial MR images showing diffuse hypointensity and avoid enhancement following contrast administration.

bone remodeling and a pattern of sinus disease reflecting ostiomeatal unit obstruction.

Typically IP is initially evaluated with a CT scan since the usual presenting symptoms suggest sinus disease. On CT, IP appears as a soft tissue density mass extending from the lateral wall of the nasal cavity, usually at the level of the middle meatus, into adjacent paranasal sinuses. Associated bone remodeling takes the form of thinning, bowing and/or sclerosis and most frequently involves the medial wall of the maxillary sinus.[22] Extensive bone destruction should raise suspicion for an associated malignancy, but this is a nonspecific finding. A cone-shaped pattern of hyperostosis has been reported as a possible predictor of the origin of IP.[23] Recurrent IP may be associated with significant hyperostosis, which should raise suspicion of a more broad focus or multiple foci of origin. Tumoral calcifications may occur and are postulated to represent remodeled

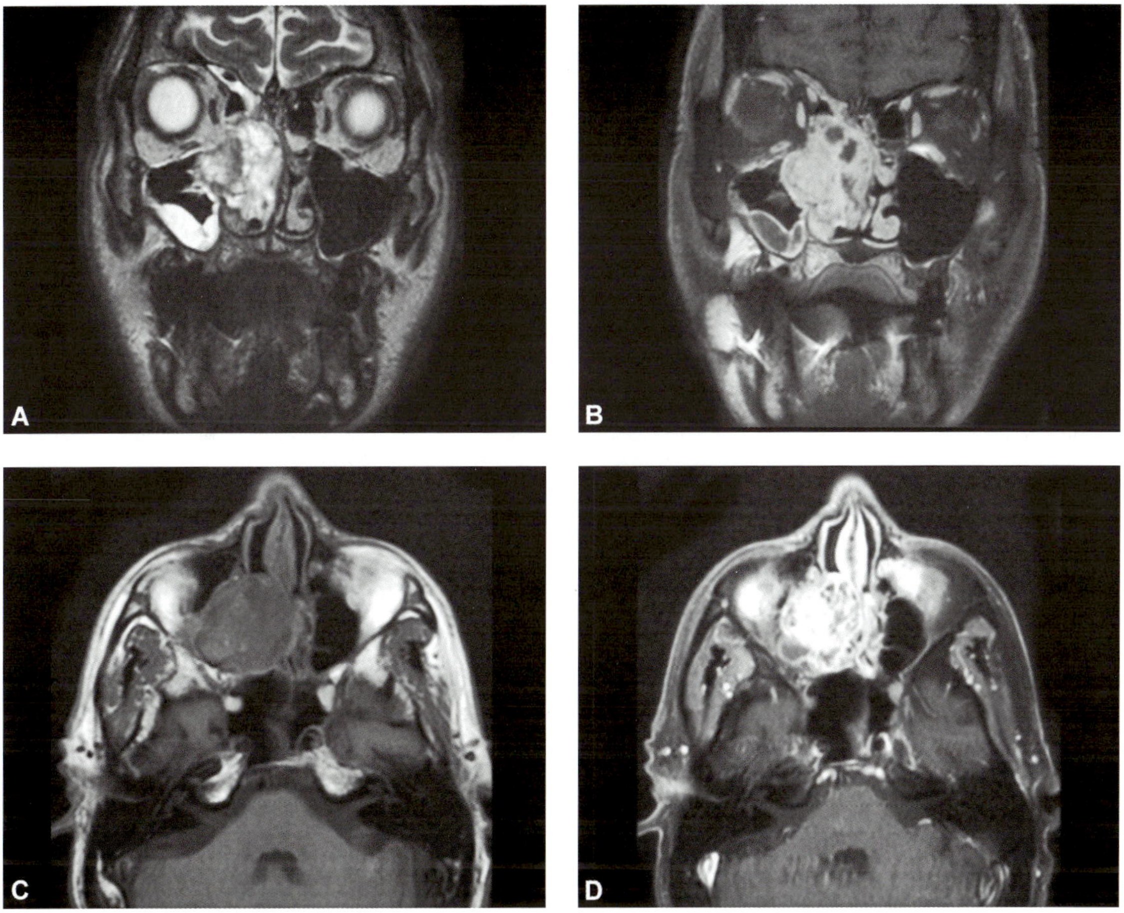

Figs 3.16A to D: (A) Pre-contrast T2-weighted; (B) Post-contrast T1-weighted fat-suppressed coronal MR images with heterogeneous, predominantly T2 hyperintense signal and avid enhancement with contrast. The mass occupies the right nasal cavity with extension into the right maxillary sinus and as a result, an obstructive pattern has developed; (C) Pre-contrast T1-weighted; (D) Post-contrast T1-weighted fat suppressed axial MR images showing T1 hypointensity and diffuse, avid enhancement following contrast administration.

or entrapped bone.[24] Enhancement patterns on CT are variable.

On MRI, IP is isointense or minimally hyperintense to muscle on T1-weighted imaging. Heterogeneity on T2-weighted images reflects a combination of viable tumor, areas of necrosis and secretions. A convoluted cerebriform pattern or septate striated appearance on T2-weighted or enhanced T1-weighted MR images have both been reported as being strongly suggestive for IP[25] (Figs 3.17A and B). However, this pattern has also been found with malignant sinonasal tumors. Focal loss of the cerebriform pattern may be an indicator of coexistent malignancy.[26]

While the possibility of using PET imaging to distinguish benign IP from those harboring coexisting malignancy has been proposed, thus far, FDG PET-CT does not appear to reliably differentiate benign IP from those associated with malignancy.[27,28]

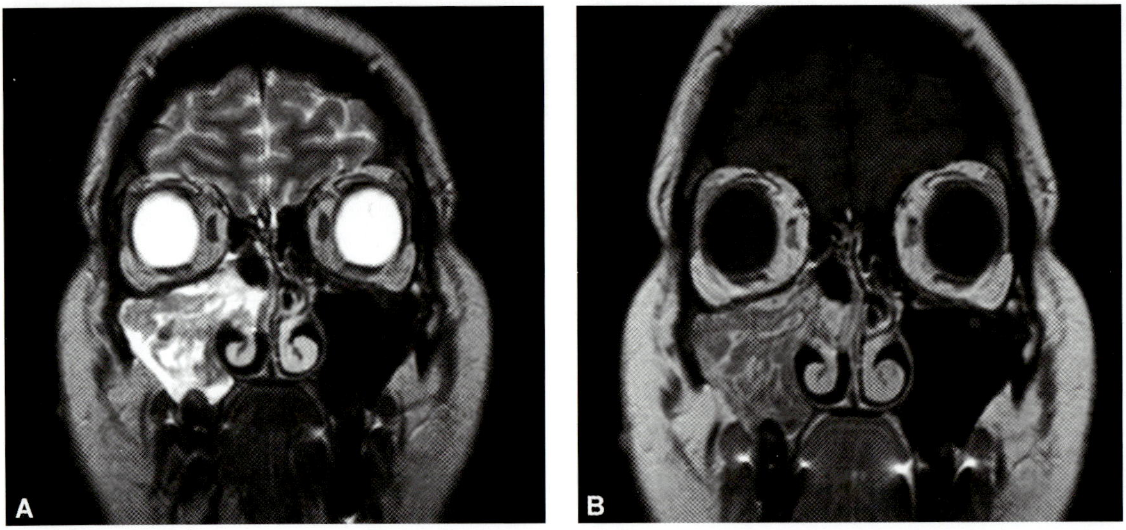

Figs 3.17A and B: (A) Noncontrast T2-weighted fat-suppressed; (B) Post-contrast T1-weighted coronal MR images. Inverted papilloma arising from the lateral wall of the right nasal cavity extending into the right maxillary sinus. Alternating hypointense and hyperintense striations throughout the tumor are consistent with the "convoluted cerebriform pattern".

Esthesioneuroblastoma

Esthesioneuroblastoma (ENB) or olfactory neuroblastoma, arise from olfactory epithelium within the superior nasal cavity along the cribriform plate. These tumors have a bimodal age distribution and are more common in the second and sixth decades. Radiographic appearance varies from small polypoid lesions to large dumbbell-shaped masses. As patients typically become symptomatic from direct extension into the adjacent paranasal sinuses, orbits or anterior cranial fossa, tumors are often large at presentation. The classic imaging appearance is a dumbbell-shaped mass centered at the level of the cribriform plate with the upper portion in the anterior cranial fossa and the lower portion in the superior nasal cavity.

On CT, these tumors are most often homogeneously-enhancing masses which cause mixed bone remodeling and destruction. MR imaging findings include hypo-to-intermediate signal intensity on T1-weighted images and intermediate-to-hyperintense signal on T2-weighted images. Cystic degeneration is known to occur. In tumors with intracranial extension, peripheral cysts along the intracranial margins are highly suggestive of this diagnosis[29,30] (Figs 3.18 to 3.20).

Sinonasal Neuroendocrine Tumor/ Sinonasal Undifferentiated Carcinoma

Both sinonasal neuroendocrine tumors (SNEC) and sinonasal undifferentiated carcinomas (SNUC) are rare tumors of the sinonasal tract which are characterized by aggressive behavior and are in the pathologic differential diagnosis for small round blue cell tumors. They can be included in the spectrum of neuroendocrine tumors, where ENB represents the most differentiated type.[31] SNEC tumors are considered a less differentiated version of ENB with more epithelial features. SNUC tumors are the least specialized of the group and have weak neuroendocrine characteristics. On imaging, these tumors are variable in appearance. They can look similar to

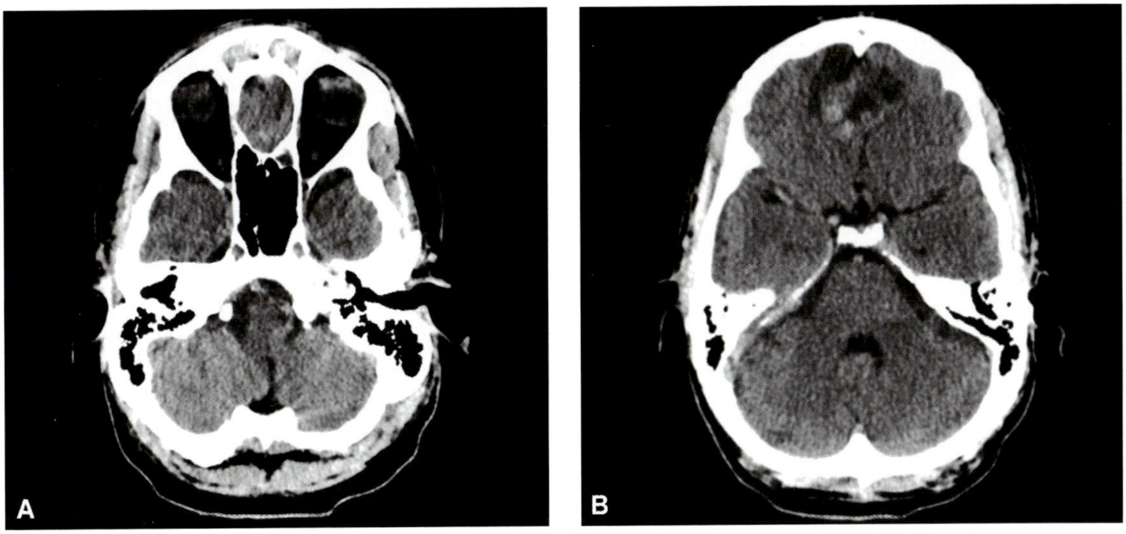

Figs 3.18A and B: Non-contrast axial CT images. (A) Esthesioneuroblastoma centered within the ethmoid air cells, extending superiorly through the cribriform plate into the anterior cranial fossa; (B) The intracranial portion is heterogeneous with multiple low density cystic components.

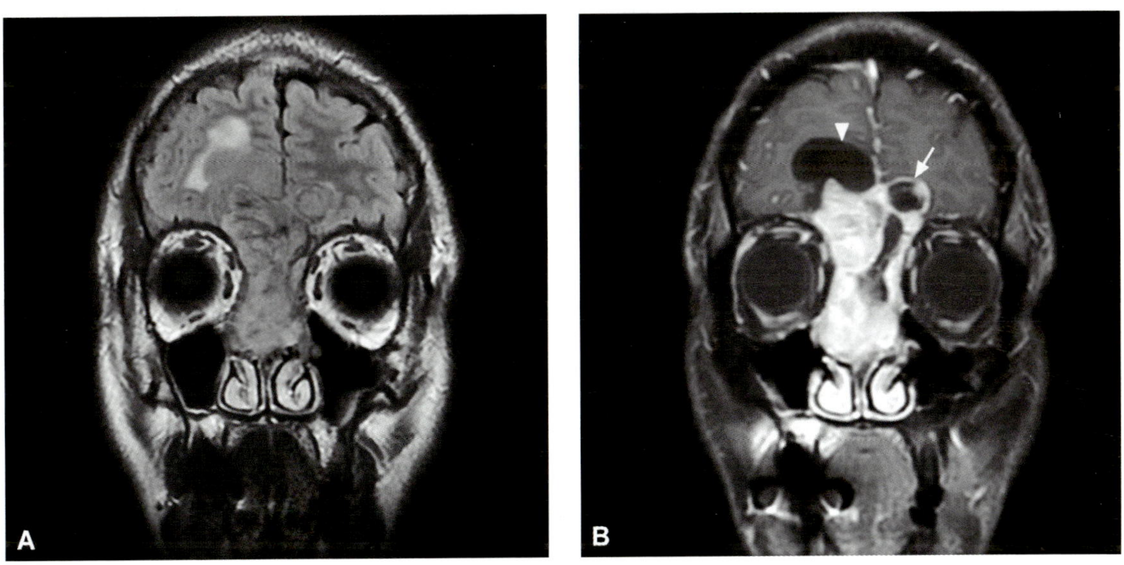

Figs 3.19A and B: (A) Pre-contrast T2 FLAIR-weighted; (B) Post-contrast T1-weighted coronal MR images of esthesioneuroblastoma. Note peripheral cysts (arrowheads).

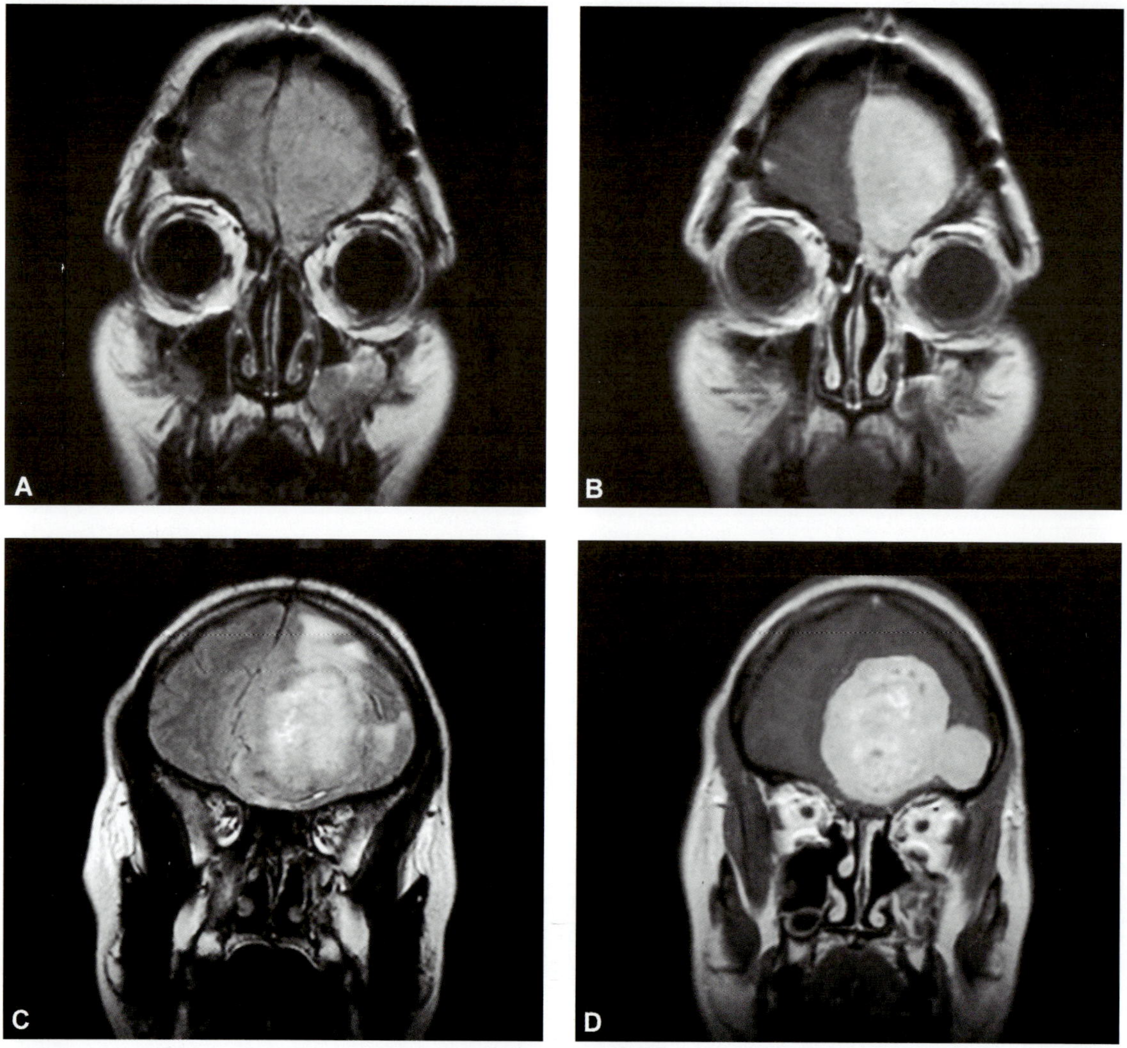

Figs 3.20A to D: (A) Pre-contrast T2-weighted FLAIR; (B) Post-contrast T1-weighted coronal MR images. T2 isointense mass extending superiorly from left ethmoid air cells through the cribriform plate with the majority of the mass situated intracranially. The mass demonstrates avid enhancement following contrast administration; (C) Pre-contrast T2 FLAIR-weighted; (D) Post-contrast T1-weighted coronal MR images. Large intracranial recurrence of esthesioneuroblastoma and evidence of prior sinonasal surgery is visible.

ENB or appear aggressive and indistinguishable from SCC (Figs 3.8 and 3.14).

REFERENCES

1. Raghavan, Phillips. Magnetic Resonance Imaging of Sinonasal Malignancies. Topics in Magnetic Resonance Imaging. 2007;18(4):259-67.
2. Kubal. Paranasal Sinuses Revisited. Seminars in ultrasound, CT and MRI. 1999;20(6):402-25.
3. Chow J, Leonetti J, Mafee M. Epithelial tumors of the paranasal sinuses and nasal cavity. Radiologic Clin N Am. 1993;31(1):61-73.
4. R Maroldi, D Farina, G Battaglia, et al. MR of malignant nasosinusal neoplasms: Frequently asked questions. Eur J Radiol. 1997;24(3):181-90.

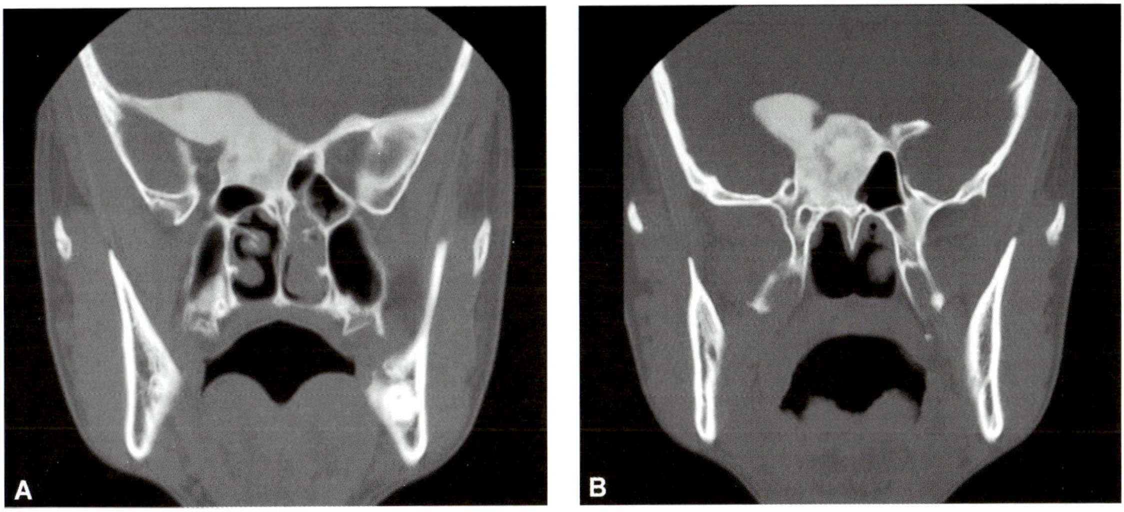

Figs 3.21A and B: (A and B) Noncontrast coronal CT images in bone windows. The lesion has characteristic benign appearing ground glass density and is consistent with fibrous dysplasia of the sphenoid bone.

5. Ginsberg LE. MR imaging of perineural tumor spread. Neuroimaging Clin N Am. 2004;14(4):663-77.
6. Maroldi R, Farina D, Borghesi A, et al. Perineural tumor spread. Neuroimaging Clin N Am. 2008;18(2):413-29.
7. Curtin HD. Detection of perineural spread: fat is a friend. AJNR. Am J Neuroradiology. 1998; 19(8):1385-6.
8. Yousem DM, Gad K, Tufano RP. Resectability issues with head and neck cancer. AJNR. Am J Neuroradiology. 2006;27(10):2024-36.
9. Soo KC, Carter RL, O'Brien CJ, et al. Prognostic implications of perineural spread in squamous carcinomas of the head and neck. Laryngoscope. 1986;96:1145-8.
10. Kim HJ, Lee TH, Lee HS, et al. Periorbita: Computed tomography and magnetic resonance imaging findings. Am J Rhinology. 2006;20(4):371-4.
11. Eisen MD, Yousem DM, Loevner La, et al. Preoperative imaging to predict orbital invasion by tumor. Head and Neck. 2000;22(5):456-62.
12. Eisen MD, Yousem DM, Mointone KT, et al. Use of preoperative MR to predict dural, perineural, and venous sinus invasion of skull base tumors. AJNR Am J Neuroradiol. 1996;17(10):1937-45.
13. Scott AM, Gunawardana DH, Bartholomeusz D, et al. PET changes management and improves prognostic stratification in patients with head and neck cancer: results of a multicenter prospective study. Journal of Nuclear Medicine: official publication, Society of Nuclear Medicine. 2008;49(10):1593-600.
14. Scho H, Yeung HWD, Kraus D, et al. Radiology Head and Neck Cancer: Clinical Usefulness and Accuracy of PET/CT Image Fusion 1. Radiology. 2004;231(1):65-72.
15. Liu T, Xu W, Yan WL, et al. FDG-PET, CT, MRI for diagnosis of local residual or recurrent nasopharyngeal carcinoma, which one is the best? A systematic review. Radiother Oncol. 2007;85(3):327-35.
16. Yen RF, Ting LL, Cheng MF, et al. Usefulness of 201TL SPECT/CT relative to 18F-FDG PET/CT in detecting recurrent skull base nasopharyngeal carcinoma. Head Neck. 2009;31(6):717-24.
17. Loevner La, Sonners AI. Imaging of neoplasms of the paranasal sinuses. Neuroimaging Clinics N Am. 2004;625-46.
18. Sklar EML, Pizarro JA. Case Report Sinonasal Intestinal-Type Adenocarcinoma Involvement of the Paranasal Sinuses. AJNR. Am J Neuroradiology; 2003. pp. 1152-5.
19. Madani G, Beale T, Lund V. Imaging of Sinonasal Tumors. Seminars in Ultrasound, CT, and MRI. 2009;30(1):25-38.
20. Licitra L, Locati LD, Bossi P, et al. Head and neck tumors other than squamous cell carcinoma. Current opinion in oncology. 2004;16(3):236-41.

21. Som P, Curtin P. Head and neck imaging. 4th Edition. Mosby Inc: St. Louis; 2003. pp: 261-373.
22. Vrabec D. The inverted Schneiderian papilloma: a 25-year study. Laryngoscope. 1994;104:582-605.
23. Lee DK, Chung SK, Dhong HJ, et al. Focal hyperostosis on CT of sinonasal inverted papilloma as a predictor of tumor origin. AJNR. Am J Neuroradiology. 2007;28(4):618-21.
24. Anari S, Carrie S. Sinonasal inverted papilloma: narrative review. J Laryngology Otology. 2010;124(7):705-15.
25. Ojiri H, Ujita M, Tada S, et al. Potentially Distinctive Features of Sinonasal Inverted Papilloma on MR Imaging. AJR. Am J Roentgenology. 2000;175:465-8.
26. Jeon TY, Kim HJ, Chung SK, et al. Sinonasal inverted papilloma: value of convoluted cerebriform pattern on MR imaging. AJNR. Am J Neuroradiology. 2008;29(8):1556-60.
27. Cohen EG, Baredes S, Zuckier LS, et al. 18F-FDG PET evaluation of sinonasal papilloma. AJR. American Journal of Roentgenology. 2009;193(1):214-7.
28. Jeon, Tae Yeon, Kim, et al. 18F-FDG PET/CT findings of sinonasal inverted papilloma with or without coexistent malignancy: comparison with MR imaging findings in eight patients. Neuroradiology. 2009;51(4):265-71.
29. Tseng J, Michel MA, Loehrl TA. Peripheral cysts: a distinguishing feature of esthesioneuroblastoma with intracranial extension. ENT. 2009;88(6):E14.
30. Som PM, Lidov M, Brandwein M, et al. Sinonasal esthesioneuroblastoma with intracranial extension: Marginal tumor cysts as a diagnostic MR finding. AJNR. American Journal of Neuroradiology. 1994;15(7):1259-62.
31. Smith SR, Som P, Fahmy A, et al. A clinicopathological study of sinonasal neuroendocrine carcinoma and sinonasal undifferentiated carcinoma. Laryngoscope. 2000;110(10 Pt 1):1617-22.

4

Surgical Approaches: Open

Carlos Perez-Mitchell, MD; Peter D Costantino, MD, FACS

INTRODUCTION

Over the last decade, there has been an overall trend towards less invasive or minimally invasive surgery (MIS). The advent of endoscopic sinus surgery (ESS), helped build the foundation for these less invasive approaches. The development of endoscopic skull base surgery, adapting and utilizing techniques well known by the otolaryngologist, has brought a new paradigm in the approach and treatment of this challenging anatomical area. Nevertheless, while these new techniques are extremely promising and have proven to be successful in the treatment of sinonasal tumors,[1-4] we cannot forget the time tested open approaches which have been in use since the early 1900s.[5] Interestingly, the first open transfacial approaches, as described by Schloeffer in 1907, was designed to access the pituitary gland area, the very same area which sparked the development of minimally invasive techniques.[6] While we seek to minimize the morbidity of treatment in choosing to perform minimally invasive techniques, we must understand the indications and, most importantly, the contraindications for such approaches. Not every patient will be a candidate for an endonasal endoscopic, minimally invasive tumor resection. Therefore, the sinonasal tumor surgeon should be acquainted not only with endoscopic techniques, but also with more invasive, conventional approaches in order to make an appropriate and safe treatment decision.

It is not our intention to describe an algorithm in order to decide whether an open or endoscopic approach should be undertaken. In this chapter, we will review the most common currently used open approaches to the sinonasal complex. Along with descriptions of popular approaches, we will define indications, enumerate the most important steps including any reconstructive efforts needed, highlight contraindications and mention the most common complications encountered while performing these procedures.

OPEN APPROACHES TO THE SINONASAL COMPLEX

Before embarking on a detailed discussion about each surgical approach, the reader should be familiar with the anatomy of the sinonasal complex and anterior skull base area as discussed in Chapter 2. The anterior cranial base is that area which extends from the frontal bones, over the orbital roof to the anterior edge of the greater wing of the sphenoid bone.[7] Note that defining precisely which anatomical area is/are being affected by the neoplastic process will help dictate the surgical approach chosen.

For example, paranasal sinus tumors can also involves the skull base in a contiguous fashion.[8] Additionally, some of the tumors involving the sinonasal area and nasopharynx could extend to the lateral middle skull base, i.e. sphenopalatine fossa, infratemporal fossa; therefore, utilizing a combination of procedures is not uncommon when addressing these entities.[9]

We cannot overemphasize the importance of an adequate preoperative evaluation, which includes sinonasal endoscopy, with or without a biopsy, and imaging in the form of both high resolution computerized tomographic (CT) scan and magnetic resonance imaging (MRI) with gadolinium enhancement on axial, coronal and sagittal views.

When deciding how to approach a sinonasal mass, having a preoperative tissue diagnosis helps define the ultimate treatment goal and can help determine the desired extent of resection. The vast diversity of pathologies involving this anatomical space can also add to the complexity of the chosen procedure.

When dealing with a benign lesion, we need to balance the need for resection versus any adverse effects of removing such a lesion.[10] For example, performing a lateral rhinotomy approach or a subtotal medial maxillectomy for fibrous dysplasia may result in greater morbidity than observation alone, i.e. epiphora, unsightly scar.[10] However, when dealing with a malignant lesion, the whole paradigm and philosophy of the treatment changes. The end point, when encountered with this situation, is complete removal and cure, sparing as much healthy tissue as possible.

Despite a trend towards minimally invasive approaches, classic open approaches to the sinonasal area are still preferred in certain scenarios, and should be understood by surgeons who operate in these areas.[9,11] As patients become more sophisticated and involved in their treatment decisions, we as physicians must consider their desired cosmetic results, but must prioritize oncological outcome when choosing a surgical approach.

Caldwell-Luc Approach (Sublabial Antrostomy)

The Sublabial antrostomy or Caldwell-Luc procedure, as it is widely known today, was described in the literature in the late 1800s. Founded by George Caldwell, an American surgeon, and Henry Luc, a French laryngologist, this procedure was first developed to access the maxillary sinus for treatment of sinus empyema. It was eventually recognized to be useful for the treatment of chronic maxillary sinusitis, mucoceles and even repair of mid facial fractures. More modern indications of the procedure include treatment of recurrent antrochoanal polyps after failed endoscopic sinus surgery, repair of oroantral fistulas, and as a corridor to approach the infratemporal and pterygopalatine fossae for control of recalcitrant epistaxis.[12]

The procedure also has a role in the armamentarium of the sinonasal tumor surgeon when dealing with lesions of the sinonasal complex. Caldwell-Luc is useful in performing biopsies or resection of small benign lesions of the lateral or anterior maxillary sinus through an inconspicuous, sublabial approach. An obvious advantage of this technique versus other transfacial approaches is the lack of facial incisions. By tailoring the size of the anterior maxillary window, we can target and excise malignant lesions that would otherwise be difficult to address through purely endoscopic techniques.

The Caldwell-Luc approach has been utilized in combination with endonasal endoscopic minimally invasive techniques. Har-El discussed and showed the feasibility and improvement of access to lesions in areas such as the lateral sphenoid sinus, pterygoid region and retrobulbar orbit utilizing a combined approach.[13] In our practice, we utilize this combined approach when dealing with lesions located lateral to the plane of the infraorbital nerve and for lesions of the lateral infratemporal fossa.

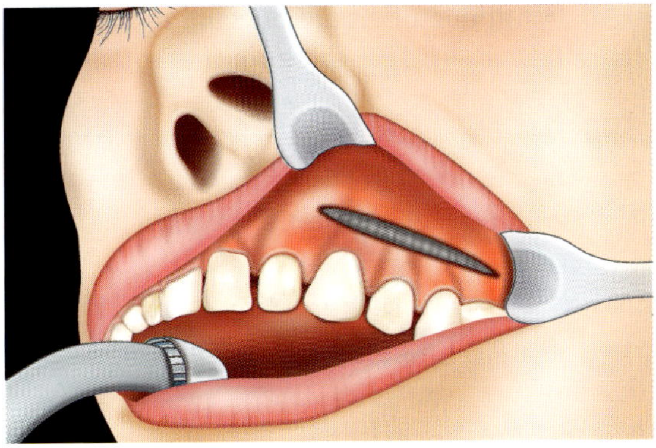

Fig. 4.1: Incision for Caldwell-Luc approach.

The surgery starts by infiltrating the gingivobuccal sulcus area using xylocaine 1% with 1:100,000 concentration epinephrine for hemostasis. An incision is then made leaving a cuff of mucosa on the gingival side in order to better approximate the tissues during later closure (Fig. 4.1). The incision can be tailored to the needed exposure, and it can be extended to the ipsilateral second molar. The surgeon should take note of the parotid duct orifice in this area. Subperiosteal elevation is performed in a cephalad direction until the canine fossa is clearly identified. At this time, the infraorbital nerve needs to be identified and preserved. Any combination of osteotomies can be used to make an anterior maxillary window, taking care not to injure the infraorbital nerve superiorly and the maxillary dental roots inferiorly. After entering the maxillary sinus, care is taken not to injure the infraorbital nerve as it runs along the orbital floor. Care also needs to be taken in order to avoid violating the thin posterior maxillary wall and injuring the internal maxillary artery.[12] After biopsy or tumor resection, an inferior meatal antrostomy may be created caudal to the inferior turbinate. The mucosa is then approximated, preferably with chromic gut sutures.

There are not many contraindications to this procedure, but one needs to be careful with its use in pediatric patients. First, there is concern for unerupted secondary teeth which could be fractured and damaged during the approach. There are also studies indicating an acquired hypoplastic maxillary effect postoperatively in children.[14] Conversely, in adults we must be aware of a hypoplastic sinus on preoperative imaging in order to prevent injury to the orbital contents.

Complications to the Caldwell-Luc procedure relate mostly to facial swelling and sensory nerve injuries. Low retrospectively studied the records of 185 patients who underwent 216 procedures and outlined the complications after Caldwell-Luc.[15] The most common complication or complaint was facial swelling (61.9%), followed by pain and/or numbness of the face (46%), and pain or numbness of the teeth and gums (30.9%). Paresthesias, which are mostly hypesthesias, are expected to resolve within three months.[16] Other rare complications reported in the literature, such as epistaxis, oroantral fistula and epiphora, occurred in less than 0.5%.[15]

Lateral Rhinotomy and Weber-Ferguson Approaches

Lateral rhinotomy is one of the older described open approaches to the sinonasal complex. First described by Michaux in 1853, it was then perfected by Moure, and popularized by Doyle in 1968.[5] This technique is suitable to access lesions of the anterior nasal cavity, medial third of the maxilla and ethmoid sinuses.[17] Lateral rhinotomy is useful in exposing the superior limit of the nasal cavity and paranasal sinuses for tumor removal when performed as part of a craniofacial approach. This is particularly helpful in the situation of malignancy or when the surgeon does not feel comfortable with craniotomy approaches to the skull base.[7]

Lateral rhinotomy can be combined with extensions through a subciliary or transconjunctival approach. These extensions are particularly helpful in assessing orbital floor involvement of tumor. The approach may also be combined with a supraciliary extension, which helps in obtaining better cephalad extension into the ethmoidal complex and when tumors traverse the skull base (Fig. 4.2).

The classic lateral rhinotomy incision begins in the medial canthal region with a W-plasty centered apically at the medial canthus (Fig. 4.3). Prior to

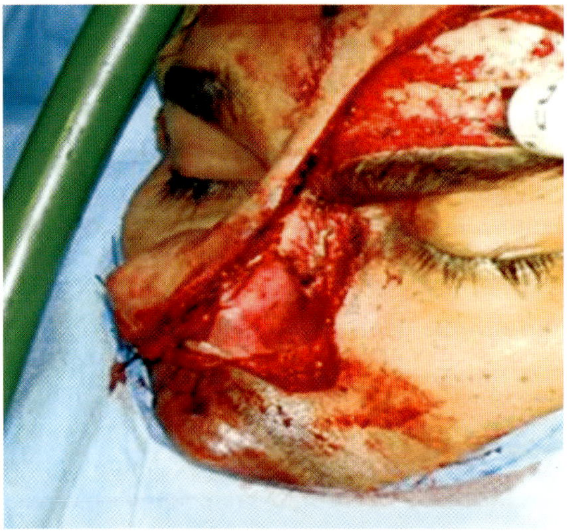

Fig. 4.2: Lateral-rhinotomy with supraciliary extension for an esthesioneuroblastoma.

Source: The illustration is the property of the department of head and neck surgery, University of Puerto Rico School of Medicine and is used with permission.

making the incision, a tarsorrhaphy suture is placed using 5-0 nylon in order to protect the orbit. The incision starts at half the distance between the medial canthus and the nasion, continuing caudal along the sidewall-cheek subunit boundary into the alar groove. Note that with the classic lateral rhinotomy approach, there is suboptimal access to the nasal cavity floor/hard palate, orbital floor, and structures lateral to the infraorbital nerve.

Weber-Ferguson Approach

The Weber-Ferguson procedure was first described in 1845 and is still widely used today. In this approach, the lateral rhinotomy incision continues inferior to the nasal sill, to the edge of the ipsilateral nasal philtrum, and into the lip/oral cavity mucosa. The incision is taken down into a deeper plane to the maxillary bone, nasal pyramid and into the nasal cavity and through its mucosa. Superiorly, the medial canthal ligament is detached from the lacrimal crests, providing better exposure to the anterior ethmoidal complex. The surgery can then be tailored to the needs of resection, i.e. medial maxillectomy, medial anterior wall maxillary resection (Fig. 4.4).

Extensions used in conjunction with lateral rhinotomy may also be beneficial in combination

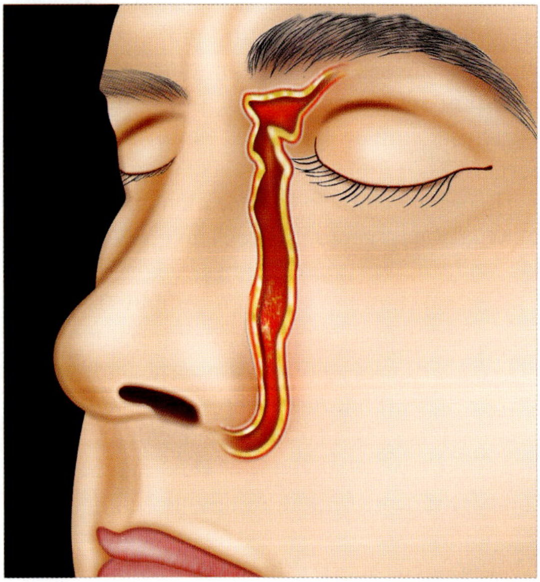

Fig. 4.3: Lateral rhinotomy incision. Note the W-plasty at the medial canthal region.

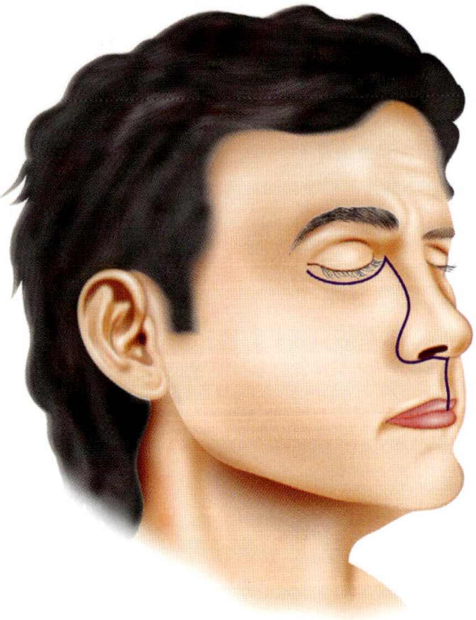

Fig. 4.4: Weber-Ferguson incision with transconjunctival extension.

with this approach. Additionally, Weber-Ferguson describes the use of a sublabial extension, which is performed by making incisions in the sublabial and gingivobuccal sulcus. Subsequently, a flap to expose the entire nasal floor and premaxillary space lateral to the infraorbital nerve may be raised.

This surgical procedure is indicated when sinonasal tumors involve bony components of the midface, i.e. subtotal maxillectomy, total maxillectomy with or without orbital exenteration (Fig. 4.5).[18]

Reconstructive and esthetic efforts should be maximized when performing transfacial incisions. For a lateral rhinotomy, in order to avoid postoperative diplopia or enophthalmos, the medial canthal tendon has to be repositioned and secured anterosuperiorly to overcompensate for gravity pull. Note that any bony midfacial reconstruction after a sub- or total maxillectomy may require the use of local flaps or free vascularized flaps. Also, the need for the use of an obturator should be addressed preoperatively and discussed with a maxillofacial prosthodontist.

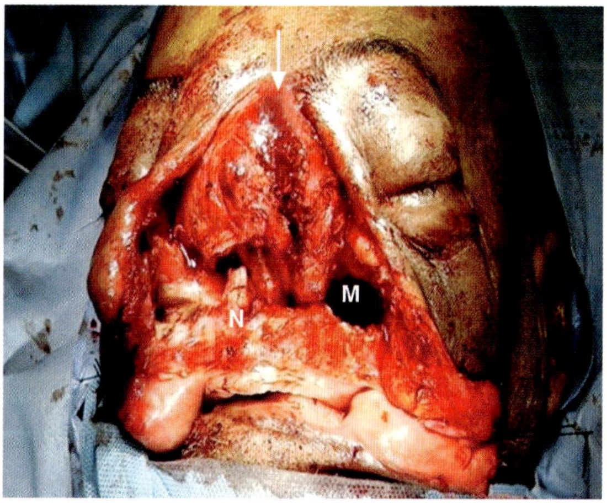

Fig. 4.5: Extensive recurrent adenoid cystic carcinoma of the ethmoid sinus complex (white arrow). Weber-Ferguson approach was used for access. maxillary sinus (M), nasal septum (N).

Source: This illustration is the property of the department of Head and Neck Surgery, University of Puerto Rico School of Medicine and is used with permission.

There is a clear consensus as to the contraindications to these procedures. First, for any case which requires facial incisions, the benefits of performing surgery on a previously irradiated patient, needs to be outweighed with the possible complications. Complications such as fistula formation, flap breakdown and non-healing wounds are common in this scenario. For lateral rhinotomy, any tumor involving an anatomical area not addressed by this procedure should be considered a contraindication. Areas of concern include the soft/hard palate, the infratemporal fossa, nasopharynx and anterior cranial fossa.[18] In the case of the Weber-Ferguson approach, contraindications further include tumors which are classified as T4b (very advanced local disease) according to the American Joint Committee on Cancer (AJCC) 2010 staging system. These areas include the lateral infratemporal fossa, orbital apex, middle cranial fossa and clivus.[19]

One of the more feared complications when resecting dorsal and caudal nasal septum is the development of a saddle nose deformity. Every effort should be made to avoid resecting 1 cm, both, superior and anterior on the nasal septal cartilage. Another complication, epiphora, can be avoided by establishing nasolacrimal drainage after resection and as a part of the reconstructive efforts. Finally, transient neuralgia could occur during retraction of the premaxillary tissues, even if the integrity of the infraorbital nerve is preserved. As previously mentioned, the neuralgia should resolve with conservative measures within three months.

Midfacial Degloving Approach

There is controversy in the literature as to who first described the midfacial degloving technique (MD).[20] It is well known that the technique evolved from a procedure described by Converse in 1950, where unilateral exposure of the midfacial skeleton was achieved via an intraoral incision with subperiosteal elevation.[21] Subsequently, the technique was extended by Casson to include a bilateral sublabial incision with elevation of the external nasal tissues via intercartilaginous and transfixion incisions, mobilizing the entire soft tissues of the midface area.[21]

The technique evolved as better and less invasive approaches were being entertained to access the midface structures. Lateral rhinotomy, with Weber-Ferguson, approaches were already established as the workhorse for approaching the midface structures and sinonasal area. As seen earlier, Caldwell-Luc approaches were utilized since the late 19th century; however, this technique bore access restrictions to certain anatomical areas. The midfacial degloving approach was developed by combining these well-known approaches with techniques used by rhinoplasty surgeons, in order to establish a procedure which offered great exposure with minimal cosmetic disfigurement. The advantage of the technique becomes obvious; nevertheless, it has received little popularity during the last decades.

Midfacial degloving was first utilized as an approach to remodel midfacial bony structures in cases of severe fibrous dysplasia. The indications were later expanded to include repair of midfacial fractures and treatment of craniofacial dysostoses.[20] Currently, indications include excision of benign and malignant lesions of the sinonasal complex, specifically the inferior maxilla and hard palate. When dealing with malignant lesions, the procedure should only be attempted when full clearance of the disease can be achieved purely via this technique. Through a MD approach we can access the bilateral midfacial structures, including bilateral nasal cavities, maxillary, ethmoid and sphenoid sinuses, nasopharynx, pterygopalatine and infratemporal fossae.[22]

Traditionally, the technique has been utilized for the treatment of inverted papilloma, replacing, in some institutions, the lateral rhinotomy as the main approach for medial maxillectomy.[21,23] For the modern sinus tumor surgeon, the technique is useful when lesions involving the bony hard palate or anterior pyriform aperture are felt to be too extensive to be addressed via a Caldwell-Luc and/or inaccessible for an endoscopic approach.[22]

The technique has also been important in the treatment of juvenile nasopharyngeal angiofibroma (JNA). Howar, et al in their cohort of 86 patients where the technique was used, reported 40 (47%) cases of angiofibromas.[21] JNA, despite its benign pathology, is a behaviorally aggressive tumor that requires the wide exposure that is particularly enabled by MD for resection. The superb exposure to the pterygopalatine fossa, also aids in vascular control by providing direct access to the internal maxillary artery. The success of this technique for treatment of JNA is further contributable to the desired cosmetic outcome of the procedure given the fact that this disease occurs in a younger patient population.[24]

The classic technique, as described by Maniglia in 1986, begins by infiltrating the gingivobuccal sulcus with xylocaine and epinephrine. Local anesthesia can also be placed in the caudal septum and columellar area as for rhinoplasty. A total of four incisions are required for this approach (Fig. 4.6). The first incision is carried in the gingivobuccal sulcus, from the first or second maxillary molar area to the contralateral counterpart, as in a Caldwell-Luc approach. When only a unilateral approach is needed, there have been modifications where the incision is carried out only to the contralateral canine.[23,25] Subperiosteal dissection is performed in a cephalad fashion to expose the

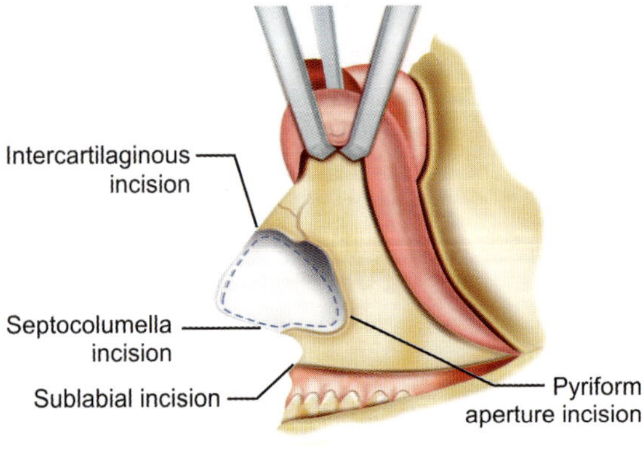

Fig. 4.6: The four basic incisions for the classic midfacial degloving approach.

anterior maxillary area to the level of the infraorbital nerve. The second incision entails a complete transfixion between the columella and septum. Bilateral intercartilaginous incisions, made as in a routine rhinoplasty, give access to the soft tissues on the nasal dorsum.[20] Finally, connecting with the previously made transfixion cuts, bilateral pyriform aperture incisions, which extend to the vestibule, are made. Modifications have been used where these pyriform circumferential incisions are avoided in order to prevent vestibular stenosis.[23,25] In the modification by Young Jeon et al, a lateral osteotomy is performed in order to mobilize the nasal pyramid and avoid the circumferential vestibular incision. Finally, the soft tissues of the premaxilla and nasal area can be degloved completely to level of the glabella, nasion and medial canthal region (Fig. 4.7).

Contraindications of the procedure are related to preoperative imaging findings. As previously mentioned, the procedure should only be performed if complete tumor removal can be achieved successfully with the approach. When this cannot be achieved, alternative or a combination of approaches needs to be entertained. The approach does not offer adequate exposure to the frontal sinus region or the anterior cranial fossa. When encountered with this scenario, a coronal approach can be added in order to complete a craniofacial resection.[24]

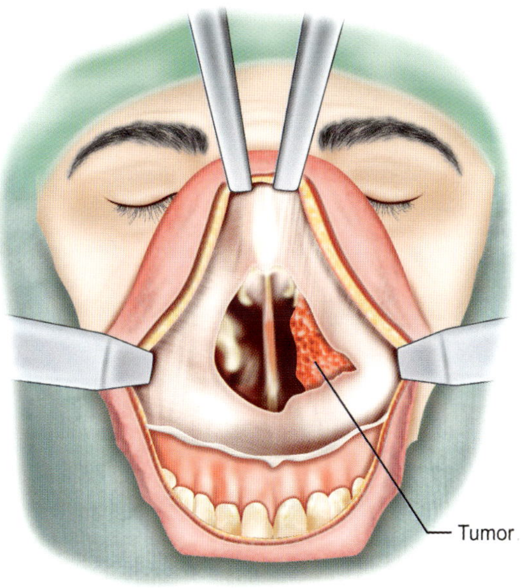

Fig. 4.7: The midfacial soft tissues can be retracted to the level of the glabella, nasion and medial canthal region.

There is always apprehension when performing radical midfacial surgery in children. Eze et al showed in their prospective cohort of nine pediatric patients, the feasibility and safety of performing midfacial degloving in this patient population.[22] This compares to previous studies where facial growth disturbances were not demonstrated on long-term follow-up.[26] The overall consensus reported in the literature is that the procedure is not contraindicated in the pediatric population. This is further supported by the fact that a majority of patients in whom the surgery is performed are young males with a diagnosis of JNA.

The most common complications of the procedure are related to extensive postoperative nasal crusting and infraorbital nerve hypesthesia.[24] Patients may require aggressive nasal saline irrigation treatments and weekly office nasal debridement. The hypesthesia is treated conservatively and should resolve within three months. The most feared complication has been vestibular stenosis; however, this complication seems to have a low incidence rate, althoug an extremely high morbidity rate whenever it occurs. Lenarz et al reported the incidence of vestibular stenosis in their series of 40 patients to be 2.5%.[27] Oroantral fistula can also occur, especially when the procedure is performed following a Caldwell-Luc approach. Howard and Lund found the incidence in their series of 86 patients to be 3.5%.[21] This may be minimized by meticulous mucosal approximation of the intranasal and sublabial incision edges during closure.[24]

Transfacial Approaches: The Facial Translocation Approach

The facial translocation approach was first described by Janecka et al in 1990, in order to access the nasopharynx, clivus and cavernous sinus.[28] Overall, transfacial approaches are a group of procedures which are indicated for benign and malignant tumors which arise extracranially and extend to the posterior maxillary sinus, pterygopalatine and infratemporal fossae, lateral sphenoid, clivus, middle cranial fossa and cavernous sinus.[29] The facial translocation approach is the method of choice in targeting extensive tumors of the nasopharynx and the infratemporal fossa, especially when the tumor involves the previously mentioned areas.[9]

Specific examples of malignant tumors that would be appropriate candidates for treating with this approach are squamous cell carcinomas (SCC), adenoid cystic carcinomas (ACC) or adenocarcinomas that arise in the posterior maxillary or ethmoid sinuses with extension into the infratemporal fossa. This approach is also ideal to address the following: adenoid cystic carcinomas with perineural spread along the trigeminal nerve to Meckel's cave, nasopharyngeal carcinomas, clivalchordomas that extend laterally and infratemporal fossa sarcomas (Fig. 4.8).[29]

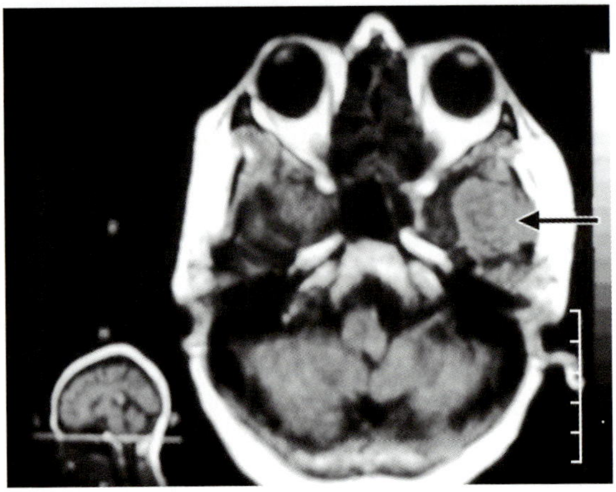

Fig. 4.8: T1-weighted skull base MRI with gadolinium enhancement showing a left infratemporal fossa lesion (Black arrow). Final pathological diagnosis showed a giant cell forming tumor.

Source: This illustration is the property of the department of Head and Neck Surgery, University of Puerto Rico School of Medicine and is used with permission.

The classic facial translocation starts with the facial incisions as shown in Figure 4.9. Note that the infraorbital nerve needs to be transected in order to be able to reflect the cheek flap completely. Reapproximation of the nerve could be performed during the reconstructive process. The osteotomies are performed in a controlled fashion utilizing a reciprocating saw. The zygomaticomaxillary unit is removed in a single unit to have access to the infratemporal fossa (Fig. 4.10A).[7] Lateral access to the infratemporal fossa can be better achieved by removal of the mandibular coronoid process (Fig. 4.10B). Note that access to the entire nasopharynx is also obtained through this approach, by removing the pterygoid processes. If needed for exposure, the orbital floor complex could be included in the osteotomized segment. Likewise, the nasal septum

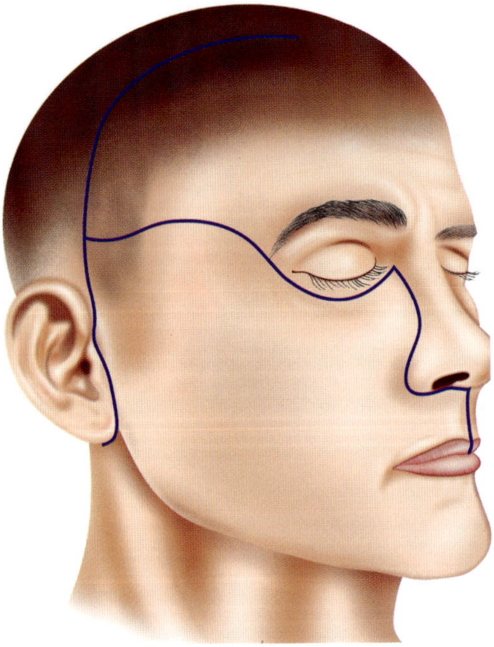

Fig. 4.9: Incisions for classic facial translocation approach.

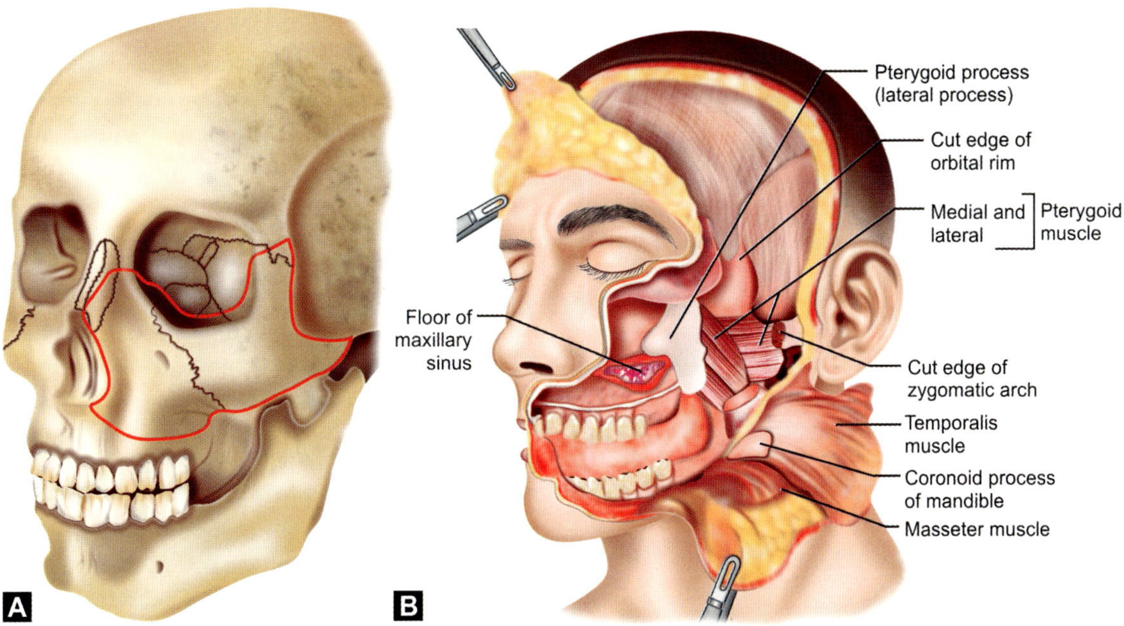

Figs 4.10A and B: (A) Osteotomies for zygomaticomaxillary unit removal; (B) Access achieved after osteotomies, with identification of the pterygoid plates and wide exposure to the nasopharynx.

can also be excised to have access to the contralateral nasal cavity. Concomitantly, a subtemporal craniectomy can be performed in order to gain access intracranially, if the tumor extends cephalad through the skull base.

A temporalis muscle flap is usually needed for reconstruction after a facial translocation, whether or not a craniotomy is performed.[7] Temporalis muscle is supplied by the deep temporal artery, a branch of the internal maxillary artery. This artery may have been compromized during tumor resection, thereby compromizing the muscle flap. When encountering this scenario a free tissue transfer becomes essential for reconstruction. A flap which provides bulk like the abdominal rectus or anterolateral thigh flap is an appropriate choice. The temporalis muscle flap is placed in the infratemporal fossa area defect and tacked into place. The bone segment is brought back into place and secured using miniplates. Sensory nerves that needed to be transected for access are reanastomosed. At this time, the lacrimal system needs to be stented, or it may be done as a secondary procedure in the form of an endoscopic dacryocystorhinostomy (DCR). Acceptable cosmetic and excellent functional results can usually be achieved after this type of reconstruction.

Suarez et al commented on results of patients in whom the defect was reconstructed with a vascularized muscle flap or in whom the translocated bone segment was kept attached to the cheek soft tissues during resection. He found that these patients did not develop bone necrosis, a possible complication of the procedure, even in patients who received adjuvant radiation therapy.[9] Hao et al found in a series of 42 patients in which the bone segment was detached during resection, that the segment became devitalized in 61% of patients who received adjuvant radiotherapy.[30]

As in other transfacial procedures which require osteotomies, facial translocation needs to be carefully considered in the pediatric population. It is well known that mid facial growth can be affected by the procedure in this age group.

Causative factors of the procedure include periosteum elevation and the use of metal plate fixation.[31]

The main disadvantage of these approaches is the need for facial incisions. Other than facial scars, the procedure can also cause ectropion, epiphora and the sequelae of sensorial nerve transection. Although frontal muscle palsy is also included in the literature as an expected result of this procedure, it is our experience that frontal branches of the facial nerve can be spared in most tumor resections.[7]

The use of the temporalis muscle, for reconstruction, results in a hollowing of the temporal fossa, creating an obvious cosmetic deformity. In our practice, we use hydroxyapatite cement® in a secondary procedure to fill the defect. This is done during a secondary procedure because of the known increased rate of infection when using alloplastic implants during primary tumor resection, especially in patients receiving adjuvant radiation therapy.[32] Meticulous reconstructive efforts should be followed for optimal results as this procedure involves temporary disarticulation of the craniofacial complex.

Anterior Craniofacial Resection

Craniofacial resection (CFR) was first introduced by Ketcham in 1963 as a technique to access paranasal sinus tumors with extension to the anterior skull base area.[3] The technique has hardly changed since its introduction and is still considered the workhorse of anterior skull base surgery. It is considered the "gold standard" for the resection of tumors involving the anterior skull base, against which other treatments must be measured.[33] Surgeons treating patients with malignancies of the sinonasal tract needs to recognize when and why choosing an open vs. endoscopic approach is the more appropriate treatment choice. Current indications for CFR include tumors arising from the nasal cavity, frontal and ethmoid sinuses, nasopharynx, and cribiform plate area with extension to or through the anterior skull base (Figs 4.11A and B). Nonneoplastic processes, like invasive fungal sinusitis, can also be an indication for a CFR.

Neurosurgical evaluation of these patients cannot be overemphasized, and intraoperative support needs to be addressed. A cranial base team, led by

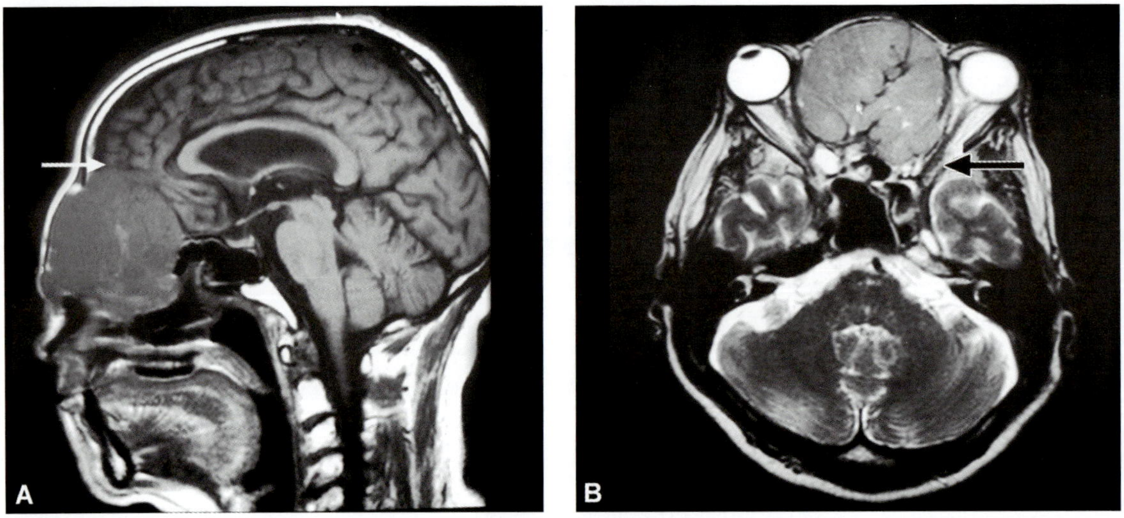

Figs 4.11A and B: Adenocarcinoma arising in the ethmoid sinus. (A) Sagittal T; (B) Axial T2 MRI scans with gadolinium enhancement showing an advanced T4 adenocarcinoma eroding through the skull base (solid white arrow). Note the extension through the left lamina papyracea into the orbital contents (black arrow).

Source: This illustration in the property of the department of Head and Neck Surgery, University of Puerto Rico School of Medicine is used with permission.

an otolaryngologist and a neurosurgeon, should be the standard of care. As previously stated, having a preoperative biopsy and diagnosis is crucial in determining the extent of resection, especially when the orbital contents are at risk.[32] Cases need to be discussed in a multidisciplinary manner and a consensus obtained prior to embarking on any surgical endeavor. After recognizing the approach to be used, plans for resection and reconstruction need to be considered. Instrumentation and equipment needs to be assessed well in advance. Communication with the neuroanesthesiologist is key to obtaining an optimal surgical field intraoperatively. It is important to position the patient adequately; our preference is supine with the head on a Mayfield horseshoe headrest, and any areas for possible autograft harvest prepped, i.e. fat, fascia lata.

The surgery begins with a bicoronal incision posterior to the hairline with enough length from the nasion and the origin of the supratrochlear vessels in order to prepare for a pericranial flap. Our method entails making an incision through all layers of the scalp, and elevating in a subperiosteal plane. Care is taken to preserve the superficial temporal arteries bilaterally as these are the main blood supply to the temporoparietal fascia. This fascial layer can later be used for reconstruction of the middle cranial base or the infratemporal fossa area.[7] The subperiosteal dissection is continued to the level of the supraorbital ridge and nasion area, taking care not to injure the supraorbital and supratrochlear vessels, which provide the main blood supply to the pericranial flap. At this time, attention is turned to the craniotomy portion of the case.

The craniotomy can be tailored to the amount of exposure needed. However, a wide craniotomy is recommended in order to diminish the amount of retraction placed on the frontal lobes. At this time, the neurosurgical team, retracting the frontal lobes posteriorly, can assess the anterior cranial fossa and its dura (Fig. 4.12).

It is our practice to perform a supraorbital bar osteotomy as a separate entity after retraction of the frontal lobes. This further enhances access and visualization of the anterior cranial base area, and in our experience obviates the need of a separate facial incision. With elevation of the frontal dura and transection of the olfactory poles, exposure can be gained as far posteriorly as the planum sphenoidale and optic chiasm.[7]

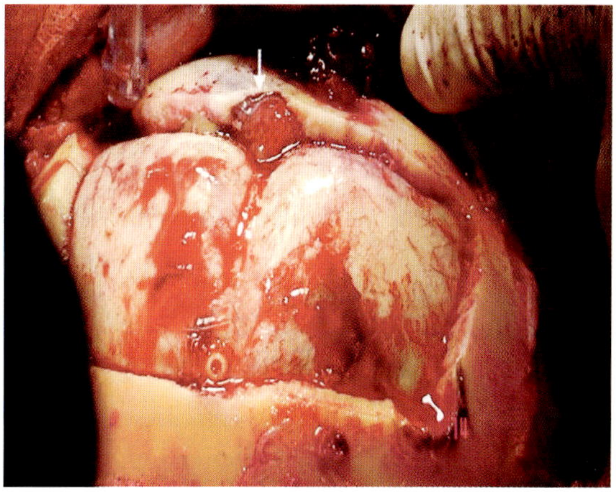

Fig. 4.12: Adenocarcinoma tumor shown intraoperatively after frontal craniotomy, the tumor can be seen as it erodes and traverses the anterior skull base (white arrow).

Source: This illustration is the property of the Department of Head and Neck Surgery, University of Puerto Rico School of Medicine and is used with permission.

Once, the area to be excised is clearly defined, osteotomies can be performed through the fovea ethmoidalis bilaterally and anteriorly, just dorsal to the posterior wall of the frontal sinus area. The posterior margin osteotomy is made at the area of the planum sphenoidale, taking care not to bypass this area as it leads to the optic chiase (Fig. 4.13). Anterior and inferior cuts are then made in the nasal septum; these can also be done at the start of the procedure and can be aided by endonasal endoscopy.[34]

When the resection is completed, margins from the anterior cranial base frontal dura, nasal septum and suspicious areas in the paranasal sinuses should be sent for frozen section analysis. The reconstructive process can begin only after biopsy proven confirmation of clear margins. The pericranial flap is the workhorse in the reconstruction

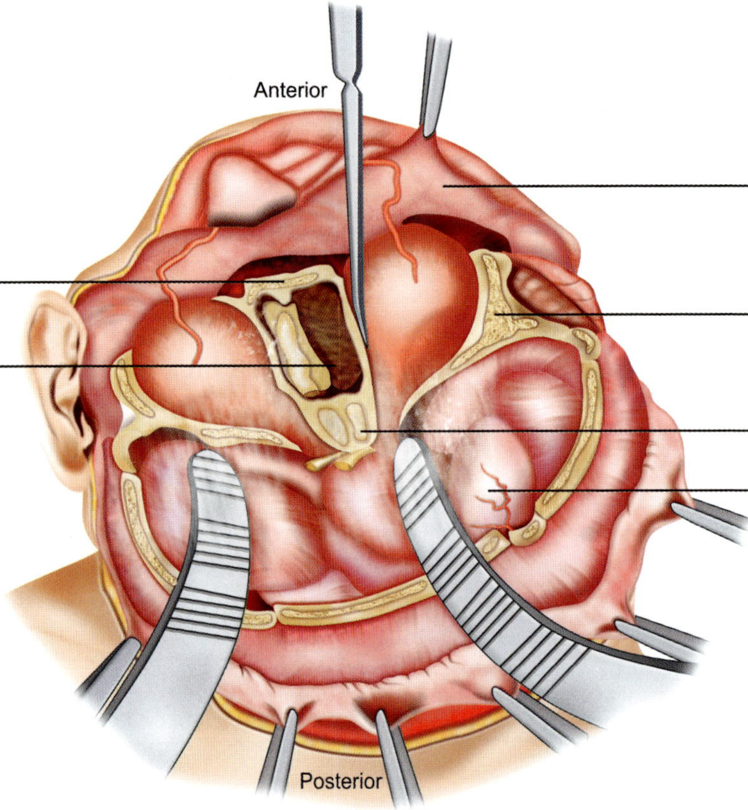

Fig. 4.13: Wide exposure after bifrontal craniotomy with posterior retraction of frontal lobe. Supraorbital ridge osteotomy was performed. The orbital roofs can be removed bilaterally and the sphenoid sinus can be entered from above when required.

of anterior skull base defects and is currently the most frequently used flap.[8] The flap is carefully harvested, making sure not to penetrate the galea aponeurotica layer. It is then placed overlying the defect, constructing a barrier between the brain and the nasal cavity. At this time, any dural tears need to be repaired, creating a watertight seal. The frontal recess needs to be plugged using either temporalis muscle or temporoparietal fascia. Note that before replacing the supraorbital ridge, a cranialization procedure, which requires the posterior table of the frontal sinus to be drilled out and the sinus completely stripped of all its mucosa, is performed. The supraorbital bar is replaced and secured using titanium miniplates, making sure the extraocular muscles do not become entrapped during the process. The flap is brought back into anatomical position and subgaleal drains are left in place. Intranasal packing should be placed under direct visualization utilizing an endoscope to avoid traversing the skull base reconstruction. Bilateral nasal trumpets are then placed, also under direct visualization, in order to bypass the flow of air through the nasal cavity and diminish the risk of pneumocephalus.

There is controversy in the literature as to whether resection of massive intraparenchymal brain disease offers any benefit for survival. Hanna et al. consider extensive brain parenchymal involvement a contraindication for the procedure. The presence of tumor extension to the cavernous sinus, internal carotid artery, optic chiasm and distant metastasis, are also considered contraindications by the MD Anderson Group.[8] In their 25 year experience with CFR, Howard et al. reported that once tumor has involved the brain, the prognosis is particularly poor with very few survivors, irrespective of histology.[33] However, there may still be a role for palliative resection, even in the presence of massive disease.

The morbidity and mortality after CFR varies considerably in the literature. Ganly et al. in their international collaborative study from 17 institutions analyzed 1,193 patients for postoperative complications. They found a complication rate of 36.3% and a mortality rate of 4.7%, deeming the procedure safe and effective.[35] Howard et al. in their cohort of 308 patients spanning 25 years divided their complications into immediate, intermediate and long-term. In the immediate cohort of patients, 2.6% developed any complications, with one death. The intermediate cohort experienced a 4.8% complication rate, with two deaths. While the long-term cohort experienced a 25% complication rate, with three deaths; most of these complications included serous otitis media, epiphora and diplopia, which where managed with relative ease.[33] The authors highlight that most of their complications occur red during the early part of their series; and that with experience in this technique, the rates of major complications decreases. Note that proponents of strictly endoscopic CFR techniques have shown evidence of complication rates between 6–19% in their series.[2,3]

Major complications, noteworthy of discussion, include cerebrospinal fluid (CSF) fistulas, meningitis, pneumocephalus and intracranial hemorrhage. The rate of CSF fistula, after major CFR, may be expected to be as high as 20%.[36] Our paradigm for treating postoperative CSF fistulas entails assessing and differentiating between a low flow and a high flow leak. High flow leaks will appear spontaneously either through the wound, the nose or the external ear canal. Low flow leaks are harder to assess and usually require some sort of ancillary test to be diagnosed, i.e. CT cisternography, β-2 transferrin analysis. A high flow leak is better treated by revision surgery as soon as it is diagnosed. Low flow leaks can be managed conservatively by placement of a lumbar drain for a maximum of five days. If the drain is unsuccessful, then surgical revision is needed.

Meningitis is a non-specific term for inflammation of the meninges. After skull base surgery, meningitis is usually either aseptic or bacterial.[7] Postoperative aseptic meningitis is due to the breakdown of blood products and the surgical manipulation itself. The rate of meningitis after CFR is reported in the literature at 5–7.7%.[37] Having a CSF leak is the major predisposing factor for the development of bacterial meningitis, therefore, in a patient diagnosed with meningeal inflammation a source of leakage should be meticulously addressed. CSF of patients with a lumbar drain should be sampled and tested daily to rule out meningitis, since patients may not develop clear signs or symptoms of the disease until later in the process. Patients should be on intravenous antibiotics with adequate CSF penetrance perioperatively and continued Postoperatively until all the drains and nasal packings are removed.

Pneumocephalus is related to the connection between the nasal cavity and intracranial compartment. While some intracranial air is expected after CFR, a problem arises when a defect acts as a one-way valve creating a tension pneumocephalus. An event such as severe straining, sneezing or coughing can precede the development of pneumocephalus. Suboptimal postoperative care, presence of lumbar drains and length of surgery can all play a role in the development of tension pneumocephalus.[4] The most frequent symptoms of tension pneumocephalus are headaches and an altered level of consciousness. Any patient with these symptoms should be evaluated further with imaging studies. A characteristic symptom that has been described in the literature is the subjective complaint of a "splashing sound" intracranially.[39] The conservative treatment for small, asymptomatic pneumocephalus consists of strict bed rest in an upright position and avoiding any straining or Valsalva maneuvers. For symptomatic cases, urgent evacuation and repair of the defect is needed.

All patients undergoing CFR surgery need a brain CT scan, without contrast, within the first 24 hours after the procedure. A baseline is needed to better assess any hematoma or collections that may subsequently develop. A postoperative hematoma can cause a mass effect with eventual brain compression, infarction and herniation.[7] The internal carotid artery is usually not at risk during CFR, but care needs to be taken when resecting posterolaterally to the area of the planum sphenoidale. The internal carotid artery could be lacerated by a bone spur during the osteotomies, which may later cause a "blowout injury."[38] Significantly, two out of the five deaths reported by Howard et al. in their series of 308 patients were secondary to hemorrhagic complications. The physician should be wary of changes in the patient's mental status as this may signal the possibility of an existing or developing vascular complication.

CONTROVERSIES

There is still controversy in the literature as to the treatment of tumor extension into the orbital contents. Suarez et al. found that orbital involvement is an important predictor of overall survival.[40] Most authors agree that preserving the orbital contents, when indicated, does not alter local recurrence or survival. When the lesion is traversing the cranial base and involving the brain, a craniofacial resection has been the treatment modality of choice for the past 25 years.[33] Craniofacial resection has become the gold standard, to which other surgical procedures, including minimally invasive approaches, must be measured. In the clinical scenario of brain involvement, the literature shows that the prognosis is poor regardless of tumor histology. Howard et al. showed on a multivariate analysis the prognostic importance of intracranial and orbital spread, emphasizing the necessity of being able to assess and resect these areas adequately.[33] More of these surgical debates will be discussed in a later chapter.

SUMMARY

In this chapter, we have summarized the most common, currently used open approaches to access the sinonasal complex. Mastering the anatomy of such an intricate area is key in achieving surgical success. It is crucial that a thorough preoperative evaluation should be entertained prior to executing the surgical approach. Discussing every case in a multidisciplinary fashion will allow for an educated, evidence based decision when choosing a treatment option. This will translate into a better overall surgical outcome, not only oncologically, but in terms of the patient's morbidity as well. Preoperative knowledge of the tumor type and of its behavior, helps not only in deciding which approach to entertain, but also in the extent of resection. Intraoperative communication between the otolaryngologist and neurosurgeon is critical in optimizing the surgical outcome. Reconstructive efforts need to be maximized and may require the use of local or free flaps to achieve an optimal functional and cosmetic result. It is important that complications are recognized early and immediate aggressive action be taken. Open approaches are still valuable in the modern sinonasal tumor practice and are useful in the right scenario, at times, becoming the preferred approach for areas that are hard to address with the endoscope.

REFERENCES

1. Luong A, Citardi MJ, Batra PS. Management of sinonasal malignant neoplasms: Defining the role of endoscopy. Am J Rhino and Allergy. 2010;24(2):150-5.
2. Nicolai P, Battaglia P, Bignami M, et al. Endoscopic surgery for malignant tumors of the sinonasal tract and adjacent skull base: a 10-year experience. Am J Rhinol. 2008;22(3):308-16.
3. Batra PS, Luong A, Kanowitz SJ, et al. Outcomes of minimally invasive endoscopic resection of anterior skull base neoplasms. Laryngoscope. 2010; 120(1):9-16.

4. Castelnuovo P, Dallan I, Battaglia P, et al. Endoscopic endonasal skull base surgery: past, present and future. Eur Arch Otorhinolaryngology. 2010;267(5):649-63.
5. Lueg EA, Irish JC, Katz MR, et al. A patient- and observer-rated analysis of the impact of lateral rhinotomy on facial aesthetics. Arcs Facial Plas Surg. 2001;3(4):241-4.
6. Jho HD, Carrau RL. Endoscopy assisted transsphenoidal surgery for pituitary adenoma. Technical note. Acta Neurochir (Wiena) 1996;138(12):1416-25.
7. Costantino PD, Ismail AS, Janecka IP. Cranial-Base Surgery. In: Bailey BJ, Johnson JT, Newland S, (Eds). Head and Neck Surgery-Otolaryngology. 4th Edition. Philadelphia, PA: Lippincott Williams & Wilkins; 2006. Pp:1827-52.
8. Hanna EY, Kupferman M, Demonte F. Surgical Management of Tumors of the Nasal Cavity, Paranasal Sinuses, Orbit and Anterior Skull Base. In: Hanna EY, Demonte F, (Eds). Comprehensive Management of Skull Base Tumors. New York, NY: Informa Healthcare USA; 2009. pp: 227-65.
9. Suárez C, Llorente JL, Muñoz C, et al. Facial translocation approach in the management of central skull base and infratemporal tumors. Laryngoscope. 2004;114(6):1047-51.
10. Harvey RJ, Sheahan PO, Schlosser RJ. Surgical management of benign sinonasal masses. Otolaryngologic Clinics of North America. 2009;42(2): 353-75, x.
11. Sharma V, Koirala K. Lateral rhinotomy vs midfacial degloving for T3 inverted papilloma of nose and paranasal sinus. Nepal Med Coll J. 2009;11(2): 115-7.
12. Lazar RH, Mitchell RB. Sublabial Antrostomy (Caldwell-Luc Procedure). In: Bailey BJ, Calhoun KH, (Eds). Atlas of Head and Neck Surgery-Otolaryngology. 2nd Edition. Philadelphia, PA: Lippincott Williams & Wilkins; 2001. pp. 918-9.
13. Har-El G. Combined endoscopic transmaxillary-transnasal approach to the pterygoid region, lateral sphenoid sinus, and retrobulbar orbit. Annals Otorhinolaryngology. 2005;114(6):439-42.
14. Lawson W, Patel ZM, Lin FY. The development and pathologic processes that influence maxillary sinus pneumatization. Anatomical Record (Hoboken). 2008;291(11):1554-63.
15. Low WK. Complications of the Caldwell-Luc operation and how to avoid them. Aus NZJ Surg. 1995;65(8):582-4.
16. Maniglia AJ. Indications and techniques of midfacial degloving. A 15-year experience. Arch Otolaryngo- Head Neck Surg. 1986;112(7):750-2.
17. Close LG. Lateral Rhinotomy. In: Bailey BJ, Calhoun KH, (Eds). Atlas of Head and Neck Surgery-Otolaryngology. 2nd Edition. Philadelphia, PA: Lippincott Williams & Wilkins; 2001. pp. 22-3.
18. Close LG. Weber-Fergusson Approach with Subtotal Maxillectomy and Total Maxillectomy with Orbital Preservation. In: Bailey BJ, Calhoun KH, (Eds). Atlas of Head and Neck Surgery-Otolaryngology. 2nd Edition. Philadelphia, PA: Lippincott Williams & Wilkins; 2001. pp. 26-9.
19. American Joint Committee on Cancer. Nasal Cavity and Paranasal Sinuses. In: AJCC Cancer Staging Book.7th Edition. New York, NY: Springer-Verlag; 2010. pp. 93-102.
20. Howard DJ, Lund VJ. The midfacial degloving approach to sinonasal disease. J Laryngol Otology. 1992;106(12):1059-62.
21. Howard DJ, Lund VJ. The role of midfacial degloving in modern rhinological practice. J Laryngol Otology. 1999;113(10):885-7.
22. Eze NN, Wyatt ME, Bray D, et al. The midfacial degloving approach to sinonasal tumours in children. Rhinology. 2006;44(1):36-8.
23. Jeon SY, Jeong JH, Kim HS, et al. Hemifacial degloving approach for medial maxillectomy: a modification of midfacial degloving approach. Laryngoscope. 2003;113(4):754-6.
24. Browne JD. The midfacial degloving procedure for nasal, sinus, and nasopharyngeal tumors. Otolaryngologic Clinics of North America. 2001;34(6): 1095-104, viii.
25. Cansz H, Tahamiler R, Yener M, et al. Modified midfacial degloving approach for sinonasal tumors. J Craniofacial Surg. 2008;19(6):1518-22.
26. Conley J, Price JC. Sublabial approach to the nasal and nasopharyngeal cavities. Am J Surg. 1979;138(4):615-8.
27. Lenarz T, Keiner S. Midfacial degloving: an alternative approach to the frontobasal area, the nasal cavity and the paranasal sinuses. Laryngorhinootologie. 1992;71(8):381-7.
28. Janecka IP, Sen CN, Sekhar LN, et al. Facial translocation: a new approach to the cranial base. Otolaryngo- Head Neck Sury. 1990;103(3):413-9.

29. O'Malley BW Jr. Transfacial approach to the infratemporal fossa, nasopharynx and middle cranial fossa. In: Long DM, Niparko JK, O'Malley BW JJ, et al. (Eds). An Atlas of Skull Base Surgery. New York, NY: The Parthenon Publishing Group; 2003. pp. 31-50.
30. Hao SP. Facial translocation approach to the skull base: the viability of translocated facial bone graft. Otolaryngo- Head Neck Surg. 2001;124(3):292-6.
31. Fagan JJ, Snyderman CH, Carrau RL, et al. Nasopharyngeal angiofibromas: selecting a surgical approach. Head and Neck. 1997;19(5):391-9.
32. Nishino H, Ichimura K, Tanaka H, et al. Results of orbital preservation for advanced malignant maxillary sinus tumors. Laryngoscope. 2003;113(6):1064-9.
33. Howard DJ, Lund VJ, Wei WI. Craniofacial resection for tumors of the nasal cavity and paranasal sinuses: a 25-year experience. Head and Neck. 2006;28(10):867-73.
34. Hatano A, Nakajima M, Kato T, et al. Craniofacial resection for malignant nasal and paranasal sinus tumors assisted with the endoscope. Auris Nasus Larynx. 2009;36(1):42-5. Epub 2008 May 16.
35. Ganly I, Patel SG, Singh B, et al. Complications of craniofacial resection for malignant tumors of the skull base: report of an International Collaborative Study. Head and Neck. 2005;27(6):445-51.
36. Sen C, Snyderman CH, Sekhar LN. Complications of skull base operations. In: Sekhar LN, Janecka IP, (Eds). Surgery of cranial base tumors. New York,NY: Raven Press; 1993. pp. 831-40.
37. Torres A, Acebes JJ, López L, et al. Complications of craniofacial resection in anterior skull base tumors. Neurocirugia (Astur). 2005;16(6):492-8.
38. Jellish WS, Edelstein SB. Anesthesia and Intraoperative monitoring of Patients with Tumors of the Skull Base. In: Hanna EY, Demonte F, (Eds). Comprehensive Management of Skull Base Tumors. New York, NY: Informa Healthcare USA; 2009. pp. 119-29.
39. Aleksander M Vitale, Andries A le Roux. Tension Pneumocephalus as a Complication of Intracranial Pressure Monitoring: A case report. Indian J Neurotrauma. 2007;4(2):115-8.
40. Suárez C, Ferlito A, Lund VJ, et al. Management of the Orbit in Malignant Sinonasal Tumors. Head Neck. 2008;30(2):242-50.

5

Surgical Approaches: Endoscopic

Vijay R Ramakrishnan, MD

INTRODUCTION

Endoscopic approaches to the sinuses and beyond have become progressively sophisticated, such that one can access nearly the entire anterior and central skull base through the transnasal route. Historically, endoscopic anterior and lateral access was limited and adjunctive external approaches were often necessary. With currently available instrumentation, the anterior aspect of the frontal and maxillary sinuses can now be reached in most patients, and lateral access to the infratemporal fossa is possible. The central skull base is accessed through the sphenoid sinus, and endoscopic transcranial dissection is now gaining acceptance.

The endoscopic approach should be sufficiently broad to accomplish the surgical goals: adequate visualization, complete tumor resection, sinus ventilation, and ability for postoperative endoscopic inspection. Simply reaching these areas is sufficient to biopsy lesions, but for a complete resection, wider exposure may be necessary for 2-handed tumor dissection. In these scenarios, one option is for the surgeon to use a static scope-holder. Our preference is a two-surgeon approach, where a 3-handed or even 4-handed technique may be utilized. A second surgeon provides more than two extra hands. Experience with a second surgeon provides valuable consultation regarding anatomy, technique, and surgical decision-making. When 3- or 4-hands are used during dissection, a binostril approach is preferred, so two instruments can be inserted in each nostril (Fig. 5.1). The endoscope and two to three instruments may potentially work through a single nostril, but collision of hands or instruments may be frustrating with this technique.

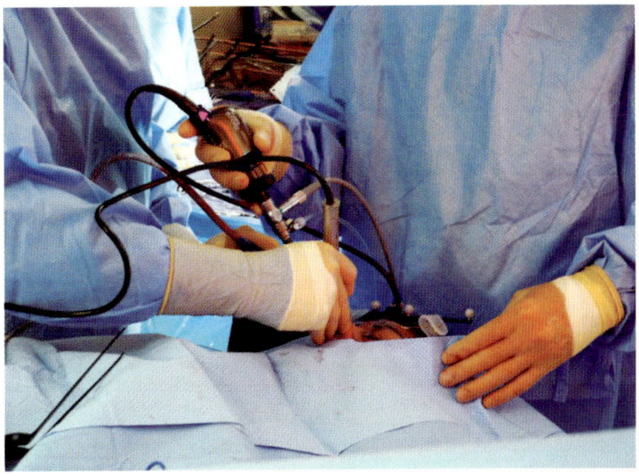

Fig. 5.1: Binostril 2-surgeon approach.

VASCULAR CONTROL

Early vascular control should be planned for most tumor resections. The location of the tumor and anatomical extent of resection will dictate which arteries need to be controlled prior to resection. The main arterial supply to sinonasal tumors is from the internal maxillary artery, sphenopalatine artery, and anterior and posterior ethmoid arteries (Fig. 5.2). Collateral blood supply is occasionally encountered from the contralateral, nasopharyngeal, or palatal arterial branches. Anteriorly, minor blood supply may come from the superior labial artery or terminal branches of the greater palatine artery through the incisive foramen. Contributions from the internal carotid circulation may occur in sphenoid neoplasms or juvenile nasopharyngeal angiofibromas (JNAs).

In the surgical excision of large sphenoid or posterior ethmoid vascular tumors, such as a JNA or hemangiopericytoma, embolization of the terminal branches of the internal maxillary artery can be performed 24–48 hours preoperatively. This is done so that the patient can be observed for potential complications from the embolization procedure and surgery is performed within 24–48 hours prior to the development of collateral arterial supply to the tumor. Digital subtraction angiography is used to selectively guide the catheter tip into the internal maxillary artery, and observe for collaterals from the ethmoid or internal carotid artery circulations. In order to avoid embolic complications, the microcatheter tip must be guided distal to such collaterals, as well as the superficial temporal, middle and accessory meningeal arteries. Gelfoam, polyvinyl alcohol particles, platinum coils, or a combination may be used for embolization. The ethmoid branches of the ophthalmic artery are typically not embolized due to risk of blindness.

Alternatively, the internal maxillary artery and its terminal branch, the sphenopalatine artery, may be controlled with ligation at the time of surgery. The sphenopalatine artery can be reached transnasally with or without creation of a large maxillary antrostomy. A vertical incision is made along the lateral nasal wall just anterior to the horizontal attachment of the middle turbinate.

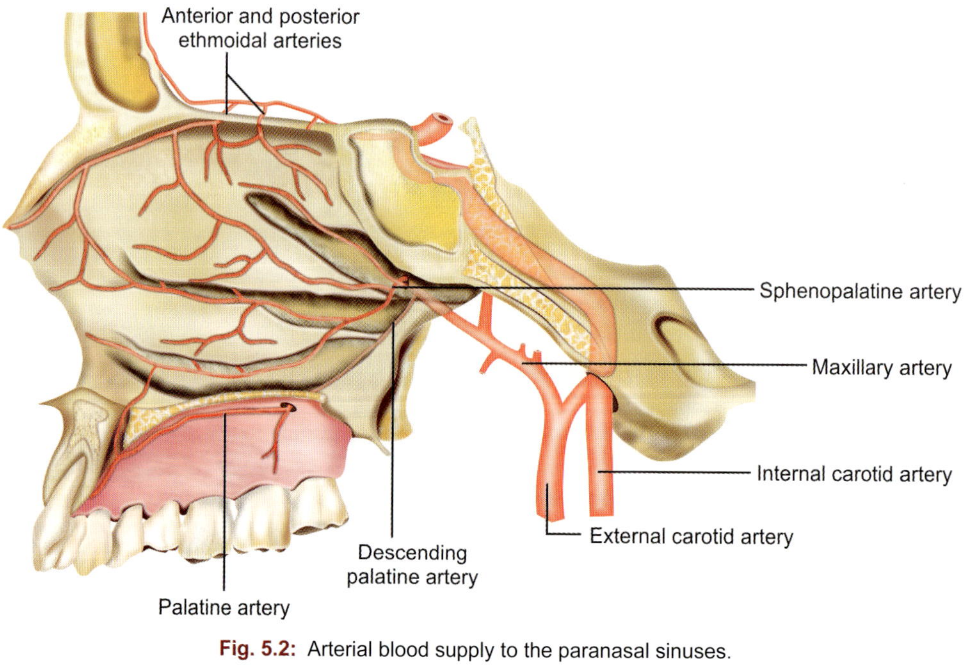

Fig. 5.2: Arterial blood supply to the paranasal sinuses.

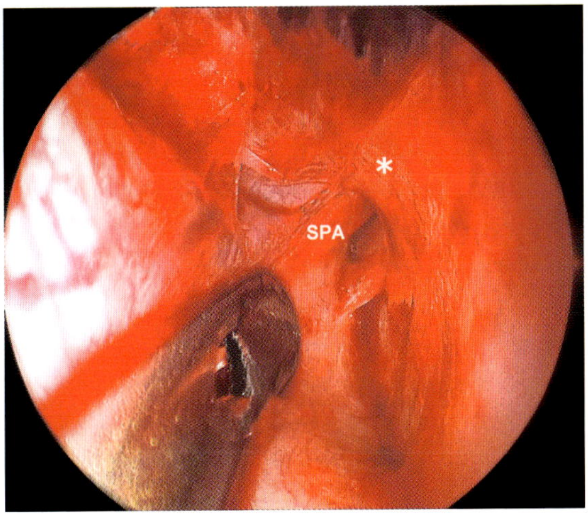

Fig. 5.3: After elevation of the mucoperiosteum, the crista ethmoidalis* and sphenopalatine artery branches are identified.

The mucoperiosteum is elevated and the crista ethmoidalis is identified (Fig. 5.3). The main branch of the sphenopalatine artery is located directly behind this consistent anatomic landmark. The crista ethmoidalis is taken down with a Kerrison rongeur or diamond drill. The artery is skeletonized with a suction elevator and probe (Fig. 5.4). The artery may then be ligated with a bipolar forceps and/or endoscopic application of a microclip. As there are frequently multiple branches of the sphenopalatine artery, these should be looked for and ligated if found.

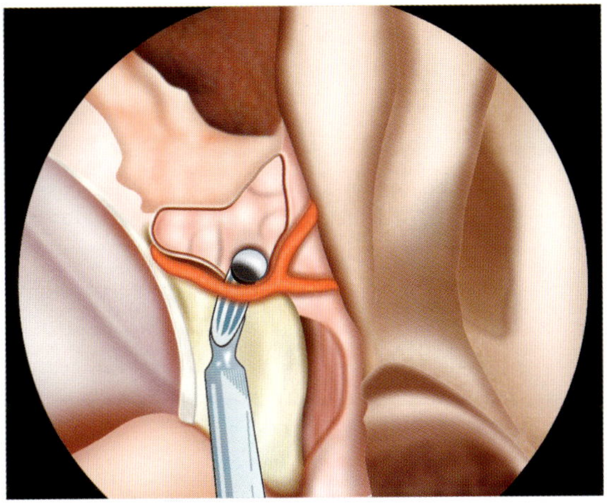

Fig. 5.4: A probe or elevator is used to isolate the artery in preparation for ligation.

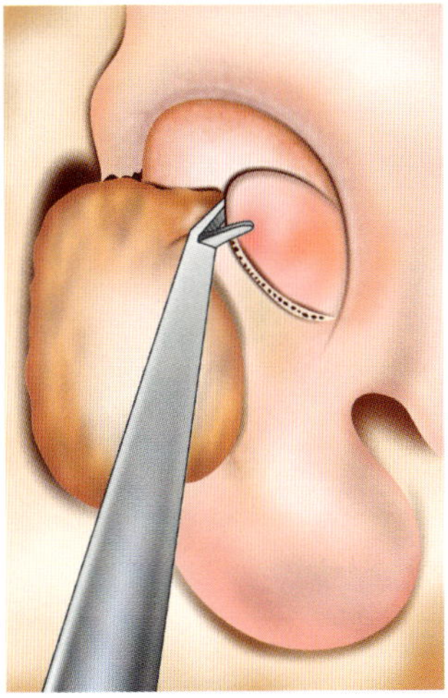

Fig. 5.5: In this schematic of a JNA, a Kerrison Rongeur is used to remove the crista ethmoidalis and a portion of the posterior wall of the maxillary sinus in order to find the internal maxillary artery.

The internal maxillary artery may be similarly ligated after its identification and isolation in the pterygopalatine fossa (PPF). A large maxillary antrostomy is first created. The mucoperiosteum is elevated anteroinferior to the horizontal attachment of the middle turbinate and the crista ethmoidalis is identified and taken down as previously described. The course of the sphenopalatine artery is then followed proximally (laterally), with removal of overlying bone and mucosa (Fig. 5.5). This is typically achieved with a Kerrison Rongeur, 15-degree diamond drill and J-curette. The periosteum of the PPF is kept intact until sufficient bone removal has occurred. The periosteum is then incised with a sickle knife and the artery is dissected from the PPF contents with a suction elevator (Figs 5.6 and 5.7). Bipolar electrocautery and/or microclip application is used to control the artery (Fig. 5.8). No reconstruction is needed, as remucosalization will occur without intervention. Occasionally, the microclip may be visible postoperatively and can

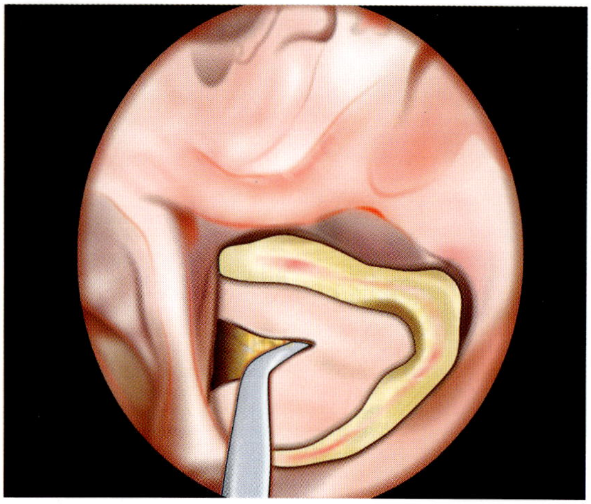

Fig. 5.6: Periosteum of the pterygopalatine fossa is incised.

be associated with minor asymptomatic mucosal edema.

In cases in which the tumor resection involves the anterior skull base, control of the anterior and posterior ethmoid arteries is recommended prior to tumor resection. The anterior and posterior ethmoid arteries can be approached endoscopically or through an external Lynch incision. The anterior ethmoid artery is typically more responsible for arterial supply of tumors than the posterior

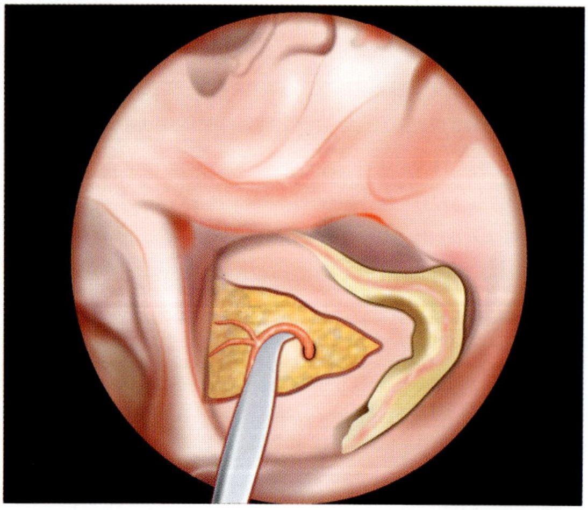

Fig. 5.7: The internal maxillary artery is dissected from the fat of the pterygopalatine fossa.

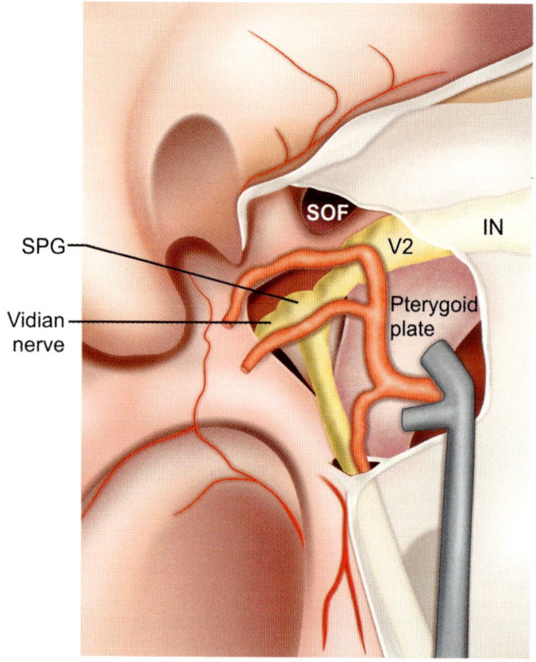

Fig. 5.8: Once isolated, the artery may be ligated with bipolar cautery or clipped.

ethmoid artery, but they may be both accessed in the same manner. The endoscopic approach requires ethmoidectomy and skeletonization of the lamina papyracea. The upper portion of the lamina papyracea is removed and the course of the anterior ethmoid artery is identified. Bipolar cautery or endoscopic microclip application will control the artery on the lateral side of the lamina (Fig. 5.9). If the artery is in a mesentery, this approach is significantly easier, and the artery may even be controlled within the anterior ethmoid sinus. If there is bulky tumor that surrounds the anterior ethmoid artery, or if the artery is embedded within the bone of the skull base, an external approach may be necessary.

The open approach to the ethmoid arteries is most often performed through a Lynch incision, a 15 mm incision placed halfway up the nasal dorsum from the medial canthus (Fig. 5.10). Subperiosteal dissection divides the medial canthal tendon, elevates the lacrimal gland, and identifies the ethmoid arteries between the periorbita and the lamina

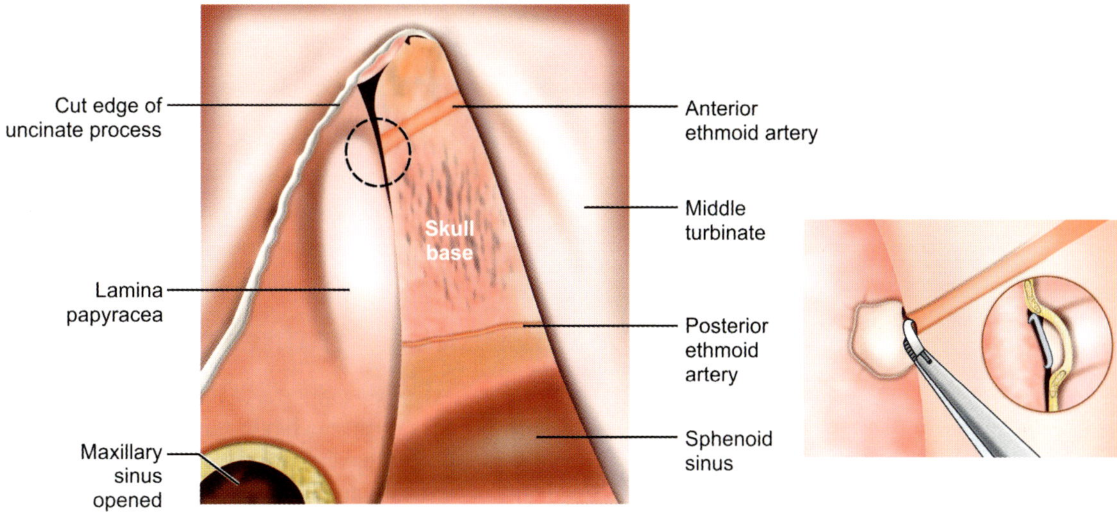

Fig. 5.9: In the endoscopic approach to the ethmoid arteries, the upper portion of the lamina papyracea is removed, and the artery may be controlled with bipolar cautery or application of a microclip.

papyracea. The anterior ethmoid artery is located 24 mm back from the anterior lacrimal crest, the posterior ethmoid artery another 12 mm back, and the optic nerve another 6 mm posteriorly (Fig. 5.11). In 23% of cadaveric specimens, the posterior ethmoid artery was found to be absent.[1] It is crucial that the surgeon not automatically cauterize and divide the next structure seen after ligation of the anterior ethmoid artery. The posterior ethmoid artery must be reliably identified as an arterial branch heading medially rather than a large neurovascular bundle heading posteromedially.

Given the associated scarring and disruption of the medial canthal anatomy, a less invasive method for arterial ligation is preferred. The same exposure provided by a Lynch incision is afforded through the medial conjunctival route.[2] A 15 mm incision is made through the caruncle, and dissection proceeds through avascular tissue planes to the posterior lacrimal crest (Figs 5.12A and B).

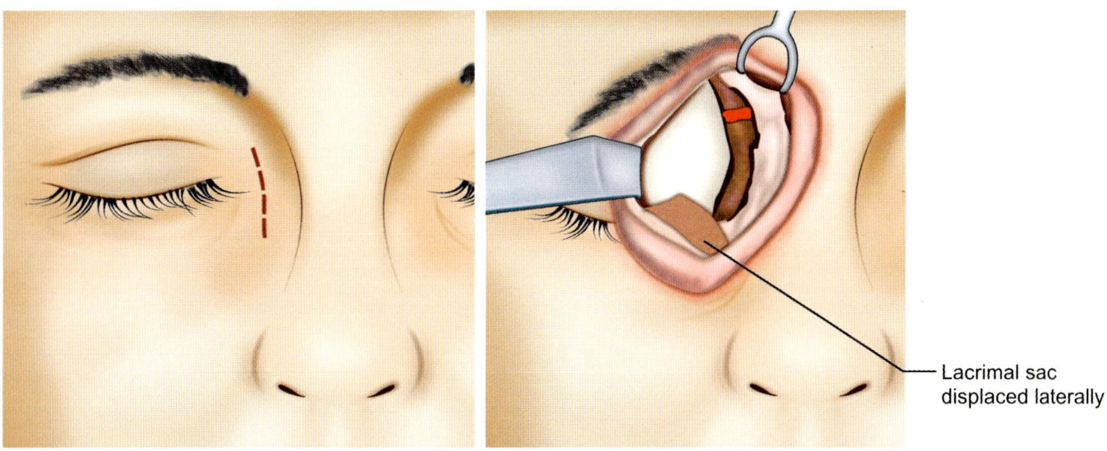

Fig. 5.10: The open approach to the ethmoid arteries may be performed through the classic Lynch incision.

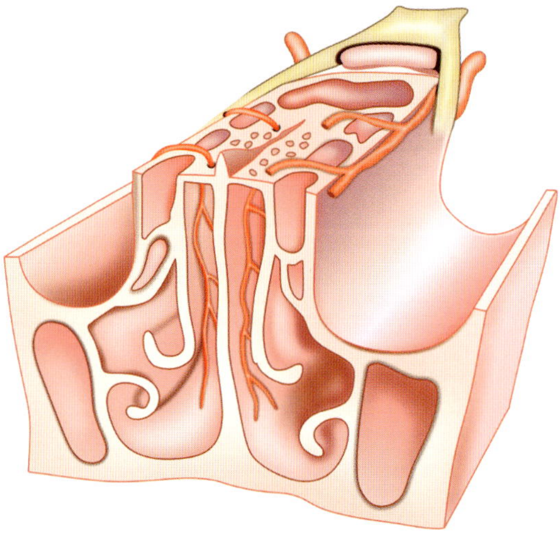

Fig. 5.11: A known anatomic relationship exists between the anterior ethmoid artery, posterior ethmoid artery, and optic nerve. It is important to realize, this relationship is variable and a posterior ethmoid artery can be missing 23%.

In this fashion, the lacrimal sac and medial canthal anatomy is left undisturbed. The periorbita is incised and the endoscope is inserted as a suction elevator opens the subperiosteal space. The anterior and posterior ethmoid arteries can be exposed and ligated with bipolar cautery or a microclip. The superior oblique and medial rectus muscles are in close proximity, so low cautery settings should be used. The incision can be loosely closed with 6–0 fast absorbing gut suture. Once vascular control is obtained, the approach for tumor resection can begin.

TRANSNASAL, TRANSETHMOID APPROACH

The transnasal approach is the simplest endoscopic approach, and provides access to the nasal floor, septum, medial aspect of the turbinates, cribriform plate, and limited access to the sphenoid sinus. Most frequently, this approach is combined with ethmoid dissection to access the ethmoid sinuses, medial orbital wall, and ethmoid skull base. Wider access to the sphenoid sinus is then possible (Fig. 5.13). The middle turbinate may be sharply

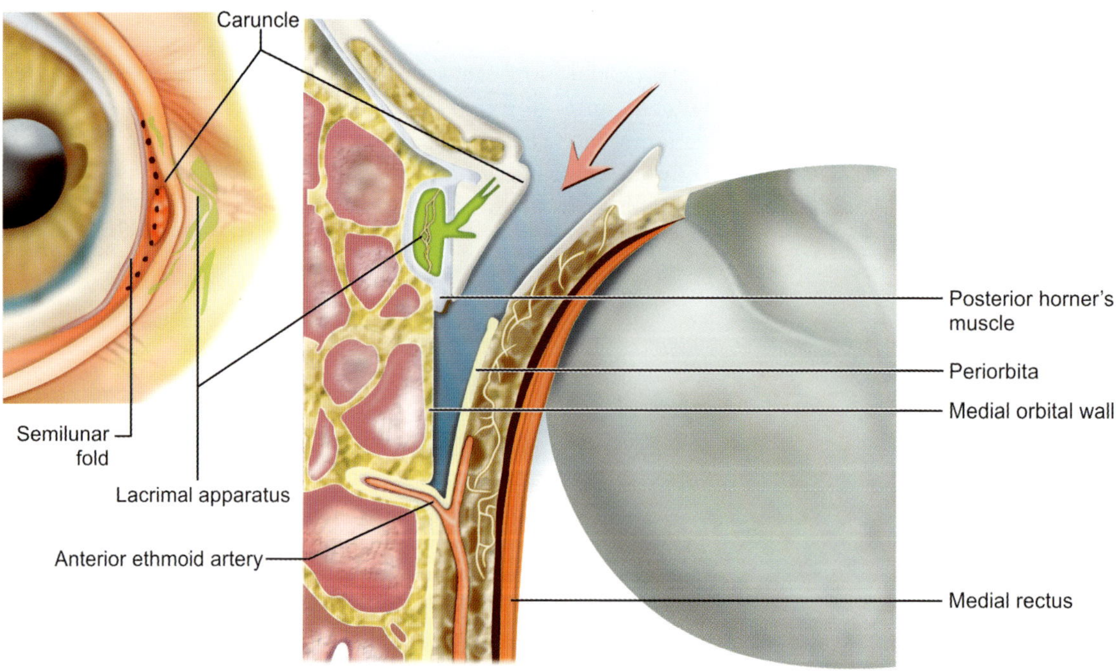

Figs 5.12A and B: (A) Placement of the transcaruncular incision; (B) The transcaruncular dissection proceeds through an avascular plane to the medial orbital wall.

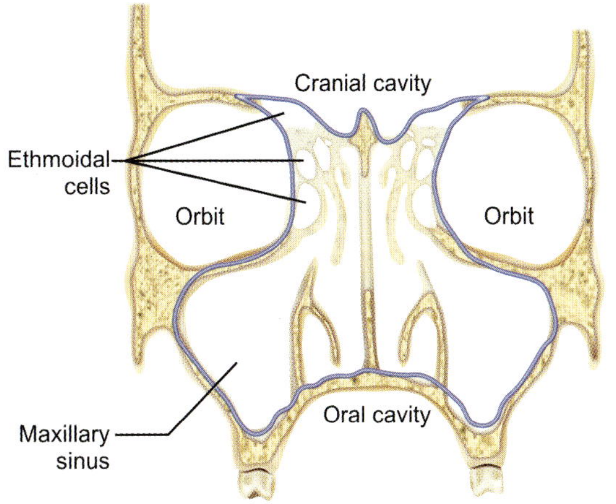

Fig. 5.13: Coronal diagram of the potential access provided by combination of the transnasal and transethmoid routes.

removed with a curved endoscopic scissor to provide wide access to the skull base, harvest graft material, or provide a flat surface for skull base reconstruction. The middle turbinate should be amputated just below the skull base rather than flush with it as the meninges may herniate into its skull base attachment (Fig. 5.14). When the middle turbinate is removed, it is prudent to cauterize the posterior stump to prevent bleeding from arterial branches of the sphenopalatine artery.

Depending on tumor location, partial septectomy may be necessary to obtain margins, or widen the operative field for binostril surgery. If a margin is needed, this should be taken sharply with a sickle knife or otologic beaver blade. The bleeding edge can then be cauterized after the specimen has been taken. The degree of septectomy needed is driven by tumor location, and if possible the anterior 1.5 cm of dorsal and caudal cartilage should be maintained. Combining transnasal and transethmoid dissections with middle turbinectomy and septectomy provides exposure of the entire ethmoid skull base from lamina papyracea to lamina papyracea (Figs 5.15A and B). Intracranial dissection can be performed after the transnasal or transethmoid dissection. Removal of the cribriform plate or ethmoid skull base can be performed with careful use of a diamond drill. Control of the anterior and

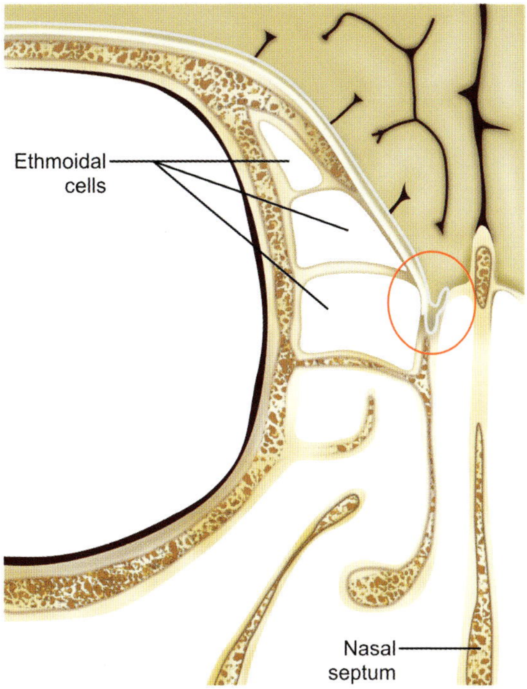

Fig. 5.14: Coronal diagram of the skull base attachment of the middle turbinate. A small amount of meningeal herniation may occur into the root of the middle turbinate.

posterior ethmoid arteries is required either prior to or during this dissection. Often, tumor presence or invasion will have demineralized the bony skull base, and dura will abut the superior aspect of the tumor.

ENDOSCOPIC ANTERIOR APPROACH

In the sagittal plane, anterior dissection is performed through the transnasal or transethmoid approach, and may be combined with frontal sinus dissection ranging from the Draf IIa to endoscopic modified Lothrop (EMLA/Draf III) approaches. The Draf IIa frontal sinusotomy may be sufficient for frontal sinus inspection and maintenance of a patent sinus postoperatively, but is rarely adequate for dissection within the sinus. The sinusotomy may be widened medially with resection of the anterior portion of the middle turbinate, and removal of the medial frontal sinus floor with aggressive punches

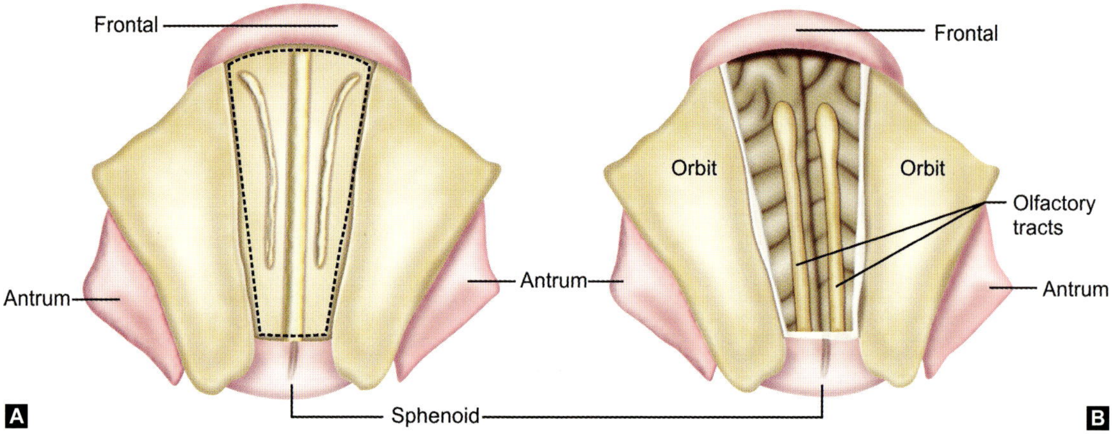

Figs 5.15A and B: Endoscopic view of exposure afforded by partial septectomy, bilateral middle turbinectomy, and bilateral total ethmoidectomy. The operative field extends from one medial orbital wall to the other, and up to the ethmoid skull base and cribriform plate.

or a diamond bur (Figs 5.16A to C). EMLA begins with bilateral ethmoidectomy and identification of the frontal sinus ostia. The frontal sinus ostia are maximally enlarged with punches as in the Draf IIb approach. The anterior aspect of the middle turbinates are removed up to the skull base, and the superior septectomy is performed with through-cutting instruments and a microdebrider. A 70-degree diamond drill is used to remove the frontal sinus floor and intersinus septum (Fig. 5.17). If the anterior-posterior distance is narrow (less than 5-10 mm), then this approach is significantly more difficult, and removal of the nasofrontal beak may provide extra access (Fig. 5.18). In this approach,

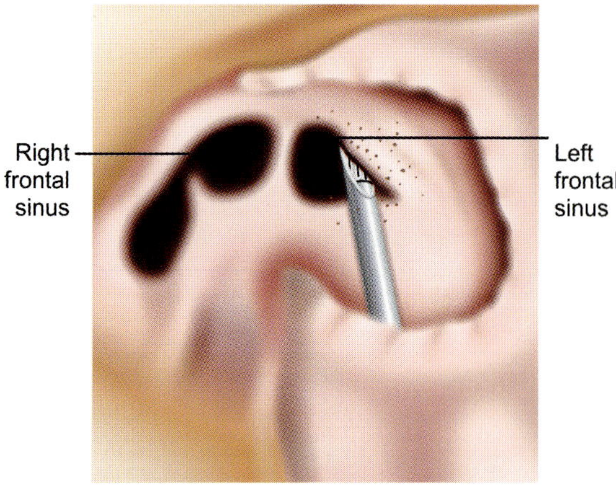

Fig. 5.17: Binostril approach facilitates drilling after superior septectomy.

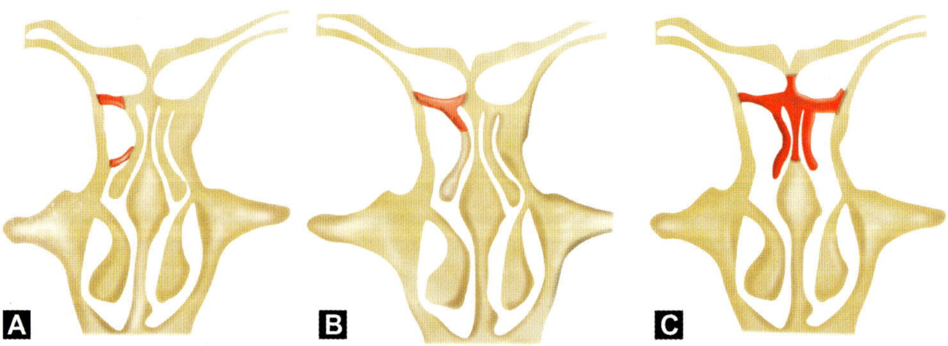

Figs 5.16A to C: Frontal dissection, according to Draf. (A) Draf IIa; (B) IIb; (C) III.

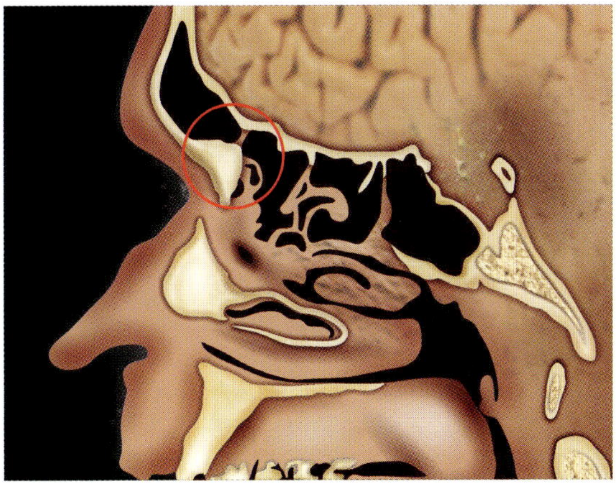

Fig. 5.18: Sagittal diagram of narrow A-P diameter due to prominent nasofrontal beak. This bone will need to be drilled away to enlarge the opening.

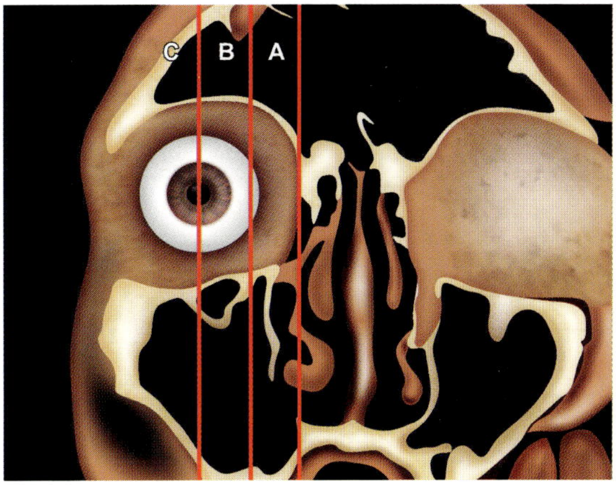

Fig. 5.19: Coronal diagram through the orbit showing access limitations at the medial orbit and midpupillary lines.

visualization within the frontal sinus is much better than instrument access. The far superior and lateral extent of well-pneumatized frontal sinuses may not be routinely accessible for surgical dissection due to limited reach of instruments. The surgeon may be able to pull tumor down from these areas if the site of attachment is lower, but through-cutting instruments, a microdebrider, or drill may not reach these areas. If this is the case, a supplementary external approach may be required. Similarly, the anterior table of the frontal sinus may be visualized but dissection along its surface is challenging. Malleable suctions and curettes are often necessary to create a more optimal angle than standard frontal sinus instruments. For fibro-osseous lesions, proposed boundaries of lateral access have been the lamina papyracea or possibly even to the mid-pupillary line.[3,4] In the latter study, the lateral aspect of the anterior and posterior walls was accessible to a 70-degree diamond bur in 95% of specimens after EMLA, but the orbital roof was significantly more difficult to access. The mid-pupillary line was accessible for dissection in 57% of specimens, and lateral to this point in only 5% (Fig. 5.19). An alternative technique to reach and remove portions of the orbital roof is to progressively remove the superomedial orbital wall, elevating and depressing the periorbita until the extent of bone removal is sufficient for that particular disease process (Fig. 5.20). In large anterior skull base tumors, the EMLA procedure provides the anterior margin of the *en bloc* skull base resection.

ENDOSCOPIC POSTERIOR APPROACHES

Endoscopic approaches to posterior sinonasal tumors combine the transnasal and transethmoid approach with supplementary exposure through the sphenoid sinus. The sphenoid sinus has been described as the gateway to the skull base for

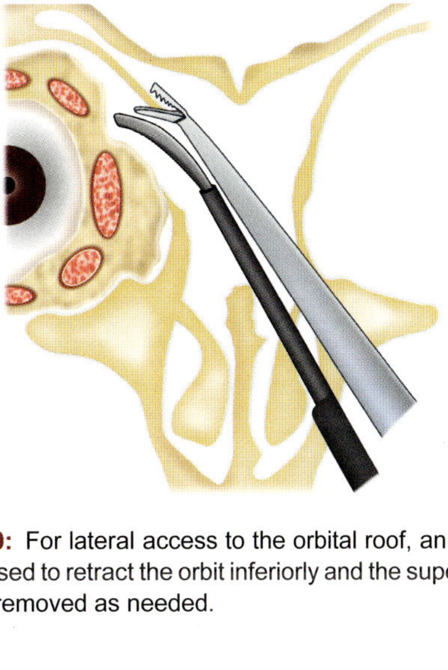

Fig. 5.20: For lateral access to the orbital roof, an elevator can be used to retract the orbit inferiorly and the superior roof may be removed as needed.

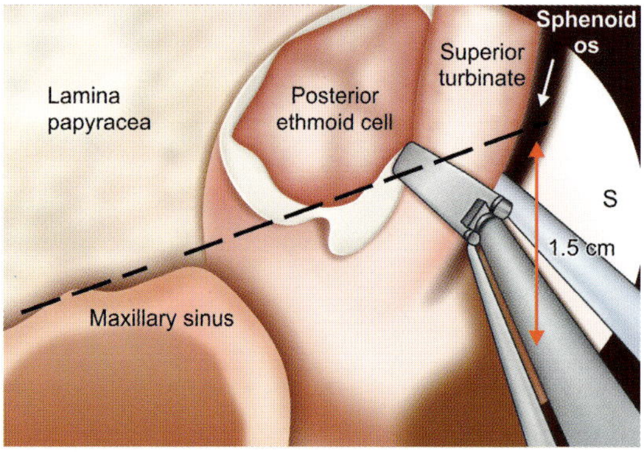

Fig. 5.21: Location of the sphenoid natural os and relationships.

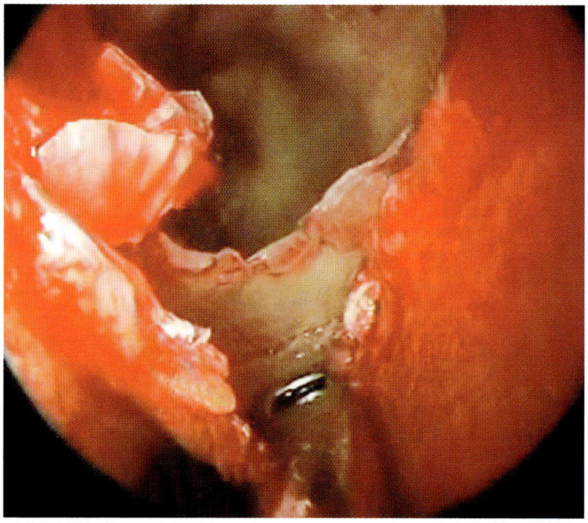

Fig. 5.22: Cottle elevator reflecting choanal arch mucoperiosteum down, protecting the artery while enlarging sphenoidotomy.

advanced endoscopic skull base surgery, and intimate understanding of the anatomy in this region is critical. The first step is a wide sphenoidotomy, either unilaterally or bilaterally. Identification of the natural ostium of the sphenoid sinus utilizes three landmarks. The natural os occurs at roughly the height of the superior maxillary sinus (orbital floor), 1.5 cm superior to the choanal arch, and usually lies medial to the insertion of the superior turbinate (Fig. 5.21). A J-curette can be inserted into the natural ostium with downfracture of the sphenoid rostrum to enlarge the opening. Serial enlargement with a mushroom punch or Kerrison Rongeur can widely open the sphenoid sinus to the level of the skull base superiorly and laterally to the medial orbit. When enlarged inferiorly, the location of the posterior septal branch of the sphenopalatine artery should be remembered, especially if a nasoseptal flap is to be preserved for reconstruction. This arterial branch will pass within the mucoperiosteum inferior to the sphenoid ostium over the arch of the choana. If violated, suction bovie electrocautery can be used in this area to control bleeding. When the sphenoid rostrum needs to be taken down for exposure of the floor of the sinus or instrument passage, but the artery needs to be preserved, the surgeon should simply elevate the nasoseptal flap and displace it into the nasopharynx or maxillary sinus. Alternatively, a Cottle elevator can be used to elevate the mucoperiosteum containing the artery and displace it inferiorly while the bone is removed with a punch, rongeur or drill (Fig. 5.22).

Bilateral sphenoidotomies can be combined with a posterior septectomy to allow for wide exposure of the sphenoid sinus and skull base. This also facilitates a two-surgeon, bi-nostril dissection. The posterior septal artery and nasoseptal flap can be protected as described above, either with early dissection and preservation of the flap(s), inferior reflection of the mucoperiosteal tissue containing the artery, or conservative septectomy (Fig. 5.23). This type of limited septectomy heals rapidly and has been shown to have no long-term effects on smell.[5] The lateral limits of this exposure are the carotid arteries, cavernous sinuses, and optic nerves bilaterally. The sella, optic chiasm, and planum sphenoidale are found superiorly. In the inferior direction, this approach can be extended to and through the nasopharyngeal soft tissues, clivus, and anterior ring of the first cervical vertebra. Further intracranial dissection can be performed with a diamond drill to "eggshell" and flake away the bony skull base. In this manner, transplanum,

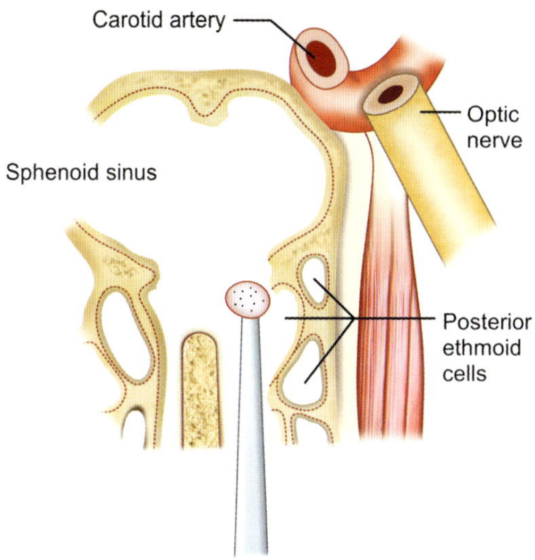

Fig. 5.23: Axial view of wide bilateral sphenoidotomies and conservative posterior septectomy. Access to the entire sphenoid skull base is provided.

transsellar, and transclival approaches can further expose portions of the anterior, middle, and posterior cranial fossae.

Transpterygoid Approach

To reach the lateral recess (pterygoid recess) of a pneumatized sphenoid sinus, a number of maneuvers can be performed. Use of angled endoscopes and curves instruments through a wide sphenoidotomy may be sufficient. Malleable instruments are helpful in this approach. Straight, or lesser angled, endoscopes and instruments may be effective from the opposite nostril through a posterior septectomy. Finally, the transpterygoid approach can help broaden the exposure. After wide maxillary antrostomy, total ethmoidectomy, and wide sphenoidotomy, the sphenopalatine artery should be controlled. The contents of the medial PPF are then lateralized with an elevator or suction. The pterygoid wedge can then be removed from a medial to lateral direction with either a large Kerrison punch or diamond drill (Fig. 5.24). This can expose the pterygoid recess lateral to V2. Without lateralization of the PPF contents, injury to the pterygopalatine ganglion or branches from V2 is possible.

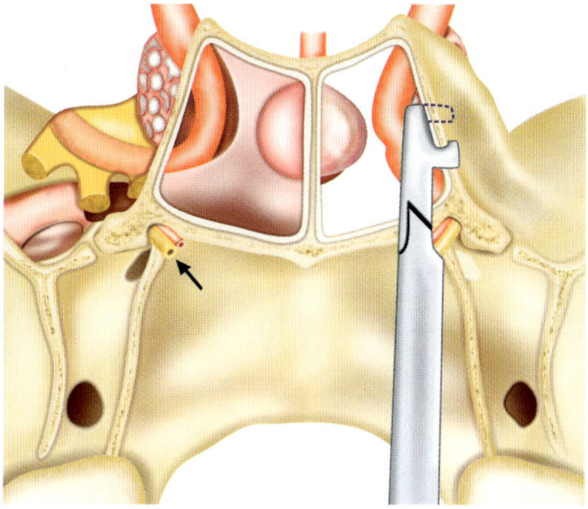

Fig. 5.24: Lateral sphenoid sinus access with a rongeur. The vidian artery and nerve are located at the inferior-lateral aspect.

ENDOSCOPIC LATERAL APPROACHES

A sequence of maneuvers may provide extended access in the anterolateral direction for surgery of the maxillary sinus, pterygopalatine fossa, and infratemporal fossa. With preoperative review of radiology, the necessary maneuvers may be predicted based on zones of access[6] (Fig. 5.25). The first maneuver is the wide maxillary antrostomy. After

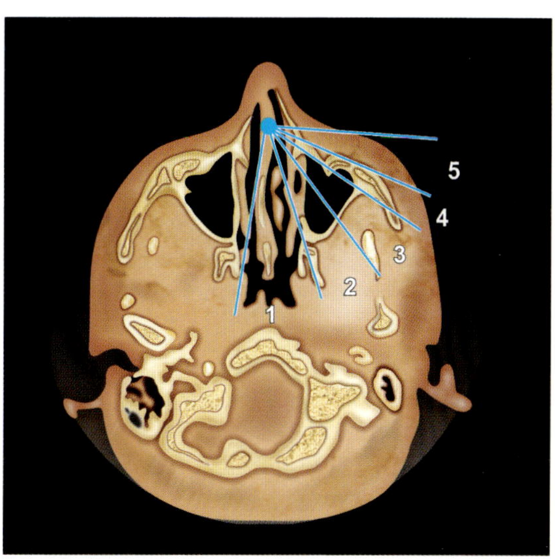

Fig. 5.25: Axial CT diagram of MUSC zones.

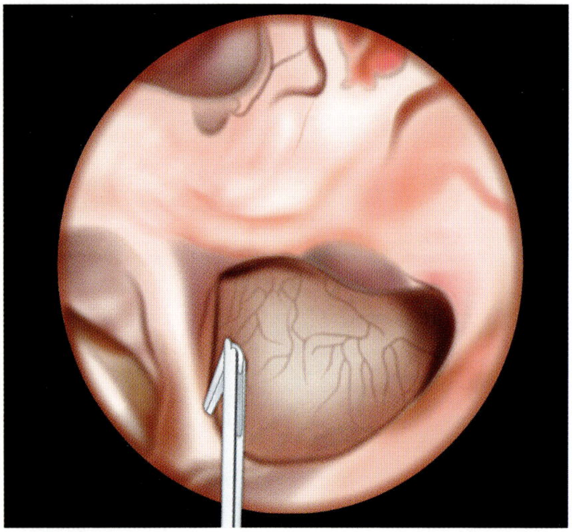

Fig. 5.26: A wide maxillary antrostomy is created with through cutting forceps, antral punch and backbiter.

uncinectomy, a 30° endoscope is used to identify the natural ostium. This is enlarged posteriorly to the posterior wall of the maxillary sinus with through cutting forceps. Use of an antral punch and/or backbiter extends the antrostomy inferiorly to the level of the inferior turbinate (Fig. 5.26).

The next maneuver is the modified endoscopic medial maxillectomy (MEMM). This technique provides improved access to the floor of the sinus and the lateral aspect of the posterior wall. In this procedure, the anterior one-third of the inferior turbinate is preserved, as is the nasolacrimal duct. The posterior two-thirds of the inferior turbinate is removed with a curved endoscopic scissor and the posterior stump is cauterized. A nasal floor flap based on the nasal septum may be created with an angled Beaver blade after injection of 1% lidocaine with 1:100K epinephrine (Fig. 5.27). This flap is reflected medially, and the remaining medial maxillary bone is removed with a 15-degree diamond drill. This is taken down to the nasal floor, and the flap is replaced over the area of exposed bone at the end of the procedure (Fig. 5.28). Extensive drilling often causes a temporary dysesthesia of the upper palate and anterior dentition postoperatively, and the patient should be made aware of this.

More anterolateral access is afforded with the removal of the anterior medial maxilla and nasolacrimal duct, in the procedure known as a total endoscopic medial maxillectomy (TEMM). After MEMM, a backbiter is used to remove the medial maxillary bone to the level of the anterior maxillary wall. Angled endoscopy and diamond bur may also facilitate this dissection. Anticipation and management of epiphora is performed according to surgeon preference: observation, silicone tube stenting, transcanalicular stenting, or endoscopic dacrocystorhinostomy. In a retrospective study, over 25% of patients suffered prolonged epiphora if nothing was done at the time of TEMM.[7] Dacrocystorhinostomy without stenting is easily performed with instruments used in TEMM, and is preferred based on anecdotal evidence. The bone overlying the nasolacrimal sac is drilled away with a 15-degree diamond bur, and the sac is incised and marsupialized (Fig. 5.29). Canalicular probing and/or stenting may be performed according to surgeon preference.

At this point, the entire maxillary sinus is easily visualized with angled endoscopes. However, proper instrumentation may not be available for dissection along the anterior maxillary wall. In this scenario, a more favorable angle of approach is necessary for use of less angled telescopes and instruments. One possibility is the addition of the Dencker maxillotomy approach, which can be performed endoscopically or through and open approach. In the endoscopic approach, an incision is made along the lateral nasal mucosa just anterior to the medial maxillary buttress. This is more simply achieved using a headlight rather than an endoscope, and using an elevator or nasal speculum to palpate the prominence of the medial maxillary buttress. A premaxillary subperiosteal plane is then dissected, and osteotomies are performed to remove the medial buttress (Fig. 5.30). This process can be associated with cosmetic consequences such as alar retraction and soft tissue collapse and may also be associated with injury to the anterior superior alveolar nerve and the canine root.

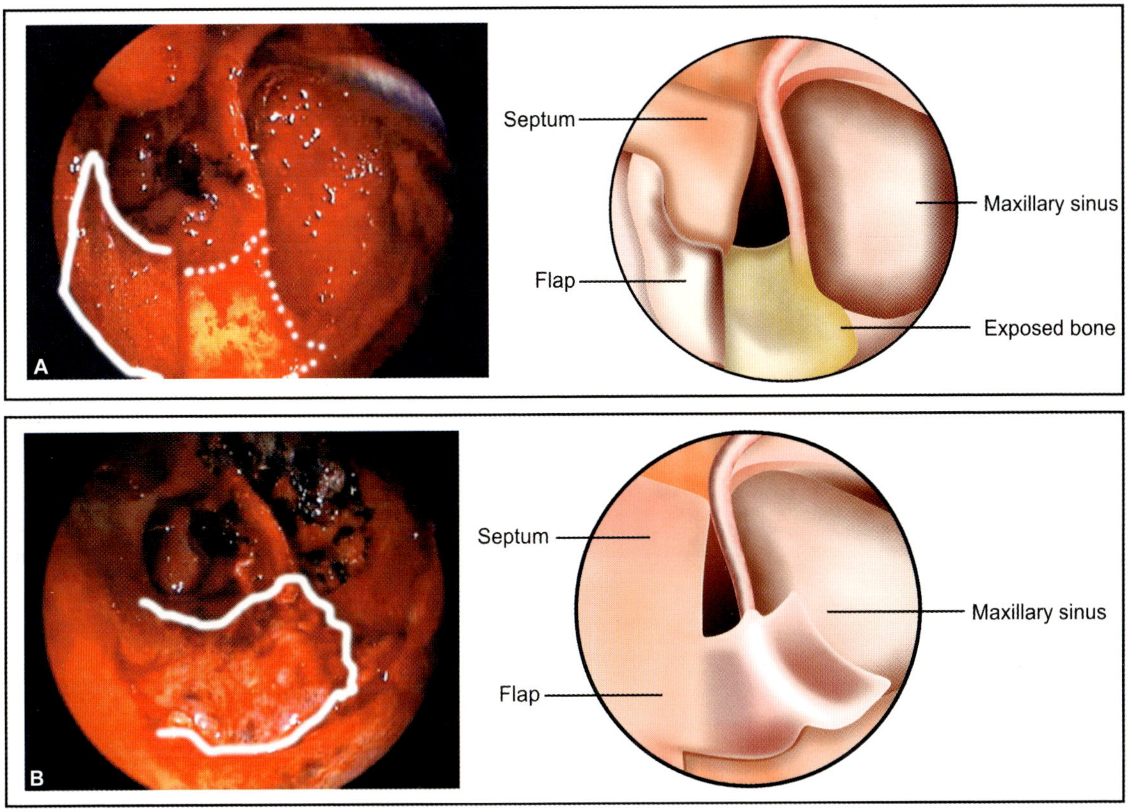

Figs 5.27A and B: Creation of the nasal floor flap for use in medial maxillectomy.

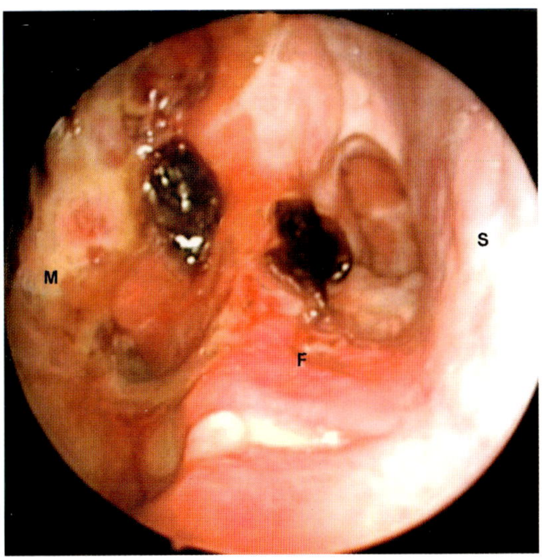

Fig. 5.28: Endoscopic appearance 2 weeks after right MEMM with replacement of nasal floor flap over exposed bone.
Key: S: septum; M: Maxillary sinus; F: Floor of nasal cavity.

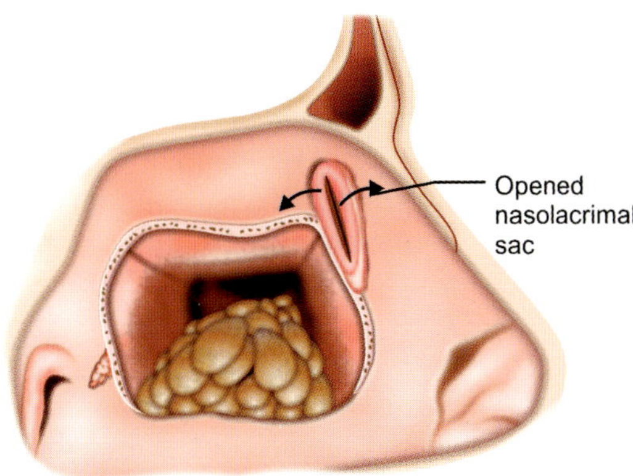

Fig. 5.29: Endoscopic appearance after TEMM with marsupialized nasolacrimal sac.

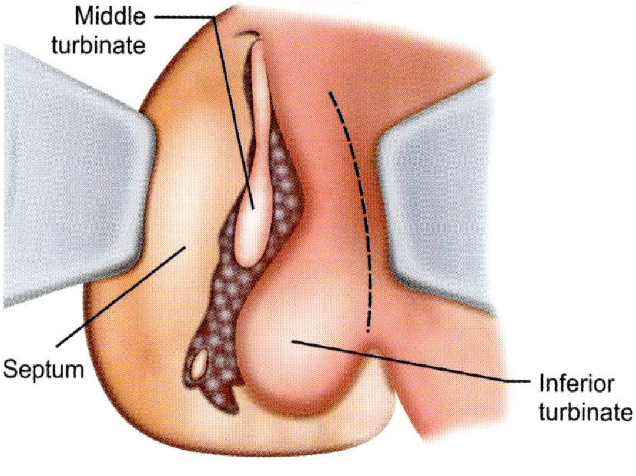

Fig. 5.30: A nasal speculum is used to palpate the medial maxillary wall, identifying the proper location for incision in the Dencker maxillotomy approach.

An alternative method for improved anterolateral access is the trans-septal approach. At this point in the serial expansion of access, the nasal septum becomes the limiting factor for anterior reach, as the shafts of the endoscope and instrument(s) are limited by the caudal septum and columella. In this procedure, a large nasoseptal flap is created on the contralateral side to the tumor. After elevation, the flap is protected by displacement into the posterior nasal cavity. A 1.5–2.0 cm window of central septal cartilage is removed, and can be replaced at the time of reconstruction. A horizontal incision is created on the ipsilateral mucoperichondrial flap, and may be modified into a U-shaped flap based on the floor of the nasal cavity (Figs 5.31A to D). A binostril approach may then be used for tumor dissection at a more favorable angle. Replacement of cartilage and meticulous suture apposition of the flaps is necessary to minimize risk of subsequent septal perforation. Upon conclusion of the procedure, thin silastic splints are placed along the septum bilaterally, and removed approximately 2 weeks postoperatively.

Rather than traversing the septum for use of straight instruments and less angled endoscopy, we have found septal dislocation to provide a similar degree of access.[8] Septal dislocation can also be used in any tumor case to maximize operative space within a single nasal cavity. This technique does not traverse the septum or mucoperichondrial flaps, but rather dissects, displaces, and replaces these structures. In this procedure, a hemitransfixion incision is made and bilateral mucoperichondrial flaps are widely elevated from the septum and nasal floor. The cartilaginous septum is sharply freed from the maxillary crest and the bony-cartilaginous junction (Figs 5.32A to D). A releasing incision can be placed superiorly in the septal cartilage, without violating the dorsal cartilaginous strut. Once mobile, the cartilaginous septum is easily displaced with introduction of instruments through the ipsilateral nostril for a more favorable anterolateral angle. This technique is simple to perform, easy to reconstruct, and virtually eliminates the risk of septal perforation found in the trans-septal approach. However, this is a one-nostril approach, which may be awkward if three- or four-handed dissection is required. In this situation, the hemitransfixion incision should be placed on the contralateral side to the lesion, and the septum dislocated and displaced from the maxillary crest as described above. A horizontal incision can then be made in the mucoperichondrial flap ipsilateral to the lesion for passage of instruments in a concept analagous to the trans-septal approach. This allows for a binostril approach and minimizes the risk of septal perforation.

Access to the pterygopalatine and infratemporal fossae is possible through the posterior and lateral wall of the maxillary sinus. The lateral extent of disease will guide how much of the medial maxillary wall needs to be removed, and if the nasal septum will need to be traversed or displaced. The approach begins as above with identification of the crista ethmoidalis, removal of the bone of the posterior wall of the maxillary sinus, and incision of the PPF periosteum. If possible, gentle blunt dissection is performed to identify the internal maxillary artery and its branches, which can be controlled with bipolar cautery and or placement of microclips. In many situations, this is not feasible. Blind biopsies, cautery, or vigorous dissection should be avoided

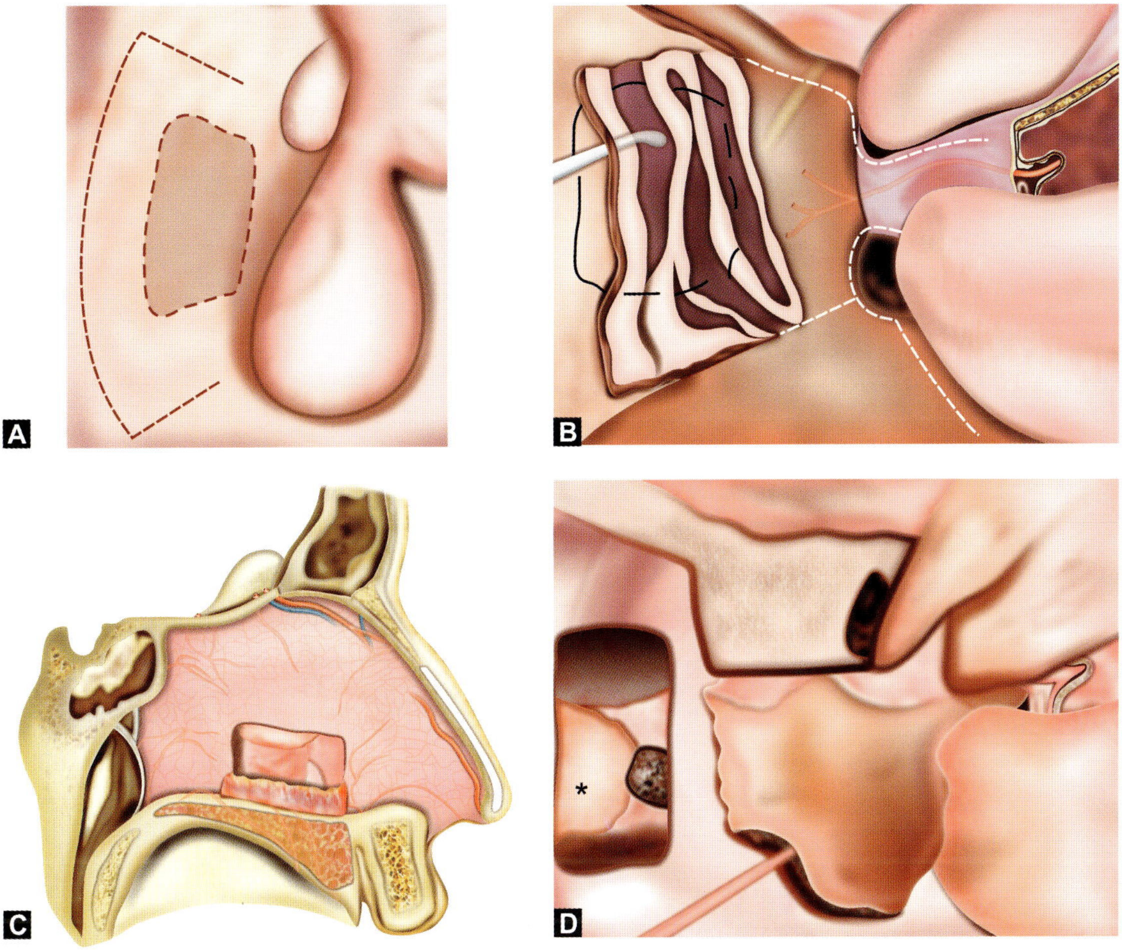

Figs 5.31A to D: Trans-septal approach. (A and B) A large left-sided nasoseptal flap is created based on the posterior nasal branch of the sphenopalatine artery; (C) A right-sided U-shaped flap is created from the nasal floor; (*, D) After displacement of the flaps, a trans-septal corridor is created to the right maxillary sinus.

superomedially in the PPF, as this is the location of the majority of neural structures. Similarly, blind dissection far laterally in the PPF may create large vessel bleeding. As a rule, the surgeon is advised to limit dissection to areas that can be reached with the available instruments, should control of vessels be required.

ENDOSCOPIC-ASSISTED APPROACHES

Minimally invasive adjuvant procedures can be beneficial for introduction of endoscopes to supplement visualization or for introduction of instruments for aid in retraction or dissection. Trephination of the maxillary sinus is a simple procedure with minimal morbidity that allows for maxillary sinuscopy or placement of instruments to aid in dissection. The sublabial, anterior maxillotomy puncture should be placed in the midpupillary line at the level of the nasal floor (Fig. 5.33). If required, an incision can be made in the gingival sulcus and this maxillotomy enlarged in the more traditional Caldwell-Luc type approach.

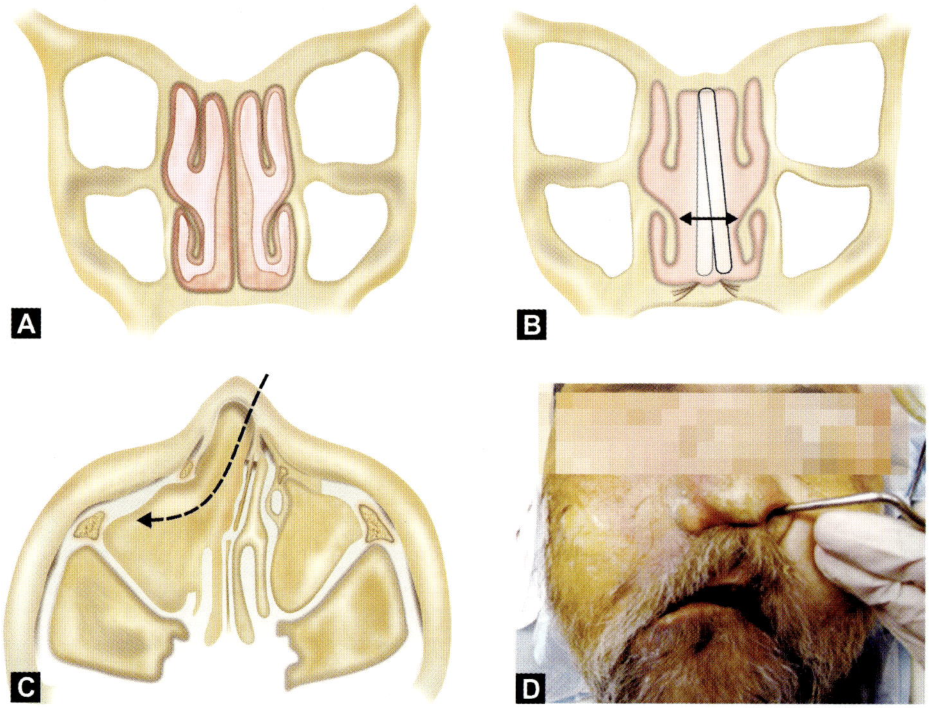

Figs 5.32A to D: Septal dislocation. (A) Generous mucoperichondrial flaps are elevated; (B) The septum is disarticulated from the maxillary crest; (C and D) Once displaced, more access is provided in the anterior and lateral direction.

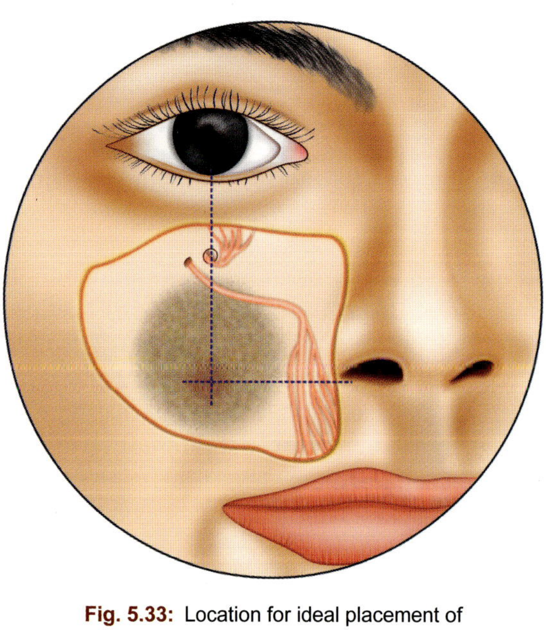

Fig. 5.33: Location for ideal placement of anterior maxillotomy.

In a similar fashion, access to the lateral aspect of the frontal sinus may require a small trephination which can be enlarged as needed for more complex dissection. An incision 1–2 cm in size can be placed in or around the brow, its location depending on pneumatization of the sinus and the purpose of the trephination (Fig. 5.34). The incision should be beveled to follow the hair follicles rather than crossing them. Meticulous reapproximation of tissues at the end of the procedure makes the scar nearly unnoticeable. Careful subcutaneous dissection should attempt to identify and preserve the supraorbital and supratrochlear neurovascular bundles. Image guidance may be helpful to confirm appropriate location of the incision and osteotomy. Alternatively, illumination of the sinus from the transnasal placement of the endoscope after frontal

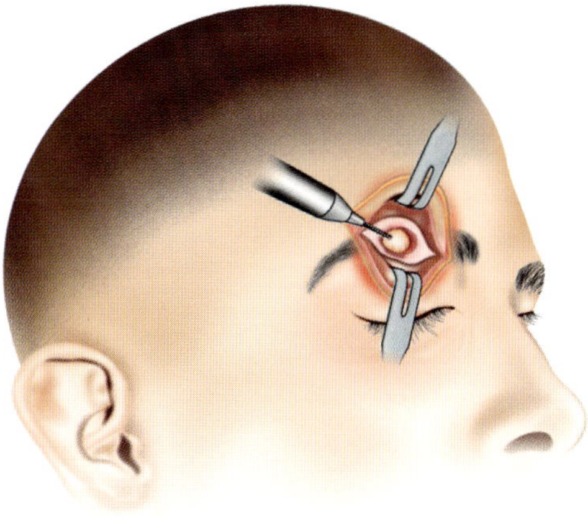

Fig. 5.34: Frontal trephine.

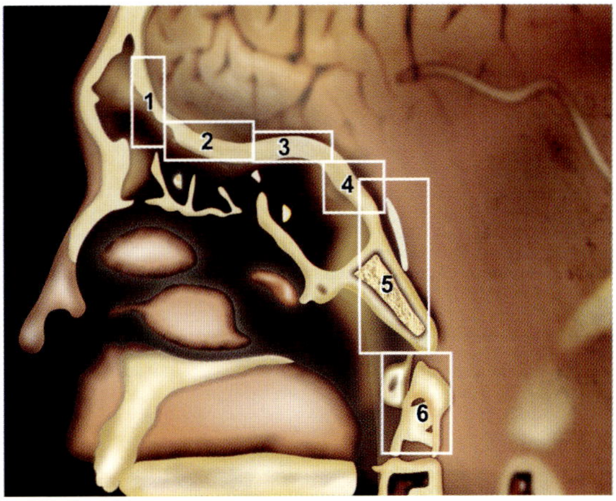

Fig. 5.35: This sagittal view illustrates possibilities for access to the central skull base.

recess dissection gives the surgeon an idea of the location of the lateral extent of the sinus, although this is not completely reliable. An "above and below" style of dissection can be performed, with instruments and the endoscope placed either through the trephination ("above") or transnasally ("below"). Known advantages of the endoscopic technique, namely enhanced illumination, magnification, and visualization suggest a role for the endoscope even in open anterior craniofacial procedures. For instance, endoscopic inspection of the cavity prior to closure or endoscopic assessment of margins is commonly performed.

CONCLUSION

The sequential addition of surgical maneuvers along with tumor debulking gradually widens the surgical exposure and facilitates tumor dissection. The ability of the surgeon to utilize these maneuvers will optimize exposure for improved tumor resection and limitation of complications. Open approaches and combined approaches should also be part of the surgical algorithm. With appropriate planning, instrumentation, and surgical decision-making, endoscopic access to the sinuses and majority of the skull base is possible (Fig. 5.35).

REFERENCES

1. Ducasse A, Segal A, Flament JB. Les arteres ethmoidales. Situation, variations. Ophthalmologie. 1993;7:361-3.
2. Ramakrishnan VR, Suh JD, Chiu AG, and Palmer JN. The utility of a minimally invasive medial orbital approach in advanced endoscopic sinoorbital surgery. Laryngoscope 2011;121(2):437-41.
3. Chiu AG, Schipor I, Cohen NA. Surgical decisions in the management of frontal sinus osteomas. Am J Rhinol. 2005;19(2):191-7.
4. Timperley DG, Banks C, Robinson D, et al. Lateral frontal sinus access in endoscopic skull base surgery. Int Forum All Rhinol 2011, epub ahead of print.
5. Hart CK, Theodosopoulos PV, Zimmer LA. Olfactory changes after endoscopic pituitary tumor resection. Otolaryngol Head Neck Surg. 2010;142(1):95-7.
6. Harvey RJ, Sheehan PO, Debnath NI, et al. Transseptal approach for extended endoscopic resections of the maxilla and infratemporal fossa. Am J Rhinol Allergy. 2009;23(4):426-32.
7. Yeo NK, Wang JH, Chung YS, et al. Contributing factors to prevent prolonged epiphora after maxillectomy. Arch Otolaryngol Head Neck Surg. 2010;136(3):229-33.
8. Ramakrishnan VR, Suh JD, Chiu AG, Palmer JN. Septal dislocation for access of the anterolateral maxillary sinus and infratemporal fossa. Am J Rhinol Allergy 2011;25(2):128-30.

6

Achieving a Cure in Sinonasal Malignancy: Prognostic Factors and Trouble Areas

Zara M Patel, MD; Jayakar V Nayak, MD, PhD

INTRODUCTION

Carcinoma of the paranasal sinuses presents unique challenges in achieving a cure. Most of these tumors present at late stages and the anatomic boundaries in this region are fraught with critical structures. Although the reported outcomes for these patients have risen on average from 5-year survival of 30–40% to 40–60% over the last decade, this is still a generally poor prognosis. As paranasal sinus (PNS) cancer only comprises 1–3%[1,2] of all head and neck cancers, the dearth of patients has also made prospective data collection and outcomes research extremely difficult. Because of this, a comprehensive review of the literature on this subject mainly includes retrospective series that utilize a variety of histologic subsets, tumor sizes, locations and treatment methods over disparate time courses. Also, as tumors arising in the frontal and sphenoid sinuses are quite rare, much of the data focuses on tumors arising from the maxillary and ethmoid sinuses as these are the most common sites of origin, 70–80% and 10–20%, respectively.[3]

Prognostic factors have been found relative to stage, site of origin, patient demographics, histopathology, modality of treatment, surgical method, and molecular characteristics.

STAGE

Multiple staging systems have been introduced into the literature over the last century. The first dates back to 1933 when Ohngren defined a plane based on an imaginary line from the angle of the mandible to the ipsilateral medial canthus in the coronal plane. When maxillary sinus tumors transgressed this plane to involve the orbit, ethmoid sinuses and pterygopalatine fossa, surgical resectability and overall prognosis both diminished.[4] Although there is still wisdom to be found in older staging systems, advances in imaging modalities and surgical techniques have provided the most widely accepted staging system by the American Joint Committee on Cancer (AJCC)[5] (Table 6.1).

American Joint Committee on Cancer staging systems has been proven to be dependable and valuable prognosticating tools over the years of treating PNS cancer. Multiple studies have verified the power of the staging system in overall and disease-specific survival.[6-11] Whereas in the past, extension into the infratemporal or pterygopalatine fossa portended a similarly bad outcome as extension to the orbit or intracranial cavity, recent studies now suggest that primarily orbital, dural, and intracranial involvement carry worsened

Table 6.1 American Joint Committee on Cancer (AJCC) staging system

Maxillary
- T1—Tumor limited to maxillary sinus mucosa with no erosion or destruction of bone
- T2—Tumor causing bone erosion or destruction including extension into the hard palate and/or the middle of the nasal meatus, except extension to the posterior wall of maxillary sinus and pterygoid plates
- T3—Tumor invades any of the following: bone of the posterior wall of maxillary sinus, subcutaneous tissues, floor or medial wall of orbit, pterygoid fossa, ethmoid sinuses
- T4a—Tumor invades anterior orbital contents, skin of cheek, pterygoid plates, infratemporal fossa, cribriform plate, sphenoid or frontal sinuses
- T4b—Tumor invades any of the following: orbital apex, dura, brain, middle cranial fossa, cranial nerves other than maxillary division of trigeminal nerve (V2), nasopharynx or clivus

Nasal cavity and ethmoid sinus
- T1—Tumor restricted to any one subsite, with or without bony invasion
- T2—Tumor invading two subsites in a single region or extending to involve an adjacent region within the nasoethmoidal complex, with or without bony invasion
- T3—Tumor extends to invade the medial wall or floor of the orbit, maxillary sinus, palate or cribriform plate
- T4a—Tumor invades any of the following: anterior orbital contents, skin of nose or cheek, minimal extension to anterior cranial fossa, pterygoid plates, sphenoid or frontal sinuses
- T4b—Tumor invades any of the following: orbital apex, dura, brain, middle cranial fossa, cranial nerves other than (V2), nasopharynx or clivus

Regional lymph nodes (N)
- N1—Metastasis in a single ipsilateral lymph node, 3 cm or less in greatest dimension
- N2—Metastasis in a single ipsilateral lymph node, more than 3 cm but 6 cm or less in greatest dimension; or in multiple ipsilateral lymph nodes, 6 cm or less in greatest dimension; or in bilateral or contralateral lymph nodes, 6 cm or less in greatest dimension
- N2a—Metastasis in a single ipsilateral lymph node more than 3 cm but 6 cm or less in greatest dimension
- N2b—Metastasis in multiple ipsilateral lymph nodes, 6 cm or less in greatest dimension
- N2c—Metastasis in bilateral or contralateral lymph nodes, 6 cm or less in greatest dimension
- N3—Metastasis in a lymph node more than 6 cm in greatest dimension

prognosis, reflecting the development of surgical approaches to access and better visualize the infratemporal and pterygopalatine regions.[7,12-15] In the largest multi-institutional, international collaborative study to date, which included over 1,300 patients from 17 different institutions, intracranial invasion specifically dropped 5 year survival to 21%. Orbital involvement also lowered survival to 44% in this analysis.[15]

Compared to other primary sites, the reported frequency of malignant regional adenopathy in the neck secondary to PNS malignancy has slightly diminished in the literature over time. Previously documented in 10–15% of patients at presentation, recent studies have suggested a rate of 8–10% for concurrent neck disease at primary presentation.[11,16] This may be due to increasingly early diagnosis of these tumors via improved imaging and endoscopy in the clinical setting, although overall the nature of clinical presentation still tends towards advanced stages of disease. Unfortunately, the presence of cervical metastases on presentation is associated with an extremely poor survival, typically less than 20%.[11,16]

Another observation regarding PNS staging has to do with a process called stage migration. As noted above, substantial advancements in imaging and examination techniques have been made over the last few decades. Stage migration occurs when these new methods of determining stage results in the upstaging of tumors previously categorized at a lower stage. During study creation, this results in an apparent improvement in outcome of lower stage cancers by moving the worst cases from lower stage groups to join with cases that were previously categorized into the advanced stage groups.[17] This must be considered when reported outcomes have appeared to shift favorably over time for patients with PNS cancer.

Site of Origin

Although much of the literature discusses these tumors under the broad umbrella term "sinonasal," certain studies have picked out site of origin as an independent prognostic factor. In particular, origin within the central nasal cavity such as the area of the nasal airway, septum, and turbinates, appears to denote a more favorable outcome than tumors originating within one of the paranasal sinuses. Harbo et al. found 5-year survival to be significantly different between nasal cavity origin (56%), maxillary origin (39%) and the other sinuses (24%).[18] Dulguerov et al. showed rates of 5-year survival of 77% for patients with tumors of the nasal cavity, 62% for patients with tumors of the maxillary sinus, and 48% for patients with tumors of the ethmoid sinuses.[19] Bhattacharyya looked separately at surveillance, epidemiology and end results (SEER) database information, a database which collects information such as incidence, prevalence and survival across the United States, on nasal cavity carcinoma and ethmoid carcinoma, and found 5 year survival to be 56.7% versus 40.3%, respectively.[8,20] Alternatively, Gil et al. found that although neural invasion was associated with maxillary sinus origin and also with positive margins, on multivariate analysis it was not an independent prognostic factor for survival.[21] Site of origin outside the nasal cavity thus appears to hold a relatively negative prognostic value. The favorable prognosis of nasal cavity malignancy over paranasal sinus malignancy may be due to earlier presentation, or may be due to the ability to more reliably resect the tumor with negative margins.[22]

Patient Demographics

Paranasal sinus cancer can affect any age group, but the majority of patients are in their fifth to sixth decades. The male to female ratio is 2:1, although this adjusts to a ratio of 1:1with increasing age.[23,24]

Younger age has been shown to be a favorable prognostic factor in multivariate analyses.[6,7] This may be due to the difficulty inherent in trying to separate out any and all comorbidities in statistical analysis. Younger age at presentation has also been shown to be a significant prognostic factor for those patients undergoing craniofacial resection (CFR), due to the same issue.[25]

Female gender has also been shown in one series to be a favorable prognostic factor.[6]

Histopathology

The majority of sinonasal neoplasms are epithelial in origin. In pooled data from 22 series including 5,578 patients, carcinomas constituted over two-thirds of all malignant neoplasms of the sinonasal tract.[2] The most common histopathologic subtype is squamous cell carcinoma (SCC), accounting for 30–75% of all PNS cancer (Table 6.2). Thus, in most studies, generalized prognostic factors are most consistently valid in this tumor population.

Table 6.2* Histopathology of sinonasal neoplasms[2]

Histologic type	*Literature review (%)*
Squamous cell carcinoma	36
Adenoid cystic carcinoma	9
Adenocarcinoma	16
Mucoepidermoid carcinoma	1
Undifferentiated carcinoma	6
Lymphoma	4
Malignant melanoma	6
Esthesioneuroblastoma	8.5
Sarcoma	8.5
Transitional cell carcinoma	<1
Other	1

*With kind permission from Springer Science+Business Media, reproduced from Khademi, B, Moradi, A, Hoseini, S, et al. Malignant neoplasms of the sinonasal tract: report of 71 patients and literature review and analysis. Oral Maxillofacial Surgery. 2009;13:191-9 (Table 5).

Adenoid cystic carcinoma (ACC) has classically been reported as the second most common tumor of the paranasal sinuses,[26] although more recent meta-analyses may have its incidence third behind adenocarcinoma (ACA). With most histologic subtypes (Table 6.2) there is a reasonably stable survival from the first 5–10 years after surgical resection. Unfortunately, as seen with ACC elsewhere in the head and neck, the propensity exists for relatively high 5-year survival followed by a dramatic decrease in 10 year survival due to a pattern of relentless locoregional and distant recurrence, presumably due to insidious spread along neural sheaths. In a large single institution series, 5-year survival was 63% with eventual drop off to equal the results for SCC at 10 years. Skull base invasion was a significant poor prognostic factor, as was T4 and stage IV categorization. When the histopathologic subtypes of ACC were compared, patients with cribiform-type tumors had the best survival and those with solid tumors had the worst, with tubular-type showing intermediate prognosis. Surgery with postoperative radiation provided the best survival compared to other treatment modalities, and primary treatment of disease with surgery at the outset versus primary radiation or chemotherapy also improved survival. Recurrences, treatment of recurrences or response to treatment of recurrence were not prognostic factors.[27]

Adenocarcinoma comprises 15% of all PNS cancer. Orvidas et al. found that histologically higher grade lesions and those with intracranial invasion conferred adverse prognostic factors, and found younger age to be beneficial for survival.[28] Choussy et al. noted that T stage, presence of malignant adenopathy and intracranial invasion provided for poorer outcomes.[29] Overall paranasal ACA shows a better 5-year survival than SCC and has improved functional outcomes.[3]

Esthesioneuroblastoma, also termed olfactory neuroblastoma, is a rare tumor of the paranasal sinuses arising from the olfactory neuroepithelium that has a significantly better prognosis than SCC, and even better prognosis than ACA. Prognostic factors for esthesioneuroblastoma are closely linked to the Kadish staging system, or extent of tumor within or beyond the paranasal sinuses, and to the Hyams grading system, taking into account tissue architecture, mitoses, nuclear polymorphism, fibrillary matrix, rosettes and necrosis. The overall survival at 5 years is generally greater than 75%.[30]

Mucosal melanoma (MM) of the paranasal sinuses is rare and has a very poor prognosis. A recent chart review of 58 patients sought to determine prognostic factors and outcomes based on recent treatment modalities. These investigators found T stage and degree of tumor pigmentation to be associated with decreased survival, while pseudopapillary architecture was associated with higher locoregional failure.[31] Penel et al. reported that clear margin status is an important prognostic factor as well.[32] This is an interesting finding as obtaining negative margins in mucosal melanoma may be quite challenging. Clinicians often question if true margin status can reliably be assessed as unrecognized spread and multifocal disease may be present. Overall, the 5-year survival for MM of the paranasal sinuses ranges from 20–35% among different series, has not changed significantly over the last several decades, and compares quite poorly against other cancers of this region.

Sinonasal undifferentiated carcinoma (SNUC) is an exceedingly rare high-grade malignancy, also with exceptionally poor prognosis. Due to its rarity, series are small and no true prognostic data for this subset of cancers can be garnered. However the overall survival can be compared to that of other tumors. Survival is generally so poor that it is not reported in 5 years, but in 2 years, terms of survival. The median overall survival at 2 years is 64%, but when reported, 5-year survival is less than 25%.[33,34]

Perineural spread may or may not confer a significant decrease in prognosis. Given the anatomic complexity of the region, it is often not possible to follow a nerve proximally to clear the margin of an involved nerve, as one-third of cases with perineural invasions will extend more that 1 cm proximal to the tumor.[21] Even if a negative neural biopsy were obtained, "skip lesions" may be present, leading the surgeon to falsely assume that the neural margin has been cleared.

It may be best to conceptualize malignant sinus tumor pathology into broad low-grade and high-grade categories according to their overall clinical behavior. Esthesioneuroblastoma, confined adenoid cystic carcinoma, hemangiopericytoma, low-grade ACA, and low-grade sarcomas carry reasonable prognoses. SCC, high-grade ACA and sarcoma, melanoma, and undifferentiated carcinomas carry much worse prognoses.

Modality of Treatment

There has been some debate in the literature about whether or not surgery alone, radiation alone, combination chemoradiotherapy, or surgery combined with radiation is the best option for treatment of PNS cancer. Many retrospective series have reported superior outcomes for patients undergoing a combined modality approach as opposed to radiation alone.[18,35] The use of radiation alone has had lower survival associated with it, usually 30–40%.[36,37] Recently, a prospective series looking at 109 patients, all-comers with the exception of maxillary sinus tumors, again showed that overall survival is superior in those patients treated with both surgery and radiation (84%) versus radiation alone (43%).[38]

The problem with traditional external beam radiation was the inability to deliver full coverage of the tumor while protecting critical structures in the path of the radiation source at the orbit and skull base. Since the advent of intensity modulated radiation therapy (IMRT), these problems have been mitigated, allowing escalation of total dose far beyond what was delivered a decade ago. A study comparing IMRT in the post-surgical treatment of PNS cancer to traditional radiotherapy found that IMRT resulted in significantly improved disease-free survival (60% vs 72%; $p = 0.02$). The use of IMRT also significantly reduced the incidence of acute as well as late side effects, especially regarding skin toxicity, mucositis, xerostomia, and dry-eye syndrome.[39]

The timing of radiation in relation to surgery has also been discussed in the literature. Some authors suggest preoperative radiation as a way to avoid resection of critical structures such as the orbit, however other surgeons advocate primary surgery to debulk the majority of tumor burden and its mass effects, before the sequela of radiation has a chance to effect the tissue planes and pretreatment margins. No significant difference has been found in survival based on pre- versus postoperative dosing.[34,40]

In cases of advanced or unresectable minor salivary gland malignancies such as ACC, compared to standard external beam radiation therapy, both neutron beam radiotherapy and gamma knife radiosurgery can be used and have provided some benefit in locoregional control.[41,42]

The role of chemotherapy in concurrent administration with radiation, although widely accepted for locoregionally advanced head and neck cancer, has not been well studied in regard to PNS cancer. Although there was initial investigation into intra-arterial cisplatin administration in addition to traditional intravenous agents, the toxicity of the dosing proved to be too high.[43] There have been promising results from selected small series looking at adding chemotherapy to the traditional management of SNUC and esthesioneuroblastoma with increased locoregional control.[44,45] We also now know that in high-risk head and neck cancer with features found on surgical pathology such as positive margins, perineural and perivascular spread and extracapsular extension, postoperative chemotherapy may improve locoregional control.[46]

Surgical Method

Two-thirds of PNS lesions arise within the area of the anterior cranial fossa, with the remainder affecting the regions of the middle and posterior fossae.[47] Dating back to 1941 when Dandy first resected an orbital tumor via an anterior craniotomy and ethmoid incision, techniques and approaches to anterior craniofacial resection (ACFR) has been developing (Fig. 6.1). Ketcham and others, in

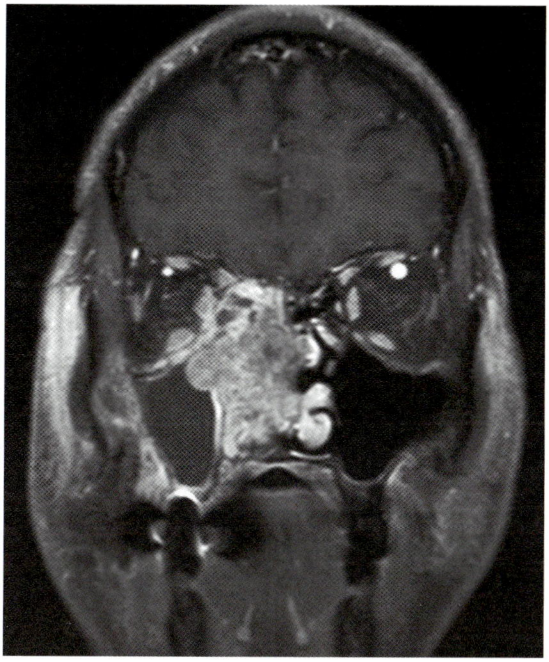

Fig. 6.1: MRI demonstrating a primary sinonasal malignancy originating from the right ethmoid skullbase. Traditionally resected via an open ACFR approach, this tumor may now be a candidate for endoscopic resection.

1963, described the craniofacial approach to the paranasal sinuses.[48,49] This open approach to the skull base has been further developed and refined through the 1970s and 1980s, and rapidly became the "gold standard" for resecting anterior skull base neoplasms.[50] Both recurrence rate (12% vs 60%) and disease-free survival (82% vs 38%) improved with the advent of ACFR.[51,52]

Casiano et al. published the first description in the literature of endoscopic CFR for an esthesioneuroblastoma in 2001.[53] Since, that time there has been increasingly heated debate in the literature surrounding the question of whether endoscopic technique is appropriate for resection of malignancy. Recently, a collection of publications have come out in support of endoscopic resection of malignancy, reporting comparable short-term locoregional tumor control and prognosis as open ACFR, with decreased patient morbidity.[54-58] While endoscopic approaches can be attractive to both patient and surgeon, it should be emphasized that sound surgical oncologic principles should be maintained with each endoscopic resection. Whichever approach is employed, the complete resection of tumor to negative margins remains the most important factor in surgically associated prognosis.[2,3,11,12,26,51]

Molecular Characteristics

Cytogenetic and molecular research is still in its infancy in relation to PNS cancer. There are few researchers and funding agencies supporting work on the treatment of these tumors, but to date an interesting array of molecular prognostic factors have been found.

There is one common finding which applies to esthesioneuroblastoma, ACA and SCC — all show complex karyotypic changes with numerous chromosomal abnormalities.[59]

A recently published study on sinonasal mucosal melanoma analyzed by comparative genomic hybridization revealed consistent alterations with chromosomal gain on 1q in 14/14 tumors and gains onto 6p and d8q in 93% and 57%, respectively.[60] Sinonasal ACAs have been investigated for the expression of the oncoprotein c-erbB-2, a putative transmembrane protein which has prognostic significance in a variety of ACAs at other sites within the human body. In a group of 28 sinonasal ACAs, 32% stained positive for c-erbB-2. Tumors which overexpress c-erbB-2 have a significantly increased risk for recurrence and distant metastases.[61]

Out of the group of tumor suppressor genes, p53 has been the most thoroughly investigated. p53, which plays a key role in DNA repair, is the most frequently mutated gene in human neoplasms. Overexpression of p53 was found in 60% of sinonasal carcinomas, including 42 SCCs and 10 ACAs, in a Taiwanese study on Asian patients. In another study, 43% of undifferentiated carcinomas stained positive for p53, while p53 overexpression was absent in olfactory neuroblastomas and malignant melanomas.[62]

Looking at other molecular factors, a strong association has been found between Ki-67 expression and microvessel density and overall survival ($p < 0.05$ and $p = 0.039$, respectively), while VEGF-C expression was a prognostic factor in SCC patients only ($p < 0.05$).[63]

Lastly, a burgeoning interest in the role of human papilloma virus (HPV) and its role in head and neck oropharyngeal cancers has ignited new research in PNS SCC. HPV has been shown to correlate with significantly better 5-year survival in patients with same site, grade and stage of PNS squamous cell tumors.[64]

CONCLUSION

The prognostic factors involved in PNS cancer are multiple and varied. The rarity of the disease has made neoplasms of this area challenging to study and has forced some extrapolation of data across histology, subsites, patient populations and institutions. Average treatment outcome, although improving, is still not an acceptable prognosis to give our patients. Impressive strides in both surgical technique and adjunctive treatments have shown promise for improved tumor control and outcomes, with advances in understanding the molecular basis of tumorigenesis of PNS actively under investigation. Hopefully it will not be long before these, and related, innovations begin to impact patient survival, and allow more reliable success in the care of patients with these challenging lesions.

REFERENCES

1. Lalami Y, Vereecken P, Dequanter D, et al. Salivary gland carcinomas, paranasal sinus cancers and melanoma of the head and neck: an update about rare but challenging tumors. Curr opin oncol. 2006;18(3):258-65.
2. Khademi B, Moradi A, Hoseini S, et al. Malignant neoplasms of the sinonasal tract: report of 71 patients and literature review and analysis. Oral Maxillofac Surg. 2009;13(4):191-9.
3. Waldron J, Witterick I. Paranasal Sinus Cancer: Caveats and Controversies. World J Surg. 2003;27(7):849-55.
4. Ohngren LG. Malignant tumors of the maxillo-ethmoidal region. Acta Otolaryngologica. Supplement. 1933;13:101-6.
5. Nasal cavity and paranasal sinuses. In: American Joint Committee on Cancer. AJCC Cancer Staging Manual. 6th edition. New York, NY: Springer; 2002. pp. 59-67.
6. Le QT, Fu KK, Kaplan M, et al. Treatment of maxillary sinus carcinoma: a comparison of the 1997 and 1977 American Joint Committee on cancer staging systems. Cancer. 1999;86(9):1700-11.
7. Bhattacharyya, N. Factors Predicting Survival for Cancer of the Ethmoid Sinus. Am J Rhinol. 2002;16(5):281-6(6).
8. Blanch JL, Ruiz A, Llucia A. Treatment of 125 sinonasal tumors: Prognostic factors, outcome, and follow-up. Otolaryngol Head Neck Surg. 2004;131:973-6.
9. Thorup C, Sebbesen L, Dano H, et al. Carcinoma of the nasal cavity and paranasal sinuses in Denmark 1995-2004. Acta Oncol. 2010;49(3):389-94.
10. Airoldi M, Garzaro M, Valente G, et al. Clinical and Biological Prognostic Factors in 179 Cases with Sinonasal Carcinoma Treated in the Italian Piedmont Region. Oncology. 2009;76(4):262-9.
11. Guntinas-Lichius O, Kreppel MP, Stuetzer H, et al. Single modality and multimodality treatment of nasal and paranasal sinuses cancer: A single institution experience of 229 patients. Eur J Surg Oncol. 2007;33(2):222-8.
12. Gullane PJ, Conley J. Carcinoma of the maxillary sinus. A correlation of the clinical course with orbital involvement, pterygoid erosion, or pterygopalatine invasion and cervical metastases. J Otolaryngol. 1983;12(3):141-5.
13. Porceddu S, Martin J, Shanker G, et al. Paranasal sinus tumors: Peter MacCallum Cancer Institute experience. Head Neck. 2004;26(4):322-30.
14. Bentz BG, Bilsky MH, Shah JP, et al. Anterior Skull Base Surgery for Malignant Tumors: A Multivariate Analysis of 27 years of experience. Head Neck. 2003;25:515-20.
15. Patel SG, Singh B, Polluri A, et al. Craniofacial Surgery for Malignant Skull Base Tumors: Report of an International Collaborative Study. Cancer. 2003;98:1179-87.
16. Robin PE, Powell DJ. Regional node involvement and distant metastases in carcinoma of the nasal cavity and paranasal sinuses. J Laryngol Otol. 1980;94(3):301-9.

17. Feinstein AR, Sosin DM, Wells CK. The Will Rogers phenomenon. Stage migration and new diagnostic techniques as a source of misleading statistics for survival in cancer. N Engl J Med. 1985;312(25): 1604-8.
18. Harbo G, Grau C, Bundgaard T, et al. Cancer of the nasal cavity and paranasal sinuses. A clinicopathologic study of 277 patients. Acta Oncol. 1997;36(1):45-50.
19. Dulguerov P, Jacobsen MS, Allal AS, et al. Nasal and paranasal sinus carcinoma: are we making progress? A series of 220 patients and a systematic review. Cancer. 2001;92(12):3012-29.
20. Bhattacharyya N. Cancer of the nasal cavity:survival and factors influencing prognosis. Arch Otolaryngol Head Neck Surg. 2002;128(9):1079-83.
21. Gil Z, Carlson DL, Gupta A, et al. Patterns and incidence of neural invasion in patients with cancers of the paranasal sinuses. Arch Otolaryngol Head neck Surg. 2009;135(2):173-9.
22. Parsons JT, Kimsey FC, Mendenhall WM, et al. Radiation therapy for sinus malignancies. Otolaryngol Clin N Am. 1995;28(6):1259-68.
23. Myers LL, Nussenbaum B, Bradford CR, et al. Paranasal sinus malignancies: an 18-year single institution experience. Laryngoscope. 2002; 112(11): 1964-9.
24. Robin PE, Powell DJ, Stansbie JM. Carcinoma of the nasal cavity and paranasal sinuses: Incidence and presentation of different histological types. Clin Otolaryngol Allied Sci. 1979;4(6):431-56.
25. Ganly I, Gross ND, Patel SG, et al. Outcome of Craniofacial Resection in Patients 70 years or Older. Head Neck. 2007;29(2):89-94.
26. Batsakis JG. Tumors of the head and neck: clinical and pathologic considerations. 2nd Edn. Baltimore, MD: Williams & Wilkins; 1979. p. 77.
27. Lupinetti AD, Roberts DB, Williams MD, et al. Sinonasal Adenoid Cystic Carcinoma. The MD Anderson Cancer Center Experience. Cancer. 2007;110(12):2726-31.
28. Orvidas LJ, Lewis JE, Weaver AL, et al. Adenocarcinoma of the nose and paranasal sinuses: a retrospective study of diagnosis, histologic characteristics, and outcomes in 24 patients. Head Neck. 2005;27(5):370-5.
29. Choussy O, Ferron C, Védrine PO, et al. Adenocarcinoma of Ethmoid: a GETTEC retrospective multicenter study of 418 cases. Laryngoscope. 2008;118(3):437-43.
30. Day TA, Beas RA, Schlosser RJ, et al. Management of Paranasal Sinus Malignancy. Curr Treat Options Oncol. 2005;6(1):3-18.
31. Moreno MA, Roberts DB, Kupferman ME, et al. Mucosal Melanoma of the Nose and Paranasal Sinuses, a Contemporary Experience from the MD Anderson Cancer Center. Cancer. 2010;116(9):2215-23.
32. Penel N, Mallet Y, Mrabel X, et al. Primary mucosal melanoma of head and neck: prognostic value of clear margins. Laryngoscope. 2006;116(6):993-5.
33. Enepekides DJ. Sinonasal undifferentiated carcinoma: an update. Curr Opin Otolaryngol Head Neck Surg. 2005;13(4):222-5.
34. Mendenhall WM, Mendenhall CM, Riggs CE, et al. Sinonasal Undifferentiated Carcinoma. Am J Clin Oncol. 2006;29(1):27-31.
35. Alvarez I, Suárez C, Rodrigo JP, et al. Prognostic factors in paranasal sinus cancer. Am J Otolaryngol. 1995;16(2):109-14.
36. Waldron JN, Os B, Warde P, et al. Ethmoid sinus cancer: twenty-nine cases managed with primary radiation therapy. Int J Radiat Oncol Biol Phys. 1998;41(2):361-9.
37. Neal AJ, Habib F, Hope-Stone HF. Carcinoma of the maxillary antrum treated by preoperative radiotherapy or radical radiotherapy alone. J Laryngol Otol. 1992;106(12):1063-6.
38. Mendenhall WM, Amdur RJ, Morris CG, et al. Carcinoma of the nasal cavity and paranasal sinuses. Laryngoscope. 2009;119(5):899-906.
39. Dirix P, Vanstraelen B, Jorissen M, et al. Intensity-modulated radiotherapy for sinonasal cancer: improved outcome compared to conventional radiotherapy. Int J Radiat Oncol Biol Phys. 2010; 78(4):998-1004.
40. Levine PA, Gallagher R, Cantrell RW, et al. Esthesioneuroblastoma :reflections of a 21-year experience. Laryngoscope. 1999;109(10):1539-43.
41. Douglas JG, Koh WJ, Austin-Seymour M, et al. Treatment of salivary gland neoplasms with fast neutron radiotherapy. Arch Otolaryngol Head Neck Surg. 2003;129(9):944-8.
42. Douglas JG, Silbergeld DL, Laramore GL. Gamma knife stereotactic radiosurgical boost for patients treated primarily with neutron radiotherapy for salivary gland neoplasms. Stereotact Funct Neurosrug. 2004;82(2-3):84-9.
43. Papadimitrakopoulou VA, Ginsberg LE, Garden AS, et al. Intra-arterial cisplatin with intravenous paclitaxel and ifosfamide as an organ-preservation

approach in patients with paranasal sinus carcinoma. Cancer. 2003;98(10):2214-23.
44. Rischin D, Porceddu S, Peters L, et al. Promising results with chemoradiation in patients with sinonasal undifferentiated carcinoma. Head Neck. 2004;26(5):435-41.
45. Licitra L, Locati LD, Cavina R, et al. Primary chemotherapy followed by anterior craniofacial resection and radiotherapy for paranasal cancer. Ann Oncol. 2003.14(3):367-372.
46. Cooper JS, Pajak TF, Forastiere AA, et al. Postoperative concurrent radiotherapy and chemotherapy for high-risk squamous-cell carcinoma of the head and neck. N Engl J Med. 2004;350(19):1937-44.
47. Ganly I, Patel SG, Singh B, et al.: Craniofacial resection for malignant paranasal sinus tumors: Report of an International Collaborative Study. Head Neck. 2005;27(7):575-84.
48. Smith RR, Kloop CT, Williams JM. Surgical treatment of cancer of the frontal sinus and adjacent areas. Cancer. 1954;7(5):991-4.
49. Ketcham AS, Wilkins RH, Vanburen JM, et al. A Combined Intracranial Facial Approach to the Paranasal Sinuses. Am J Surg. 1963;106:698-703.
50. Lund VJ, Harrison DF. Craniofacial resection for tumors of the nasal cavity and paranasal sinuses. Am J Surg. 1988;156(3 Pt 1):187-90.
51. Biller H, Lawson W, Sachdev V, et al. Esthesioneuroblastoma: surgical treatment without radiation. Laryngoscope. 1990;100(11):1199-201.
52. Suárez C, Llorente JL, Fernandez De Leon R, et al. Prognostic Factors in Sinonasal Tumors Involving the Anterior Skull Base. Head Neck. 2004;26(2):136-44.
53. Casiano RR, Numa WA, Falquez AM. Endoscopic resection of esthesioneuroblastoma. Am J Rhinol. 2001;15(4)271-9.
54. Eloy JA, Vivero RJ, Hoang K, et al. Comparison of transnasal endoscopic and open craniofacial resection for malignant tumors of the anterior skull base. Laryngoscope. 2009;119(5):834-40.
55. Hanna E, DeMonte F, Ibrahim S, et al. Endoscopic Resection of Sinonasal Cancers With and Without Craniotomy. Oncologic results. Arch Otolaryngol Head Neck Surg. 2009;135(12):1219-24.
56. Batra PS, Luong A, Kanowitz SJ, et al. Outcomes of Minimally Invasive Endoscopic Resection of Anterior Skull Base Neoplasms. Laryngoscope. 2010;120(1):9-16.
57. Ong YK, Solares CA, Carrau RL, et al. New developments in transnasal endoscopic surgery for malignancies of the sinonasal tract and adjacent skull base. Curr Opin Otolaryngol Head Neck Surg. 2010;18(2):107-13.
58. Lund VJ, Stammberger H, Nicolai P, et al. European position paper on endoscopic management of tumours of the nose, paranasal sinuses and skull base. Rhinol Suppl. 2010;1(22):1-143.
59. Jin Y, Mertens F, Arheden K, et al. Karyotypic features of malignant tumors of the nasal cavity and paranasal sinuses. Int J Cancer. 1995;60(5):637-41.
60. van Dijk M, Sprenger S, Rombout P, et al. Distinct chromosomal aberrations in sinonasal mucosal melanoma as detected by comparative genomic hybridization. Genes Chromosomes Cancer. 2003; 36(2):151-8.
61. Gallo O, Franchi A, Fini-Storchi I, et al. Prognostic significance of c-erbB-2 oncoprotein expression in intestinal-type adenocarcinoma of the sinonasal tract. Head Neck. 1998;20(3):224-31.
62. Gotte K, Hormann K. Sinus Malignancy: What's New? Otorhinolaryngol. 2004;66(2):85-97.
63. Airoldi M, Garzaro M, Valente G, et al. Clinical and Biological Prognostic Factors in 179 Cases with Sinonasal Carcinoma Treated in the Italian Piedmont Region. Oncology. 2009;76(4):262-9.
64. Alos L, Moyano S, Nadal A, et al. Human papillomaviruses are identified in a subgroup of sinonasal squamous cell carcinomas with favorable outcome. Cancer. 2009;115(12):2701-9.

7

Perioperative Considerations in the Management of Sinonasal Tumors

Vijay R Ramakrishnan, MD; David W Kennedy, MD

INTRODUCTION

Operative management of sinonasal tumors requires thorough planning and execution. There is no standard "routine," as preoperative planning is directed by tumor histology, disease burden and location, and patient-specific factors. In general, it is better to be overprepared than to be surprised with an issue that could have been avoided or mitigated with proper foresight. Surgical success is related to a number of factors beyond patient disease and surgeon skill. Proper preoperative planning is critical to success but is too often overlooked and frequently bypassed during lectures and presentations on sinonasal tumor management. Surgery for sinonasal tumors can be extremely rewarding when a successful surgical result is obtained with minimal morbidity, but can be frustrating when complete tumor removal is not achieved, or devastating when major complications are encountered. Proper perioperative care will help both patients and surgeons achieve their goals.

PREOPERATIVE PLANNING

Prior to surgery, it is preferable to have a tissue diagnosis. Biopsy may be performed in the clinic or operating room setting, based on degree of tumor vascularity, instrument availability, and physician and patient preference. For malignancies, a metastatic workup is necessary, and should at least consist of physical examination, computed tomography (CT) imaging of the neck, and chest X-ray or CT depending on level of suspicion for pulmonary metastasis. We have found ^{18}FDG-PET scanning to detect metastatic lesions in 22% of our sinonasal malignancy patients, and are now using this modality as part of our preoperative workup (unpublished data).

Bloodwork and Imaging

Preoperative planning for sinonasal tumor surgery should never be considered routine. The magnitude of the surgery planned and patient co-morbidities should guide the extent of the preoperative laboratory workup.[1] Healthy patients undergoing limited elective procedures do not require routine preoperative laboratory evaluation, as abnormal laboratory values in surgical patients without comorbidities do not predict adverse outcomes.[2] In the setting of a large vascular tumor, or if intracranial surgery is entertained, risks of surgery warrant a more thorough preoperative workup. If significant blood loss is expected, complete blood count (CBC), prothrombin time and international normalized ratio (PT/INR), partial thromboplastin time (PTT), and type and screen should be performed. The presence of malignancy may be associated with hematologic disorders such as anemia, thrombocytopenia, or coagulation abnormalities. The best screening test for coagulation abnormalities is a thorough history, and further laboratory workup for coagulopathy can be pursued if needed. Nearly all coagulopathies can be adequately managed if identified preoperatively. Medications known to contribute to surgical hemorrhage, including herbal medications, should be identified and stopped preoperatively. If blood transfusion is anticipated, communication with the blood bank should occur as early as possible in preoperative planning and again on the morning of surgery. For particularly vascular tumors, appropriate blood products should be made available prior to surgery, and patients should be given the option of autologous donation. Liver function tests (LFTs) are indicated in the patient with advanced liver disease, as abnormal values may be associated with perioperative infection, hemorrhage, and poor wound healing. The presence of active pulmonary disease warrants a chest X-ray, and potentially pulmonary function tests and arterial blood gas examination depending on disease severity. Patients with a history of coronary or peripheral artery disease should undergo further workup prior to surgery.

Preoperative imaging should be thoroughly reviewed prior to surgery, and be readily available in the operating room. Image-guided surgical navigation is helpful for all but the simplest tumor cases. CT scans should be performed in a compatible algorithm, and may be merged with magnetic resonance imaging (MRI) for tumors that extend into the soft tissues surrounding the sinuses (Fig. 7.1). CT scans with intravenous contrast may be used to reliably establish the relationship of the carotid artery and cavernous sinus if this is unclear. Multiplanar images are reviewed preoperatively for examination of tumor location and extension, relevant surgical anatomy, and dehiscence of bony boundaries. Thorough preoperative review can identify safe areas for dissection, problem areas, and reliable intraoperative surgical landmarks. The surgeon may anticipate which maneuvers may be necessary for access, and plan for subsequent reconstruction. Intraoperative changes may occur with tumor debulking, especially when surrounding soft tissue prolapses into the surgical field, as is expected to occur with bony dehiscence or erosion of the orbit, skull base, pterygopalatine or infratemporal fossae. Image guidance should never be solely relied upon, especially in this setting. The registration accuracy should be checked repeatedly during the surgery, using fixed intranasal landmarks such as the nasal floor, nasal septum, posterior wall of the maxillary sinus, choanal arch, lamina papyracea, and skull base. Application of intraoperative CT and MRI is currently under study. Real-time image guidance updates appear to be useful to assess extent of tumor resection, especially in benign fibroosseous lesions, or when anatomic changes occur intraoperatively (Figs 7.2A and B).

Surgical Consent

When discussing risks and benefits, it is prudent to consider endoscopic removal of tumors more like classic head and neck tumor surgery, and less like functional endoscopic sinus surgery. In the setting of malignant tumors, and most benign tumors, total tumor removal with negative margins is the ultimate goal. As such, the possible need for an open approach or second stage for complete tumor removal should be discussed, and permission obtained for an open approach whenever a tumor "*might*" have an attachment which could not be drilled away or excised through a transnasal route. The need for an open approach should always be discussed in the event of uncontrollable bleeding or significant intraoperative complication. Permission for blood transfusion is often sought, although it is uncommon for blood transfusions to be required for anything other than large vascular tumors.

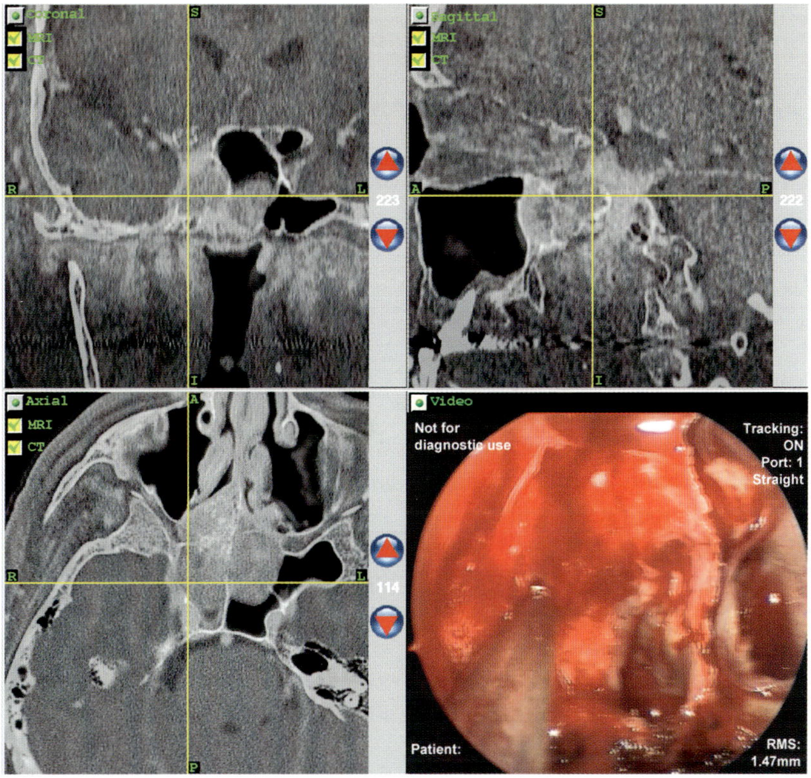

Fig. 7.1: CT-MR fusion for a skull base chondrosarcoma. Bony boundaries, the location of the carotid artery and cavernous sinus and intracranial structures are all visible.

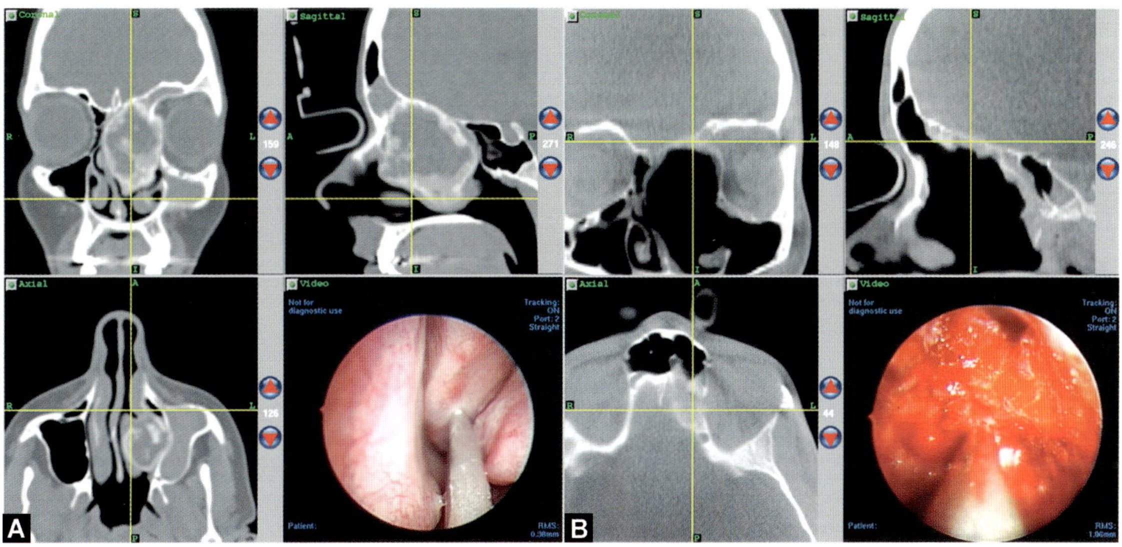

Figs 7.2A and B: (A) Real-time IGS update for fibroosseous lesion. Initial use of IGS based on the preoperative scan; (B) Is later based on an intraoperative scan to assess how much tumor is left on the skull base.

Standard risks of paranasal sinus surgery are discussed, including pain, bleeding, infection, crusting, facial/palatal hypesthesia, epiphora, diplopia, vision loss, cerebrospinal fluid leak, meningitis, anosmia, and need for additional surgery. Other patient specific factors may need to be discussed, such as: dry eye, stroke, carotid injury, blindness, need for radiation, reconstructive graft harvest, lumbar drain placement, use of intrathecal fluorescein, and possible second stage surgery. The availability of other surgical services should be considered prior to undertaking a large tumor surgery, and consent obtained for those concurrent procedures as well. These teams may include neurosurgery, ophthalmology, plastic and reconstructive surgery, and interventional radiology.

Tumor size, need for intraorbital or intracranial dissection, duration of surgery, patient comorbidities, and availability of emergency care may factor into the decision of outpatient versus inpatient surgery. If there is any doubt, the surgeon should err on the conservative side and observe the patient overnight for pain control, oral intake, risk of hemorrhage, and serial neurologic or ophthalmologic examination.

POSTOPERATIVE CONSIDERATIONS

Malignant tumors should be presented in a multidisciplinary tumor board setting to assess the need for adjuvant therapy. If postoperative radiation is a possibility, then certain reconstructive goals must be met if a skull base defect is created. Preoperative planning for reconstruction of the anticipated defect must be performed, as preservation of particular flaps, i.e. nasoseptal flap, may be among the first operative steps, prior to margin assessment and tumor removal. (Skull base reconstruction is described in chapter 9).

OPERATIVE CONSIDERATIONS

Anesthesia

A healthy working relationship with the anesthesia team is mandatory for sinonasal tumor surgery. Surgeons require access to the entire face, and the displacement of the anesthesiologist away from the airway mandates appropriate communication. An operative field free of anesthesia circuitry is necessary, and smooth emergence is ideal upon completion of the surgery. Typical the endotracheal tube is secured at the left oral commissure and taped to the left cheek, with the upper lip free from attachment. If binostril surgery is planned, an oral RAE tube is preferred, and is taped centrally to the lower lip. Oral RAE tube placement is unfavorable for extensive frontal sinus surgery, as the surgeon typically lowers his hands to achieve the necessary angle and will frequently collide with the tube.

The use of total intravenous anesthesia (TIVA) has become popular in functional endoscopic sinus surgery (FESS) due to its intraoperative hemostatic benefits, quicker arousal, and decreased postoperative nausea.[3,4] However, depth of anesthesia may be difficult to gauge if the anesthetist has little experience with this technique. A Bispectral index (BIS) monitor is often not utilized as the image guidance apparatus may obscure placement of the monitor on the forehead. Continuous infusion of a muscle relaxant may be administered if there is concern over patient movement during critical portions of the procedure. Obviously, muscle relaxant is not administered when neuromonitoring is performed. Relative bradycardia has also been shown to improve the surgical field during FESS, and may be employed during tumor cases as well.[5] Premature emergence from anesthesia should be avoided to prevent straining and coughing on the endotracheal tube. Nuisance bleeding from mucosal edges may occur, but the real worry is for intraorbital or intracranial bleeding if these areas were accessed intraoperatively. Patients undergoing lengthy procedures, often combined with neurosurgical dissection, may remain electively intubated overnight.

Appropriate fluid management is assessed with an optimal urine output of 0.5–1.0 ml/kg/hr. Vigorous administration of IV fluids may be unfavorable. Endoscopic sinus surgery does not expose body cavities to the environment, and thus insensible losses are not on the same level as open surgical cases. Excessive fluid or vasopressor administration should be avoided if a potentially tenuous reconstruction is performed, as flap edema or ischemia may compromise the repair.

Careful continuous estimation of blood loss is a team effort. Irrigation fluid should be recorded, as blood loss is calculated from the total of multiple suction canisters which include blood, manual irrigant, and irrigant from the debrider and drill. If significant blood loss is encountered, the surgeon must communicate with the anesthesiologist to make sure appropriate IV lines are in place, fluid is being administered, and hemoglobin levels are being checked. Volume loss causing decreased cardiac preload is initially treated with administration of isotonic fluid, either lactated Ringer's solution or normal saline. In the setting of decreased hemoglobin concentration, administration of packed red blood cells (pRBCs) should be considered. Transfusion will improve preload, oxygen carrying capacity and oxygen transport. In the setting of severe hemorrhage, replacement of more than one blood volume can result in a dilutional coagulopathy, necessitating the administration of platelets and fresh frozen plasma (FFP) for restoration of surgical hemostasis.

If a laser is used, appropriate laser safety precautions must be followed. A warning sign should be posted outside the room that a laser is in use, the patient's eyes and facial skin should be protected with wet gauze, operating room personnel should wear appropriate goggles, and the laser should be kept in standby mode when not in active use. The anesthesia team should be made aware that a laser will be used during the case, so that FiO2 may be lowered to the minimum level necessary, nitrous oxide will be avoided, water soluble ointments will be used rather than petroleum-based ointments, and a laser safe tube can be used, even though the laser is not likely to be directly aimed at the tube. Both the surgeon and anesthesiologist should understand the algorithm for management of an airway fire if a laser is to be used.

Use of intravenous antibiotics is not indicated for sinus surgery based on the literature, but nonetheless many surgeons practice this routine.[6] However, in head and neck tumor cases in clean-contaminated regions, antibiotic prophylaxis is recommended.[7] Our practice is to administer prophylactic intravenous antibiotics for all tumor cases. Preoperative administration of antibiotics is modified if intracranial penetration is expected. Unasyn 3gm IV every 6 hours is given for sinus and orbital prophylaxis and a combination of Ceftriaxone 1gm IV every 12 hours, Vancomycin 1gm IV every 12 hours, and Flagyl 500 mg IV every 6 hours, is given for intracranial prophylaxis.

Lumbar Drain and Intrathecal Fluorescein

If intracranial dissection is planned, preoperative placement of a lumbar drain is considered. Cerebrospinal fluid (CSF) leaks in these patients are associated with tumor-related skull base erosion and/or creation of a skull base defect during resection. CSF decompression for a few days after surgery may allow the reconstruction time to adhere, and is one advantage of a lumbar drain. However, these patients typically do not have intracranial hypertension, and postoperative drainage may not be necessary. If symptoms of a CSF leak occur within the days after surgery, a lumbar drain could then be placed, and low-level drainage (5–10 ml/hr) for a few days may provide the opportunity for the defect to seal. The use of intrathecal fluorescein in tumor surgery may be helpful to identify suspected leaks, or, in the setting of a large defect, reassure the surgeon that a water-tight seal has been created. The use of intrathecal fluorescein is not Food and Drug Administration (FDA) approved, and as such, the surgeon ought to have sufficient reasoning for its use. Careful consent and discussion of risks of paresthesias and seizures must be disclosed to the patient preoperatively. These risks appear to be dose dependent. No serious adverse effects have been encountered in over twenty years of use at low concentrations and slow administration. The surgeon should withdraw 0.05–0.1 ml of 10%

aqueous, sterile, preservative-free fluorescein in a tuberculin syringe, mix it in 10 ml of CSF or sterile saline, and administer slowly over 15 minutes. This may be followed with another 10 ml of CSF or sterile saline to clear the fluorescein remaining in the tubing. Fluorescein is metabolized by the kidneys, and it has been suggested that it should not be used in patients with renal insufficiency, or should be used in smaller doses. Intraoperative use of a blue light filter will facilitate visualization at lower concentrations (Figs 7.3A and B). Lumbar drains are associated with significant side effects, including headache, back pain, infection, and retained catheter fragments, and potential for rare catastrophic events such as over drainage leading to pneumocephalus and herniation. The incidence of lumbar drain complications in endoscopic skull base surgery was found to be over 13% in one study.[8] Therefore, routine use is not recommended for tumor surgery, but its use in selected cases may prove beneficial.

Positioning and Preparation

The operating room must be sufficiently large to accommodate the surgical team and the extensive equipment necessary, including monitors, image guidance system, surgical drill, monopolar and bipolar cautery, and possibly neuromonitoring. The operating table should be reversed such that the patient's head is located at the foot of the bed. This allows more room underneath the bed for the surgeon and a number of foot pedals, and allows the surgeon to sit, if preferred. In general, room setup is similar to routine endoscopic sinus surgery (Fig. 7.4). The surgeon sits or stands along the patient's right side, with a monitor across the bed at an ergonomic height (slightly lower than eye level). The image guidance apparatus is placed at the head of the bed. Two-team approaches may require placement of the second surgeon to the left of the primary surgeon near the head of the bed, or across the bed operating through the left nostril. In two-surgeon approaches, a shared monitor may be placed at the head of the bed, or a second monitor may be used, if available (Fig. 7.5).

Patient positioning is similar to that used for routine sinus surgery. The head of the bed is elevated 20–30 degrees to aid in hemostasis. Laser Doppler study has shown this position to decrease blood flow measured at the inferior turbinate by

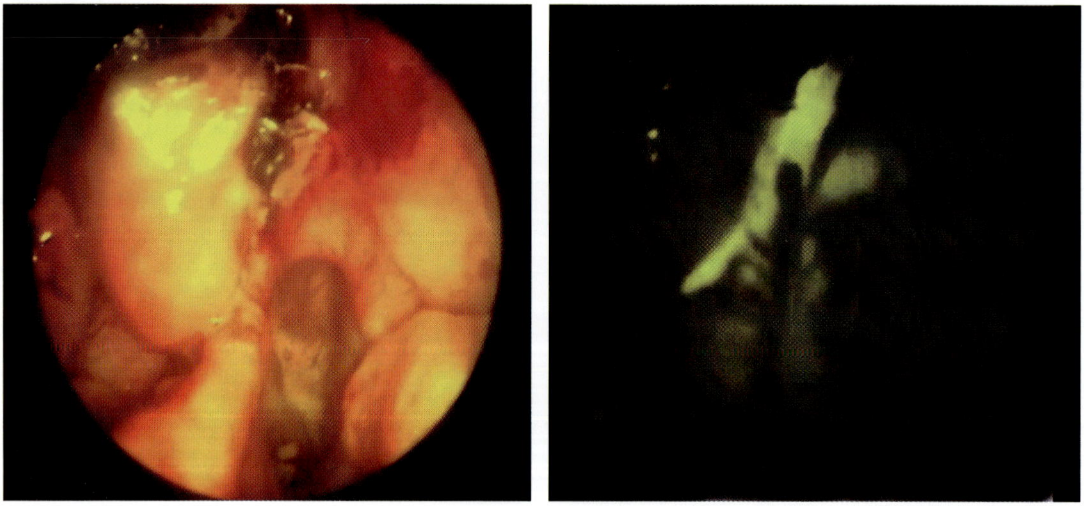

Figs 7.3A and B: Bluelight filter use in repair of a delayed postoperative CSF leak after skull base surgery. (A) Left Fluorescein is not seen endoscopically; (B) Right with the addition of the bluelight filter it is clearly seen.

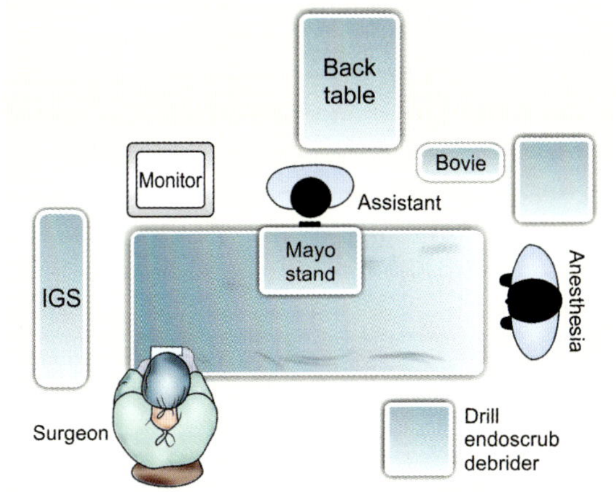

Fig. 7.4: Room setup for endoscopic tumor surgery.

38%.[9] Multiple studies have shown decreased central venous pressure at 5–25 degrees of reverse Trendelenberg position.[10,11] Sequential compression devices are placed on the lower extremities for prevention of deep vein thrombosis. Multiple intravenous lines are placed; larger-bore intravenous lines and an arterial line are placed if significant blood loss or intracranial dissection is expected. Rapid administration of fluid and blood is then possible, as is accurate continuous assessment of

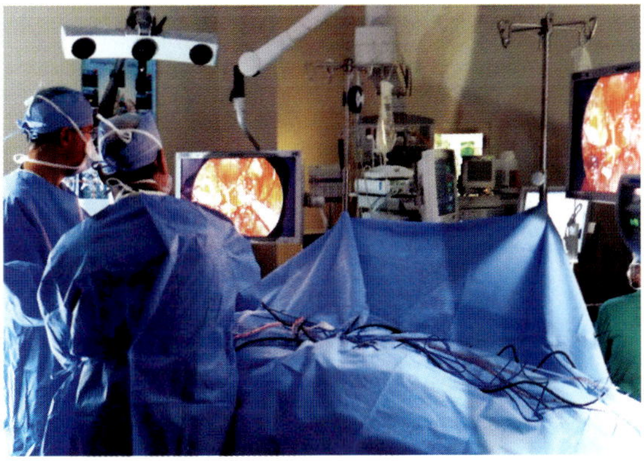

Fig. 7.5: Two-surgeon, three- or four-handed, binostril approaches may be necessary. Here, two surgeons perform a three-handed approach, sharing the same side of the bed and the same monitor. Alternatively, the surgeons may stand on opposite sides and view a common monitor at the head of the bed, or personal monitors.

blood pressure, and availability of blood samples for hemoglobin measurement. A Foley catheter is placed if duration of surgery is expected to exceed four hours. Lines, catheters, and cords are brought off the bed at the patient's feet. Attention must be paid to body positioning and padding of pressure points, especially if a long duration of anesthesia is anticipated.

When combined neurosurgical dissection is planned, a pinion headholder (e.g. Mayfield design) may be preferred by the neurosurgical team. We have found this to be unnecessary in the vast majority of sinonasal tumor cases, as communication with an attentive anesthesiologist will prevent any possible patient motion during surgical dissection. We do not routinely employ intraoperative neuromonitoring, although this has been used by some groups when extensive orbital or skull base dissection is planned. This requires coordination with an experienced neuromonitoring team and adequate space in the operating room for required equipment.

After positioning the patient as previously described, the face may be prepared with dilute betadine solution or baby shampoo. This is performed if dural entry is expected, but not necessary for routine tumor surgery. As there is no manner of complete sterilization of the nasal cavity and sinuses, the facial preparation is used to decrease bacterial load and prevent introduction of skin flora into the wound bed as instruments, cottonoids, or reconstructive grafts are inserted into the nose. Lubrication of the eyes and lateral taping is preferred, such that palpation of the globe and pupil examination may be easily performed during surgery. Placement of the image guidance apparatus over the forehead precludes the use of a BIS monitor, unless this can be fashioned around the headband.

Instruments

Proper instrumentation is crucial to successful tumor surgery. Different instruments are needed for exposure, tumor debulking, fine dissection, hemostasis, management of complications, and conversion to open surgery if necessary. Visualization for endoscopic tumor surgery requires both zero degree and angled telescopes. Thirty and forty-five degree telescopes are sufficient for most cases. Seventy-degree telescopes are helpful for far-reaching lesions of the frontal sinus, and extreme anterior or lateral visualization within the maxillary or lateral recess of sphenoid sinuses. Exposure to these areas can always be broadened such that less angles telescopes are sufficient. Maxillary sinuscopy or frontal mini-trephination instruments alternatively provide visualization in these difficult areas. Most of the dissection can be performed with instruments from routine sinus surgery sets. Curved turbinate scissors are helpful when turbinectomy is needed, although this can be performed with a number of other instruments. Kerrison Rongeurs and drills are used for bone removal. Drill bit attachment to the microdebrider platform simplifies equipment setup and provides constant suction and irrigation. More extensive bone removal can be rapidly achieved with the use of high-speed drills. Angled burs and those with longer shafts should be made available based on tumor location.

Tumor dissection generally begins will central debulking of the tumor. Except with vascular tumors, this is most frequently performed with a microdebrider. The continuous suction offered by this instrument allows for rapid debulking with continuous visualization. A number of surgeons have described the utility of coblation for tumor surgery. This has been shown to decrease blood loss in tumor surgery and provides good visualization after tumor debulking.[12] However, it does not allow for collection of tissue for complete pathologic analysis. Suction elevators can be used to dissect tumor planes, such as would occur between the tumor and the periorbita. Fine dissection after tumor debulking may be performed with instruments common to most endoscopic sinus sets or otologic sets. It is helpful to have sharp sickle knives or beaver blades to make margin incisions. Fine through cutting instruments and suctions of various diameters and lengths facilitate two-handed dissection along critical structures. Neurosurgical instruments with longer shafts may be necessary for sphenoid and skull base tumors.

Adequate hemostasis is frequently cited as a limiting factor for successful endoscopic tumor surgery. Appropriate planning and availability of supplies is critical to achievement of hemostasis. Suction monopolar electrocautery and bipolar forceps are always present on the surgical field. A number of endoscopic bipolars exist, and may be selected based on surgeon preference or tumor location. An endoscopic clip applier is helpful for ligation of the ethmoid arteries or branches of the internal maxillary artery. Bleeding directly from tumor or surrounding mucosa is managed with application of topical epinephrine or thrombin soaked pledgets. Cottonoids of various sizes (1 × 3 cm, 0.5 × 3 cm, 0.5 × 0.5 cm) should be available. Gelfoam may be applied as a sponge or a paste by mixing its powder formulation with thrombin. Gelatin-thrombin mixtures have been similarly been used, and are easily applied through an angiocatheter. Microfibrillar collagen can be topically applied as a "sandwich" within a cottonoid, or as a slurry by angiocatheter (Fig. 7.6). Bone marrow bleeding or small vessels within bone may be controlled with electrocautery, use of a diamond drill,

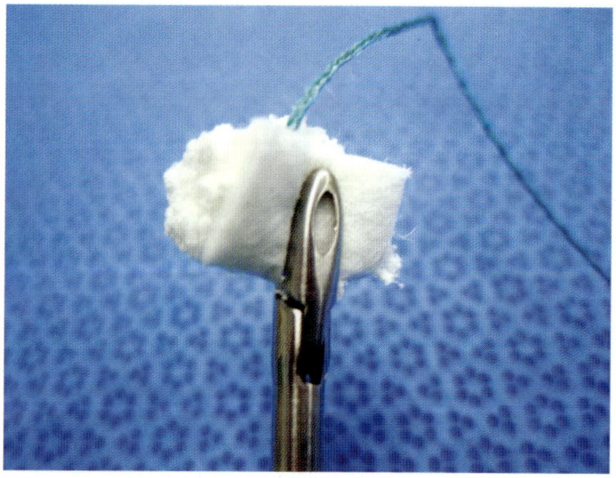

Fig. 7.6: Microfibrillar collagen can be focally applied as a "sandwich" within a pledget.

or application of bone wax. Placement of surgical over raw surfaces upon completion of the case may also be considered.

Efficient diagnosis and management of complications relies on preparation and availability of supplies. A tonopen should be available, and the surgeon should know how to use it, as measurement of intraocular pressure may affect management of orbital complications. Lateral canthotomy and inferior cantholysis can easily be performed with available instruments. CSF leaks can be sealed in a number of ways according to surgeon preference. The equipment used for CSF leak repair should be readily available, such as dural substitute, fibrin glue, and gelfoam. If autologous fat or fascia is the preferred method of closure, this should be discussed with the patient preoperatively, and the surgical site should be prepared prior to draping. Instrument sets should be available for the conversion to open surgery, either in the setting of complication, for completeness of tumor resection, or reconstruction with grafting from a second surgical site.

Hemostasis and Estimating Blood Loss

Optimal hemostasis begins with anesthetic technique and patient preparation. Total intravenous anesthesia (TIVA) has been shown to improve the surgical field in FESS cases, and similar mechanisms can be expected to carry over for endoscopic tumor removal. Anesthetic principles to be considered are attention to initial catecholamine surges associated with intubation, and avoidance of volatile inhaled anesthetics, which are known to cause peripheral vasodilation and platelet dysfunction. Heart rate and mean arterial pressure should be kept within optimal ranges.

If sinus obstruction and associated infection or inflammation is present, a preoperative course of steroids and antibiotics may aid intraoperative hemostasis. Patient preparation begins with the administration of topical decongestants. Placement of intranasal cottonoids should be done with care, as tumor bleeding can easily occur. Transoral sphenopalatine injections are placed through the greater palatine foramina for added vasoconstriction. Transnasal infiltration of mucosa around the tumor with local anesthetic and epinephrine may also be attempted. Warm saline irrigation has been found to help facilitate vasoconstriction and clotting, and also serves to keep the tip of the endoscope clean if an Endoscrub apparatus is not used during surgery.[13] When used, irrigation is most easily administered by an assistant or second surgeon.

Early ligation of arterial supply is recommended for vascular tumors. Arterial contribution is determined by the type of tumor, its location, and its size. The internal maxillary and anterior ethmoid arteries are generally the main contributors. Larger tumors along the skull base may obtain further supply from the internal carotid artery, posterior ethmoid artery, or direct pial collaterals. If possible, endoscopic ligation of the sphenopalatine branches or internal maxillary artery may be performed. However, approaches to these areas may be limited by obstructing tumor presence. Preoperative embolization is employed for juvenile nasopharyngeal angiofibromas (JNA), unless they are radiographically limited to the nasal cavity and nasopharynx. In these smaller JNAs, the surgeon and patient must weigh the risks and benefits for embolization. Endoscopic endonasal ligation of the anterior ethmoid artery has been studied in cadavers, and is only feasible in approximately 20% of cadaver specimens.[14,15] The endoscopic approach to ethmoid artery ligation is even more clinically limited with tumor presence obstructing access. Alternatively, the ethmoid arteries may be approached from ligation through the Lynch transcutaneous incision or the medial transconjunctival approach.[16]

Once tumor bleeding has begun, direct monopolar cautery with a suction bovie may be focally applied. Suction bipolar cautery may be similarly used. Near the skull base, orbit, or neural structures, focused bipolar application is recommended over monopolar cautery. Transmission of monopolar cautery has been known to cause dural disruption and associated CSF leak, vision loss, diplopia, eye pain, and cranial nerve dysfunction. In these areas, avoidance of cautery altogether may be possible with the topical application of oxymetazoline or epinephrine, thrombin, gelfoam, gelatin-thrombin mixtures such as Floseal (Baxter Intl, Deerfield IL) and Surgiflo (Ethicon Inc, Somerville NJ), or microfibrillar collagen (Avitene, Davol, Warwick RI). Oxymetazoline, 1:1000 epinephrine, and thrombin are applied focally with pledgets, and excess liquid should be squeezed from the pledget prior to placement. Topical epinephrine is preferred given its function at both alpha-1 and alpha-2 receptors, and better safety profile when compared to topical preparations of cocaine. Use of topical epinephrine is avoided, if there is any intracranial exposure. In children, the elderly, or patients with a cardiac history, topical epinephrine should be avoided or used at a lesser concentration. Gelfoam sponge squares soaked in thrombin can be placed, or powder gelfoam can be reconstituted in thrombin and applied. Direct application of gelatin-thrombin mixtures or microfibrillar collagen in a cottonoid sandwich or slurry form serves a similar purpose. It is important to realize that instant hemostasis is rarely achieved with topical medications, but usually these mechanisms are successful with gentle pressure and patience.

Again, accurate estimation of blood loss requires constant attention from the surgeon, scrub nurse, circulating nurse, and anesthetist. Multiple suction canisters and cottonoids should be examined to accurately estimate blood loss throughout the case. Administration of blood products is generally based upon overall health status, hemoglobin measurements, and cardiovascular parameters. However, the surgeon should have a preoperative estimation of acceptable blood loss. If that level is reached, the procedure may then be aborted, staged, or continued with the administration of blood products. This calculation is based on body weight, preoperative hemoglobin level, and patient comorbidities. Preoperatively, the surgeon should recognize the lowest tolerable hemoglobin concentration for that patient, 7–10 g/dL in most patients. Total estimated blood volume (EBV) is calculated as ideal body weight (kg) x average blood volume. Average blood volume in adult women is 65 ml/kg and men 75 ml/kg. Allowable blood loss can then be determined as [EBV x (initial hematocrit—final hematocrit)] / initial hematocrit.

Surgical Techniques

If pedicled flaps are to be used for reconstruction, these are dissected first, and placed into the nasopharynx or maxillary sinus and covered by a cottonoid. If the flap borders are near the tumor margin, it is prudent to send a frozen section of the margin to ensure that residual tumor is not present in the flap. Accessible tumor margins should be sent early in the case to allow the pathologist adequate time for analysis, and allow the surgeon the opportunity to send revised margins without slowing down the remainder of the dissection (Fig. 7.7).

The keys to tumor surgery are the optimization of exposure and visualization. A number of surgical

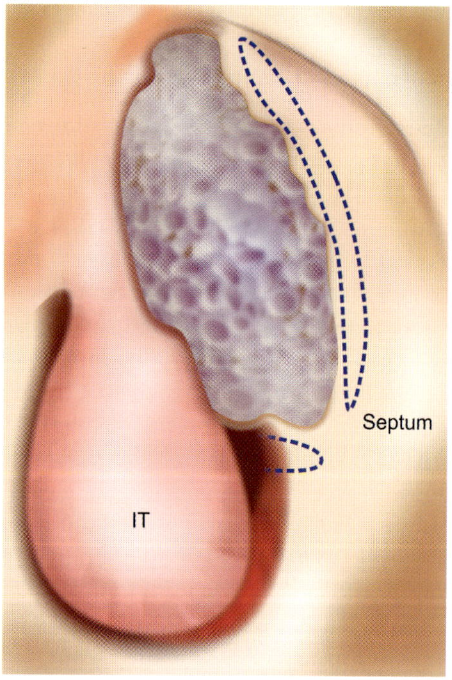

Fig. 7.7: A sharp sickle knife or beaver blade is used to take margins around the tumor.

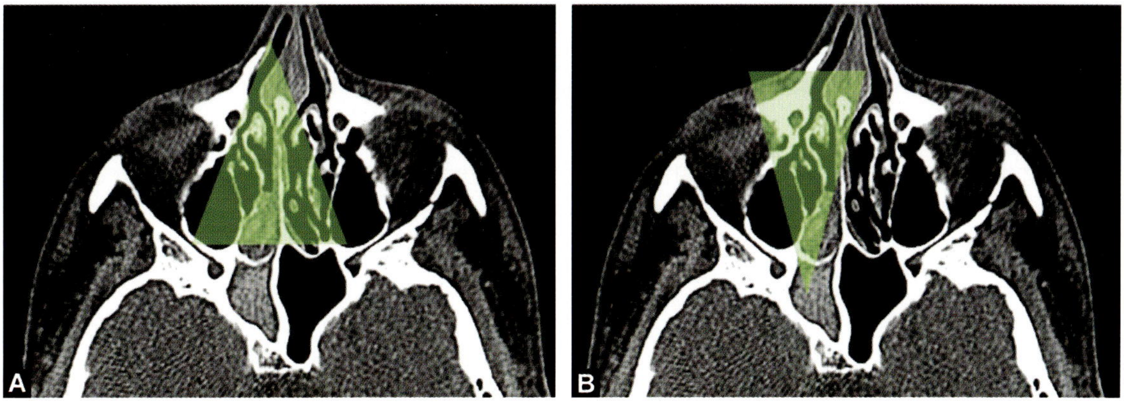

Figs 7.8A and B: (A) The endoscopic approach to skull base tumors affords a progressively wide view during deeper dissection (left), whereas; (B) A traditional open approach provides a progressively limited view (right).

approaches and intraoperative maneuvers are available to maximize exposure through a single- or binostril approach (Figs 7.8A and B). The surgeon should be comfortable with these maneuvers, and understand that the emphasis on tissue preservation in FESS for chronic rhinosinusitis is less applicable in tumor surgery. Mucosal and turbinate preservation may help facilitate recovery, but this principle should not compromise exposure. Commonly used maneuvers include: wide maxillary antrostomy or sphenoidotomy, middle or inferior turbinectomy, medial maxillectomy, posterior septectomy, Draf III approach, and septal dislocation. These maneuvers are discussed in detail in Chapter 5: Endoscopic Surgical Approaches. Optimal visualization and instrumentation is contingent upon this wide exposure. Use of the least angled endoscope allows the surgeon a wider array of instruments, including those used for fine sharp dissection. As more angled endoscopy is required, not only is the visualization more distorted, but the instruments available to the surgeon become progressively limited with regards to length, angle, size, and strength.

When approaching the tumor, establishing the location of origin is imperative. Careful blunt dissection around the visible tumor may identify tissue planes that delineate the tumor from surrounding normal structures (Fig. 7.9). This is followed by central debulking of the tumor, with displacement of the peripheral tumor into the central cavity, providing the opportunity for sharp dissection around the tumor and identification of margins (Fig. 7.10). All removed tumor should be sent for pathologic analysis. It must be remembered that if a microdebrider is used for the majority of the tumor resection, a filter or "sock" should be applied to the suction so that debrided tissue is given to the pathologist. Once the majority of the tumor has been debulked, dissection around the base of the tumor will identify its origin. In this step, it should be remembered never to "pull" at tissue that may

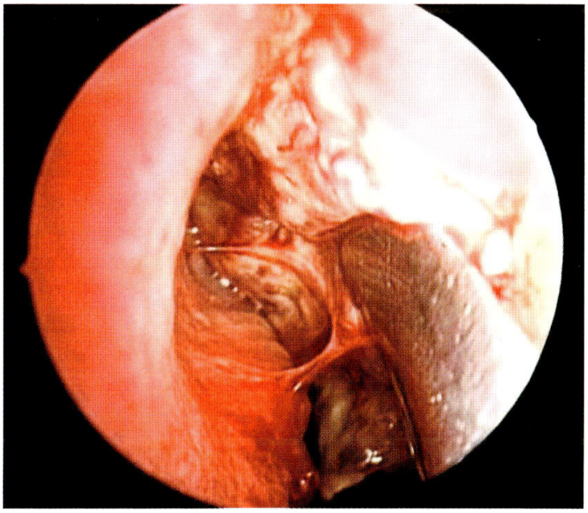

Fig. 7.9: A Freer elevator is used to delineate the tumor border along the neighboring septal mucosa, which appears uninvolved.

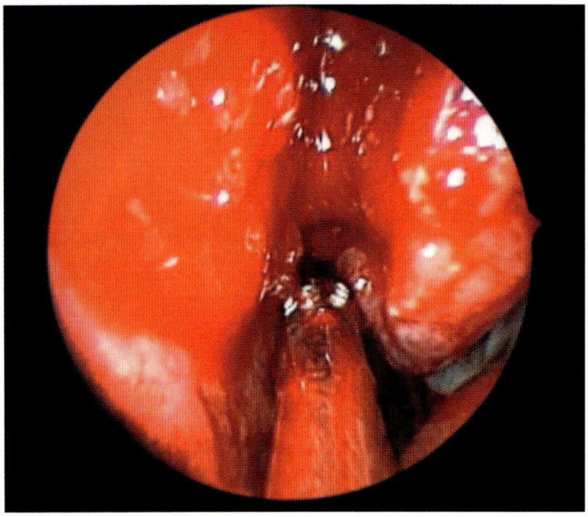

Fig. 7.10: The tumor is centrally debulked with a microdebrider to provide room for further dissection.

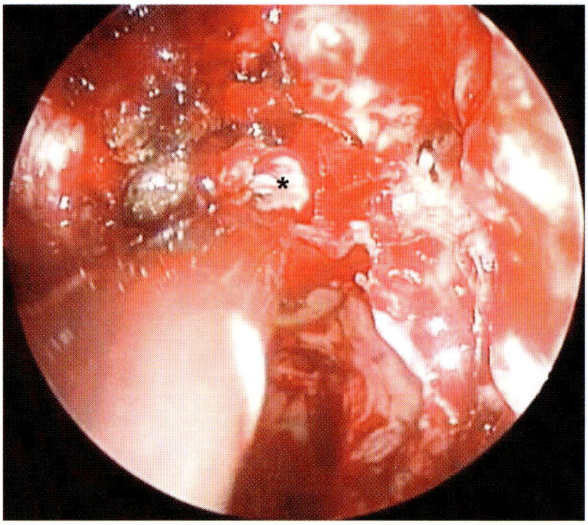

Fig. 7.11: After removal of the tumor, the skull base and dura (*) are encountered. The surgeon must decide whether to stop at this point, drill down the skull base further, or take a dural biopsy for a deep margin.

have connections intraorbitally, intracranially, or to major neurovascular structures. It is at this stage that sufficient working room for multiple instruments is finally available, and sharp dissection is always preferred.

Once the tumor is grossly removed, ideally the origin of the tumor will have been well defined. Frozen section margins should be taken from the lateral and deep aspects, if possible. Although tumor cells may gain access to bone by direct invasion or along neural pathways, bone destruction is thought to occur by host osteoclasts stimulated by local tumor-derived mediators.[17] In the setting of moth-eaten bone neighboring tumor, this is ideally removed for pathologic analysis. If that is not possible, or risks injury to critical structures, the irregular bone should be drilled down as much as possible. It is the final step of obtaining deep margins that ultimately determines if total resection with negative margins has been obtained (Fig. 7.11).

The final cavity should be fashioned such that endoscopic visualization in the postoperative clinic setting allows for adequate surveillance. Often, surveillance imaging may not sufficiently distinguish scarring from tumor regrowth, and endoscopic examination is relied upon. Additionally, debridement of crusting can be performed and patient irrigation will have sufficient penetration.

Frozen Section Margins

The surgeon should plan to send labeled specimens for margin analysis early in the surgery. Direct communication with an experienced head and neck pathologist is stressed. Serial margin specimens may be necessary for adequate tumor clearance, and waiting until the end of tumor resection to send these specimens wastes time waiting for results prior to moving on to the reconstruction. Large studies in head and neck tumor patients have shown a 96% reliability of frozen section diagnosis when compared to final pathologic diagnosis. This was found to be more reliable in the nose and sinuses than the nasopharynx.[18] However, if the pathology of a tumor is unknown, it is most often prudent to wait for a final diagnosis rather than proceeding with an extensive surgery based on a frozen section diagnosis. Errors in pathologic diagnosis are most commonly attributed to misinterpretation of the specimen, inadequate sampling, technical problems, or poor communication between the surgeon and the pathologist.[19]

Some areas of tumors may not have a true margin for assessment, such as the inferomedial border of an ethmoid sinus tumor. The pathologist and tumor board must be made aware that this does not represent a positive margin or unassessed margin. In other cases, it may not be possible to obtain a true margin, such as in the case of an ethmoid tumor in which lamina papyracea is absent but the periorbita is completely intact. In other areas, such as the sphenoid sinus, the surgeon may not be able to take a margin biopsy without serious vascular or neurologic risk.

Although frozen section analysis is reliable for many tumors, there may be an instance where the final diagnosis shows a positive margin despite negative frozen sections margins obtained intraoperatively. In this difficult scenario, the patient, surgeon, and tumor board must decide if it is warranted to go back and re-resect that margin, or proceed with observation or adjuvant therapy.

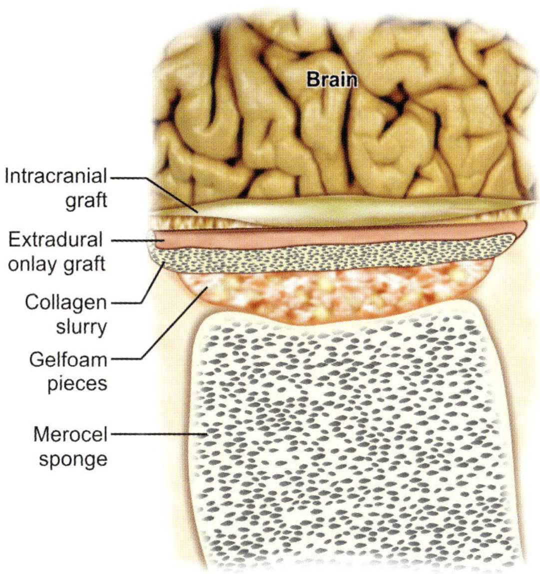

Fig. 7.12: Coronal diagram showing the layers of reconstruction of a skull base defect.

Nasal Packing

In tumor surgery, benefits of nasal dressings and packing generally outweigh the associated side effects. Patient discomfort and adhesion formation are two common reasons for avoiding packing and dressing in routine sinus surgery. However, in tumor surgery, packing presence and removal may be less painful than having the tumor itself. Merocel or finger-glove packs are cut to size and placed underneath a "breakaway layer" of gelfoam pieces or microfibrillar collagen slurry, so that removal does not alter the underlying repair (Fig. 7.12). If used, packs should be placed under endoscopic visualization to ensure proper placement. Adhesion formation is of lesser concern in these patients, as they rarely have associated chronic sinusitis, and scarring may actually be beneficial in the area of reconstruction or repair. Dressings and packing may provide a hemostatic benefit, and may be placed electively depending on vascularity of the tumor or blood loss incurred during the case. Placement of hemostatic material, such as microfibrillar collagen slurry, gelatin-thrombin mixtures, chitosan gel, hyaluronic acid formulations, or fibrin glues, along the wound bed is more frequently used in tumor surgery than FESS, as granulation and adhesion formation is less concerning in these patients. Once packing is removed, debridement is simplified, as large obstructing crusts do not fill the nasal cavity. Nasal crusting appears to be the major nasal morbidity of these approaches, and tends to resolve in 3–6 months in most cases.[20,21] Removal of these obstructing crusts early in the postoperative phase is less than ideal, as their manipulation can be painful and may disrupt the reconstruction. Depending on location, packing or dressings may facilitate keeping the sinuses open. For instance, the posterior aspect of a pack may be placed in the sphenoid sinus, preventing scar closure in an area where postoperative debridement may be contraindicated (Fig. 7.13).

POSTOPERATIVE FOLLOW-UP

Once discharged from the hospital, patients are restricted to limited activity, avoid straining and nose blowing, and begin saline sprays or gentle

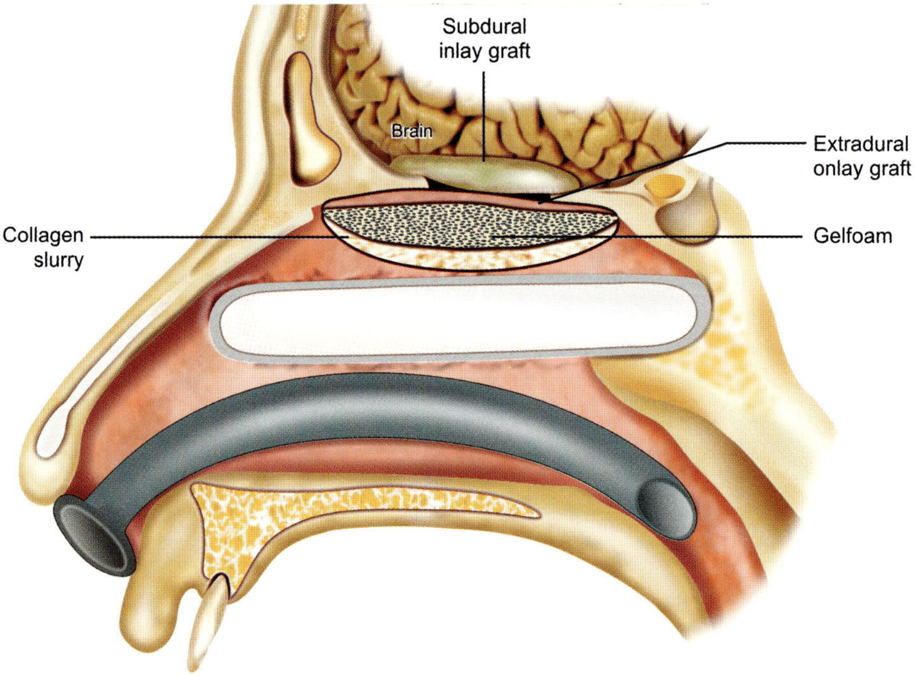

Fig. 7.13: Sagittal diagram demonstrating the placement of a finger-glove merocel pack where the posterior aspect is placed within the sphenoid. A nasopharyngeal trumpet may be placed beneath the pack for extra support and proper direction of airflow, potentially decreasing the risk of progressive pneumocephalus after skull base reconstruction.

saline rinses. Patients are given narcotic pain medications, and asked to take stool softeners, with the plan of weaning to acetaminophen as soon as tolerated. Antibiotics are prescribed for two weeks after surgery, either amoxicillin/clavulanate or the combination of clindamycin and bactrim. While on antibiotics, patients are instructed to take over-the-counter probiotics.

Anything more than minor nuisance bleeding should be brought to the surgeon's attention, and should be appropriately evaluated. Fortunately, proper surgical technique and hemostasis at the conclusion of the case makes postoperative bleeding a rare occurrence. Patients are made aware of the symptoms and signs of potential complications, such as clear nasal drainage, worsening headache, nausea, vomiting, neck stiffness, photophobia, and altered mental status. Orbital complications may be recognized early by the patient as eye pain, ecchymosis, loss of color vision, or decreased visual acuity. The surgical team must be available for prompt evaluation and management of suspected complications, as these can occur at anytime in the postoperative period and necessitate immediate attention.

The first postoperative visit generally occurs one to two weeks postoperatively, at which time packing may be removed and limited debridement is performed. Subsequent follow-up is dictated by the disease process and extent of resection and reconstruction. Plans for overall management, including adjuvant therapy and tumor surveillance, are addressed in subsequent chapters.

CONCLUSION

The perioperative management of patients undergoing sinonasal tumor surgery is critical to the short and long-term success of our procedures. Proper preoperative work-up, "tips and pearls" to limit intraoperative bleeding, and proper technique in obtaining tumor margins are just some of the examples of important things to consider in the perioperative period.

REFERENCES

1. Schein OD, Katz J, Bass EB, et al. The value of routine preoperative medical testing before cataract surgery. N Engl J Med. 2000;342:168-75.
2. Dzankic S, Pastor D, Gonzalez C, et al. The prevalence and predictive value of abnormal preoperative laboratory tests in elderly surgical patients. Anesth Analg. 2001;93(2):301-8.
3. Ahn HJ, Chung SK, Dhong HJ, et al. Comparison of surgical conditions during propofol or sevoflurane anaesthesia for endoscopic sinus surgery. Br J Anaesth. 2008;100(1):50-4.
4. Wormald PJ, van Renen G, Perks J, et al. The effect of the total intravenous anesthesia compared with inhalational anesthesia on the surgical field during endoscopic sinus surgery. Am J Rhinol. 2005;19(5):514-20.
5. Nair S, Collins M, Hung P, et al. The effect of beta-blocker premedication on the surgical field during endoscopic sinus surgery. Laryngoscope. 2004;114(6):1042-6.
6. Chandra RK, Conley DB, Kern RC. Prophylactic i.v. antibiotics in functional endoscopic sinus surgery: trends and attitudes of the American Rhinologic Society membership. Am J Rhinol Allergy. 2009;23(4):448-50.
7. Simo R, French G. The use of prophylactic antibiotics in head and neck oncological surgery. Curr Opin Otolaryngol Head Neck Surg. 2006;14(2):55-61.
8. Ransom ER, Palmer JN, Kennedy DW, et al. Assessing risk/benefit of lumbar drains in endoscopic skull base surgery. Presented at the American Rhinologic Society Meeting. Las Vegas, NV, 2010.
9. Gurr P, Callanan V, Baldwin D. Laser-Doppler blood flowmetry measurement of nasal mucosa blood flow after injection of the greater palatine canal. J Laryngol Otol. 1996;110(2):124-8.
10. Soonawalla ZF, Stratopoulos C, Stoneham M, et al. Role of the reverse- Trendelenberg patient position in maintaining low-CVP anaesthesia during liver resections. Langenbecks Arch Surg. 2008;393(2):195-8.
11. Iwabuchi T, Sobata E, Suzuki M, et al. Dural sinus pressure as related to neurosurgical positions. Neurosurgery. 1983;12(2):203-7.
12. Kostrzewa JP, Sunde J, Riley KO, et al. Radiofrequency coblation decreases blood loss during endoscopic sinonasal and skull base tumor removal. ORL J Otorhinolaryngol Relat Spec. 2010; 72(1):38-43.
13. Kassam A, Snyderman CH, Carrau RL, et al. Endoneurosurgical hemostasis techniques: lessons learned from 400 cases. Neurosurg Focus. 2005;19(1):E7.
14. Floreani SR, Nair SB, Switajewski MC, et al. Endoscopic anterior ethmoidal artery ligation: a cadaver study. Laryngoscope. 2006;116(7):1263-7.
15. Solares CA, Luong A, Batra PS. Technical feasibility of transnasal endoscopic anterior ethmoid artery ligation: assessment with intraoperative CT imaging. Am J Rhinol Allergy. 2009;23(6):619-21.
16. Ramakrishnan VR, Suh JD, Chiu AG, et al. Addition of a Minimally Invasive Medial Orbital Approach in the Endoscopic Management of Advanced Sino-orbital Disease: Cadaver Study with Clinical Correlations. Laryngoscope. In press.
17. Carter RL, Tanner NSB, Clifford P, et al. Direct bone invasion in squamous tumors of the head and neck: pathological and clinical implications. Clin Otolaryngol. 1980;5(2):107-16.
18. Remsen KA, Lucente FE, Biller HF. Reliability of frozen section diagnosis in head and neck neoplasms. Laryngoscope. 1984;94(4):519-24.
19. Saltzstein SL, Nahum AM. Frozen section diagnosis: accuracy and errors; uses and abuses. Laryngoscope. 1973;83(7):1128-43.
20. Pant H, Bhatki AM, Snyderman CH, et al. Quality of life following endonasal skull base surgery. Skull Base. 2010;20(1):35-40.
21. de Almeida JR, Snyderman CH, Gardner PA, et al. Nasal morbidity following endoscopic skull base surgery: a prospective cohort study. Head Neck. 2011;33(4):547-51.

8

Skull Base Reconstruction: Open

Darshni Vira, MD; Jeffrey D Suh, MD; Keith E Blackwell, MD

INTRODUCTION

The proven reliability of microvascular free flaps and increasing experience with endoscopic repair of skull base defects have lead to significant advances in skull base surgery. Skull base surgeons now routinely treat a wide variety of both benign and malignant tumors of the nasal cavity, paranasal sinuses, and nasopharynx using open and, more recently, endoscopic techniques with excellent results. As the approaches to these tumors have evolved, similarly have the approaches for reconstruction. The development of reliable reconstructive methods has greatly facilitated the ability to remove tumors that were previously considered unresectable or unrepairable.

The goal of anterior skull base reconstruction is to separate the cranial cavity from the sinonasal cavity with a watertight seal, to provide a lining for the nasal cavity, to remove dead space, and to restore a three-dimensional facial contour. Choosing the manner in which to reconstruct is largely based on the size, location of the defect, and surgeon experience. However, additional factors must also be considered when choosing a reconstruction method, including prior radiation treatment, planned postoperative radiation treatment, prior surgery in the donor site, and medical comorbidities. In this chapter, we will focus on the different open techniques for skull base reconstruction.

RELEVANT ANATOMY OF THE SKULL BASE

The skull base separates the brain from the remaining structures of the face, and can be divided into the anterior, middle, and posterior cranial fossa. The five bones that make up the skull base are the ethmoid, sphenoid, occipital, paired frontal, and paired parietal bones. The anterior skull base is bounded by the posterior wall of the frontal sinus anteriorly, the roof of the sphenoid sinus posteriorly, the frontal bone laterally, and the frontoethmoid suture line inferiorly. The most important structures below the anterior cranial fossa are the orbits and the paranasal sinuses (Fig. 8.1). Above the skull base, the dura mater attaches anteriorly at the frontal crest and crista galli to form the flax cerebri, which transmits the superior and inferior sagittal sinuses. Table 8.1 lists some of the more frequently used methods of anterior skull base reconstruction.

The boundaries of the middle cranial fossa include the posterior wall of the maxillary sinus

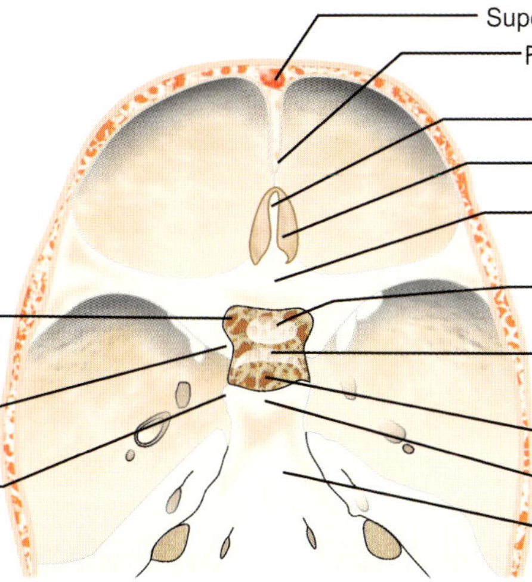

Fig. 8.1: Skull base anatomy and landmarks (Anterior cranial fossa and body of sphenoid).

Table 8.1 Most common flaps used for anterior skull base defects

- Pericranial
- Temporoparietal fascia
- Radial forearm free tissue transfer
- Anterolateral thigh free tissue transfer
- Rectus abdominus free tissue transfer
- Latissimus dorsi free tissue transfer
- Endoscopic nasoseptal
- Endoscopic turbinate

anteriorly, greater wing of the sphenoid bone laterally, and the petrous portion of the temporal bone posteriorly. Within the middle cranial fossa lie the superior orbital fissure, foramen spinosum, foramen rotundum, and foramen ovale. The superior orbital fissure transports the oculomotor nerve (CN III), trochlear nerve (CN IV), the ophthalmic nerve (CN V1), abducens nerve (CN VI), and ophthalmic veins. Foramen spinosum transmits the middle meningeal artery. The maxillary division of the trigeminal nerve (CN V2) passes through the foramen rotundum, and the foramen ovale transports the mandibular division of the trigeminal nerve (CN V3), lesser superficial petrosal nerve, and the accessory meningeal artery. It also houses the body of the sphenoid, sella turcica in which the pituitary

Table 8.2 Most common flaps used for middle cranial fossa defects

- Temporoparietal fascia
- Temporalis muscle

gland lies, middle meningeal artery, Meckel's cave, which houses the trigeminal (Gasserian) ganglion, greater superficial petrosal nerve, and the cavernous sinus. Tables 8.2 and 8.3 list different reconstructive methods for middle fossa and lateral skull base defects that are illustrated later in this chapter.

The posterior skull base is bounded at its anterior limit by the clivus and the lateral occipital bone and posterior portion of the petrous temporal bone form its lateral limit. It contains the opening of the internal auditory canal (porus acousticus), the jugular foramen through which CN IX, X, and

Table 8.3 Most common flaps used for lateral skull base defects

- Temporoparietal fascia
- Temporalis muscle
- Radial forearm free tissue transfer
- Anterolateral thigh free tissue transfer
- Rectus abdominus free tissue transfer
- Latissimus dorsi free tissue transfer

XI pass, the hypoglossal foramen where the hypoglossal nerve (CN XII) traverses, and the vertebral arteries.

OPTIONS FOR ANTERIOR SKULL BASE RECONSTRUCTION: OPEN

During the past decade, a variety of new techniques have evolved for endoscopic resection and reconstruction of anterior skull base tumors. As a result, the frequency of open skull base resection and the need for open skull base reconstruction have diminished. However, certain defects still necessitate open reconstruction.

Careful preoperative planning is essential for the successful reconstruction of skull base defects. The primary goal of reconstruction of any defect is to restore, as closely as possible, the "normal" and in the process, minimize the deformity and morbidity of the donor site. The optimal reconstructive effort does address both functional and esthetic results. The selection of the optimal reconstruction method is critical, and if chosen incorrectly, will lead to failure and frustration. The purpose of this chapter will be to discuss the most common open techniques used in skull base reconstruction.

Local Vascularized Pedicled Flaps

General Considerations

Most defects of the anterior skull base can be reconstructed with local vascularized pedicled flaps. Some of the available local flaps are listed in Table 8.4. Local flaps involve the transfer of vascularized tissue to an adjacent site. Skull base defects with a cerebral spinal fluid leak are most commonly reconstructed with a variety of local pedicled flaps, including the pericranial flap, galeal flap, temporalis muscle flap, and temporoparietal fascia flap. Advantages of local flaps are (i) location within the operative field of skull base procedures, (ii) relative ease of dissection, and (iii) generally, little donor site morbidity. Unfortunately, well-vascularized local flaps for cranial base region are sometimes in short supply. This situation is particularly true for larger defects located deep within the skull base and for defects that include significant resection of skin. These defects often require microvascular free flap reconstruction, which is described later in this chapter.

Table 8.4 Local vascularized pedicled flaps

- Galeal
- Pericranial
- Temporoparietal fascia
- Temporalis muscle
- Modified temporoparietal fascia

Local flaps are centered on vascular pedicles from which they derive their blood supply. Fairly large defects up to 15 cm can be closed reliably using these flaps. With the exception of the temporalis muscle flap, local flaps used for anterior skull base reconstruction are generally thin and do not create a significant facial contour deformity. Local flaps cannot always be used reliably in patients with a history of previous surgery in the area of the flap donor site, and they are less reliable after prior radiation therapy.

Pericranial Flap

The pericranial flap, first described by Wolfe in 1978, is versatile local flap useful for repairing central anterior cranial defects.[1] Pericranial flaps are the most commonly used local flap for open reconstruction of defects of the anterior cranial base. The pericranial flap has been used as a sling to support the brain, as a dural seal to prevent CSF leakage, as vascularized tissue to eliminate empty dead space, and as a barrier to separate the nasal, middle ear, and skin flora from the brain.[2] The flap typically utilizes an anteriorly-based pedicle that receives its blood supply from the supraorbital (SoA) and supratrochlear (StA) arteries. In cases when orbital and frontal bar resection compromises that integrity of the SoA and StA, a laterally based pericranial flap can be designed that is perfused by branches of the superficial temporal artery (Figs 8.2 and 8.3).

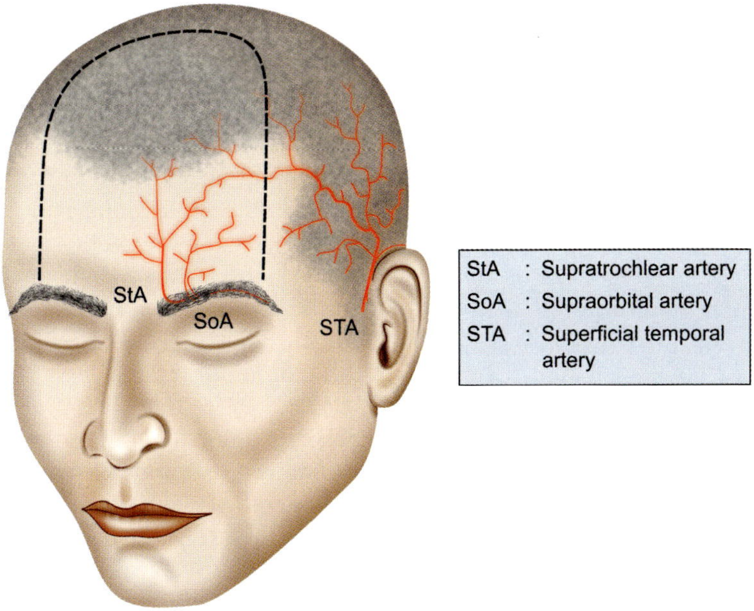

Fig. 8.2: Blood supply of the pericranial flap.

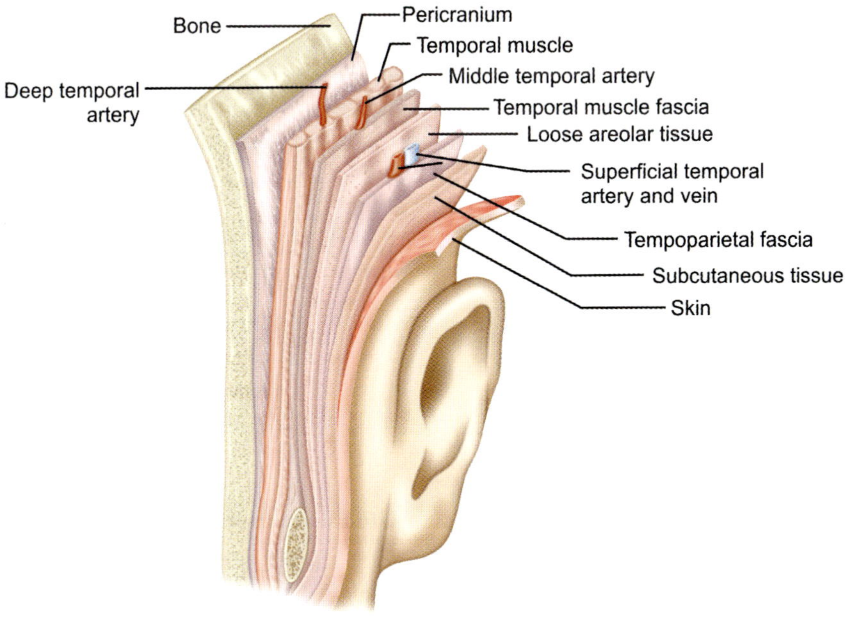

Fig. 8.3: Temporal area anatomy.

A standard bicoronal incision is used to harvest the anteriorly based pericranial flap. The scalp (including the pericranium) is then elevated from the skull to the level of the orbital rims. The StA and SoA are identified on the undersurface of this bicoronal flap and preserved on both sides, if possible. The pericranial flap is then separated from the overlying galea and frontalis muscle and left pedicled anteriorly. A skin graft can be used on the nasal surface of the flap, or more commonly the nasal surface of the graft can be left to remucosalize. After the neoplasm is resected, the flap is then rotated through the craniotomy to fill the surgical defect. The flap is then sutured to the dura at the posterior margin of the defect. This flap can be harvested up to 10 cm wide and 15 cm long and can reach as far as the clivus posteriorly.

Snyderman et al.[3] reconstructed 30 patients with defects in the anterior cranial base using lateral and anteriorly based pericranial, galeo-pericranial, and galeal scalp flaps. Nineteen of these patients were reconstructed with pericranial flaps alone. Of the 30 patients, 57% received prior therapy of surgery and/or radiation therapy. The median follow-up time was 13 months. The authors experienced only three transient (2–3 days) CSF leaks, all resolving without surgical intervention. They reported no cases of postoperative meningitis. The nasal surfaces of all flaps mucosalized uneventfully without the use of skin grafts. In contrast to the low complication rate in this study, Neligan et al.[4] reported on a series of 90 patients with skull base defects reconstructed with local, pedicled, and free tissue transfers. Pericranial flaps were used in 25% of the patients. The complication rate for local flaps was reported as 20.4%, including 14.8% with CSF leak, 3.7% with meningitis, and 9.3% with abscess formation.

Galeal Flap

Galeal flaps, like pericranial flaps, are readily available, easily harvested, and can also be used to repair a variety of dural defects. However, galeal flaps are suboptimal for use after radiation therapy or previous scalp surgery. The galeal flap is thicker than a pericranial flap. It can be raised as an anteriorly based (galeofrontalis) flap, a posteriorly based (galeo-occipitalis) flap or a laterally based (unilateral or bilateral) flap. The galeofrontalis flap has the disadvantages of producing visible irregularities on the forehead and leaving the forehead skin very thin and vulnerable to breakdown secondary to forehead and scalp skin necrosis. The galeo-occipitalis flap is not suitable to cover the anterior or middle cranial fossa. Anterior or laterally based flaps are more commonly used.[5] They can also cause functional and cosmetic complications, including sensorimotor loss and regional alopecia. In general, galeal flaps are used less commonly for anterior skull base reconstruction. Instead, the galea, loose areolar tissue, and pericranium are harvested together to create the galeal-pericranial flap. This flap is harvested by dissecting between the subcutaneous tissue of the scalp and forehead and the galea and relies on the supraorbital and supratrochlear vessels as the vascular pedicle. As described in the previous section, both the pericranial and galeopericranial flap are effective for reinforcing dural repairs. Galeopericranial flaps are more reliable than pericranial flaps after prior radiation, but may be associated with an increased risk of skin necrosis.[6] In addition, this flap is slightly thicker and adds more bulk to the reconstruction defect.

Temporoparietal Fascia Flap

In 1898, the temporoparietal fascial flap was first described for head and neck reconstruction.[7,8] The flap is thin and pliable, and it readily accepts a skin graft. Temporoparietal flaps can drape into concavities and over convexities, and they are highly vascular and resistant to infection. This reliability, particularly in the setting of trauma and devascularized tissue beds, has been one of the reasons it has been used in skull base reconstruction. Briefly, the anatomy of the temporal region is described in the Figure 8.3. The temporal region contains skin, subcutaneous fat, the temporoparietal fascia, temporalis muscle fascia, and the temporalis muscle. The blood supply in this region is mainly derived from the superficial temporal artery, which is the terminal branch of the external carotid artery. The temporoparietal fascia flap is adjacent and continuous with the galea, and flaps as large as 16 cm in length and 10 cm in width are available. The flap has been described to fill defects of the nasopharynx, orbit, anterior and middle cranial fossa, and lateral defects of the skull base. Temporoparietal flaps also can be harvested for use after endoscopic surgery. They can be used to reinforce dural defects, and they particularly useful in filling defects of the sphenoid sinus as well. Another advantage that this flap offers is that it leaves no contour deformity. The main risk of temporoparietal flap harvest is alopecia and temporal scalp skin necrosis.

A temporal scalp incision is made and the skin is carefully elevated just deep to the level of the hair follicles while not disrupting the underlying branches the superficial temporal artery and vein. The temporoparietal fascia is then elevated from the underlying temporalis muscle fascia. The temporoparietal flap can be used in conjunction with the temporalis muscle flap (Fig. 8.4). Because the temporalis muscle flap receives its blood supply from the anterior and posterior deep temporal arteries arising from the internal maxillary system, both the temporal muscle and temporoparietal fascia can be harvested based upon independent vascular pedicles on the same side for reconstruction. Inclusion of the temporalis muscle flap is advantageous in cases when additional bulk is of necessity. Reconstruction using combined temporoparietal and temporalis flaps is particularly useful in defects of the infratemporal fossa, orbital floor, and cribriform region.

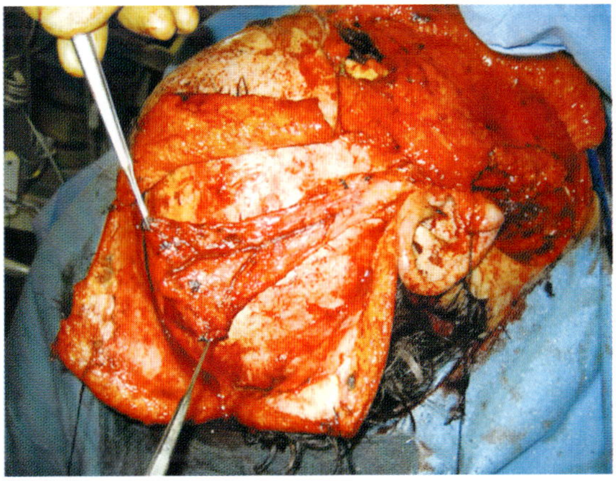

Fig. 8.4: Temporoparietal fascia flap: The temporoparietal fascia flap is perfused by the superficial temporal artery and vein, which enter the base of the flap near the zygomatic process of the temporal bone.

Modified Temporoparietal Fascia Flap

Occasionally, open reconstructive techniques are useful for reconstruction of defects that arise after endoscopic anterior skull base resection. For larger defects especially after endoscopic surgery, the temporoparietal fascia flap can be transferred into the defect using a transpterygoid technique. This approach, first described by surgeons at the University of Pittsburgh, is particularly useful for larger defects involving the sphenoid sinus and the pterygopalatine fossa.[9] This flap can be considered when the nasoseptal flap cannot be used or is unavailable, as in patients who have undergone a posterior septectomy, which will be described later in this chapter. The flap is harvested using the traditional temporal scalp incision but is advanced into the defect using an endonasal approach. The posterior wall of the maxillary sinus is removed allowing access to the pterygopalatine fossa. The infratemporal fossa is also visualized by removing part of the lateral wall of the maxillary sinus. Dissection continues by fully mobilizing the internal maxillary artery and establishing a view of the pterygoid plates. Subsequently, the temporoparietal fascia from the ipsilateral side is harvested as described earlier in the previous section. A lateral canthotomy incision must then be made to allow for adequate transposition of the flap. This incision also allows for the creation of a tunnel between the temporal, infratemporal, and pterygopalatine fossa. Serial dilation using tracheotomy dilators over a guide wire passing intranasally under endoscopic visualization is then conducted until the tunnel is sufficiently widened to transpose the temporoparietal fascia flap. The flap is then used to cover the resultant postoperative defect. Disadvantages of this flap include the need for an external incision, risk of damage to the frontal branch of the facial nerve, and the risk of alopecia.

Temporalis Muscle Flap

The temporalis muscle flap may be used alone or in combination with other flaps for reconstruction of the anterior and middle cranial fossa, the infratemporal fossa, and lateral skull base defects. For anterior skull base reconstruction, the flap arc of rotation is limited to the midline, so it is more suited for reconstruction of defects of the orbital roof rather than for defects of the ethmoid fovea that may extend beyond the midline. It has also been described for the surgical treatment of intraoral and maxillary sinus defects. The flap was first described by Golovine for the reconstruction following orbital exenteration to fill dead space.[10] Advantages for reconstruction include providing significant bulk for a local pedicled flap as well as being used for more lateral defects which other local flaps are unable to reach. The primary disadvantage of using this flap is the temporal donor site hollowing that is seen after flap transfer. This flap is primary perfused by branches of the internal maxillary artery with a secondary blood supply provided by branches of the superficial temporal artery, and can be harvested as a muscle flap or a myofascial flap. The temporalis muscle graft is harvested typically using a bicoronal or hemicoronal incision. The scalp flap is elevated in the subgaleal plane deep to the level of the temporoparietal fascia to preserve the frontal branch of the facial nerve (Fig. 8.5). The flap is elevated off of the zygomatic arch, and the attachment of the masseter muscle is freed (Fig. 8.6). The zygomatic arch is then removed after anterior and posterior osteotomies are made. Subsequently, the temporalis muscle is then elevated off of the temporal bone and rotated to the site of the defect. The temporal hollowing defect is generally reconstructed using a temporal fossa implant like porous polyethylene (Medpor), and the zygoma is secured back in place using titanium miniplates and screws.

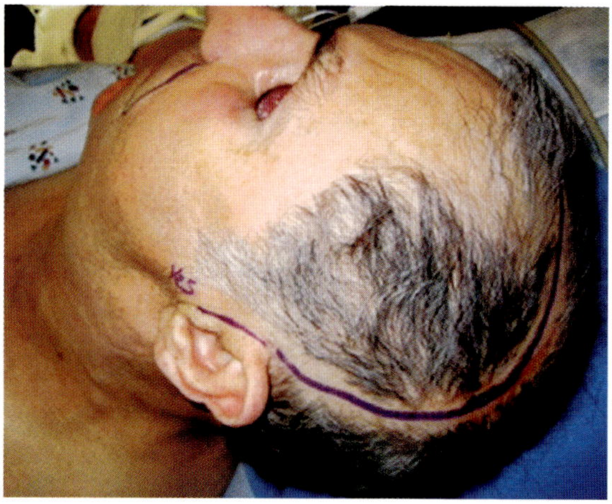

Fig. 8.5: A hemicoronal incision is designed for harvest of a temporalis muscle flap.

Estellés Ferriol et al.[11] found that the most serious complication associated with this flap was a 32% (7/22 patients) incidence of paresis of the frontal branch of the facial nerve, with four cases being permanent. There was an 18% rate of suture

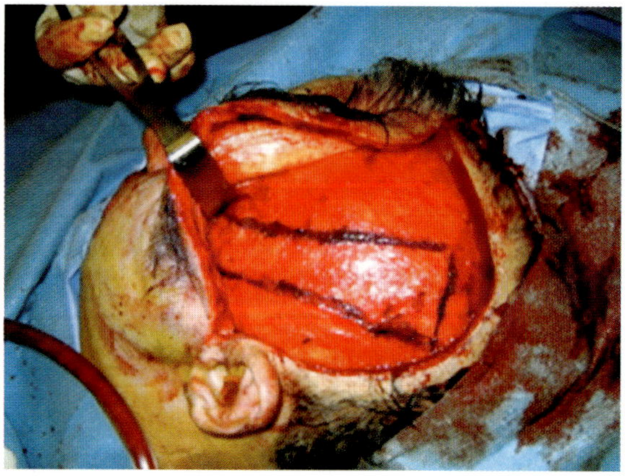

Fig. 8.6: The temporalis muscle has been exposed. A portion or the entire temporalis muscle may be used, depending upon the volume of the defect. In this case, central third of the temporalis muscle will be used.

dehiscence from partial necrosis at the recipient site, which was treated with revision surgery.

CONCLUSION: LOCAL FLAPS

The use of these flaps depends highly on preservation of the vascular supply during tumor resection. In addition, prior treatment with radiation affects local flap reliability. Pericranial flaps are the workhorse method for open reconstruction of defects of the anterior skull base. Galeal flaps should be used with caution if the patient has had prior radiation treatment due to a higher risk of forehead and scalp skin necrosis. Local flaps are may not be reliable or feasible when skull base defects are larger than 25 square centimeters, when there is a large dead space to fill, when prior surgery disrupts the vascular pedicle of local flaps, or when there are significant cutaneous defects of the scalp, forehead, or orbit. When this occurs, free microvascular tissue transfers are often needed for reconstruction.

MICROVASCULAR FREE FLAP RECONSTRUCTION

With large defects that involve the paranasal sinuses, anterior cranial floor, and facial or scalp skin, free tissue transfer may be necessary. Another indication of free tissue transfer is patients with prior treatments using surgery and/or radiation therapy that may make local flap reconstruction unreliable. Free flaps have become more widely accepted as a means of reconstruction for larger and more complex skull base defects without compromising rates of complication. Success rates for microvascular surgery have approached 99%; however, specialized training is often required to perform these complex surgeries compared to other reconstruction methods.[12] Commonly used microvascular free flaps for skull base reconstruction include radial forearm flaps, anterolateral thigh flaps, rectus abdominus flaps, and latissimus dorsi flaps. These flaps all offer a long vascular pedicle that can usually reach recipient blood vessels in the upper neck without needing vein grafts.

The type of flap that is used depends on the size of the defect, the nature of the defect, and patient body habitus. Low volume or small to moderate cutaneous defects are frequently reconstructed using radial forearm flaps. High volume defects that require a large amount of soft tissue bulk and/or reconstruction of significant cutaneous defects are frequently reconstructed using anterolateral thigh flaps, latissimus dorsi flaps, or rectus abdominus flaps. Composite soft tissue and bone defects that include resection of the maxilla or frontal bar are occasionally reconstructed using scapula flaps, fibula flaps, or iliac crest flaps. For the microvascular anastomoses, the preferred recipient blood vessels are the superficial temporal vessels in the temporal fossa or branches of the external carotid artery, external jugular vein, or internal jugular vein in the upper neck. A study by Chiu et al.[13] surveyed 70 patients who underwent microvascular free flap reconstruction of anterior and middle skull base defects. The rectus flap was used in the majority of cases. CSF leak was observed in 7% of cases, which resolved without further surgical intervention. The authors concluded that the overall rate of complications was low, with good functional results when a maxillectomy was performed. Table 8.5 illustrates free flaps as part of the overall reconstructive algorithm.

Table 8.5 Open reconstruction modalities for anterior skull base defects

Type of defect	*Reconstructive modality*
Minimal dural tear	Primary closure, endoscopic repair
Small dural defect	Temporalis fascia
Moderate to large dural defect	Fascia lata, free flaps
Bony defect: orbital wall, nasal and frontal bones	Calvarial bone graft, titanium mesh, free flaps
Posterior sinus wall, intact	Frontal sinus obliteration with abdominal fat
Posterior sinus wall, involved	Frontal sinus cranialization
Orbital exenteration	Temporalis muscle flap, free flaps
Orbitomaxillary resection	Free flap and obturator

Source: Adapted from Gil et al.[14]

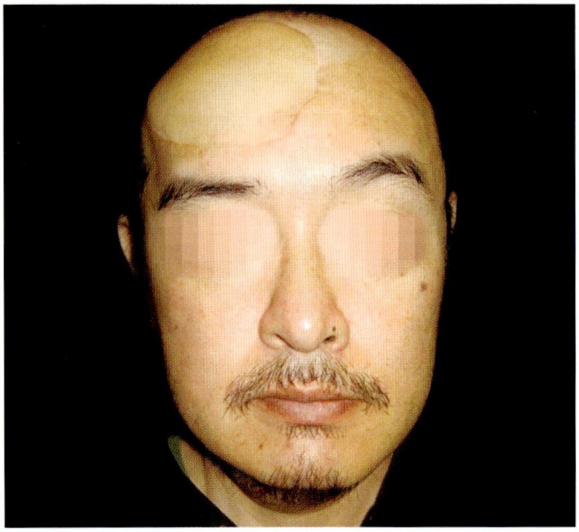

Fig. 8.7: Twelve-month postoperative appearance after right forehead reconstruction using a fasciocutaneous radial forearm free flap. When compared to other cutaneous free flaps that are commonly used for anterior skull base reconstruction, the radial forearm flap often offers a superior match to facial skin with regards to flap skin color, thickness, texture and actinic changes.

Radial Forearm Flap

The radial forearm free flap is a thin flap that is often used for low volume defects that do not require a bulky reconstruction. This flap can be harvested as a fascial or fasciocutaneous flap. Very thin fascial flaps can be used to resurface the floor of the anterior cranial fossa in cases where pericranial flaps may be unavailable or unreliable due to prior surgery or radiation. Radial forearm flaps are often useful for reconstruction of small to moderated cutaneous defects of the forehead in patients being treated for advanced facial skin cancer, since the forearm skin often offers a better match with regards to skin color, thickness, and actinic changes when compared to other free flap donor sites (Fig. 8.7).

Anterolateral Thigh Free Flap (ALTFF)

The anterolateral thigh free flap is useful for reconstruction of large cutaneous defects or high volume defects, when a radial forearm free flap would not provide sufficient tissues. Of note, vascularized fascia lata can be harvested for use in dural repair. The thickness of subcutaneous tissues that are available in anterolateral thigh free flaps varies considerably according to body habitus, but flap volume can be increased in thin patients by harvesting a myocutaneous flap that contains the vastus lateralis muscle (Figs 8.8A to C). Another advantage of anterolateral thigh flaps arises from their very low potential for significant flap door site morbidity. Disadvantages of the anterolateral thigh free flaps include an increased incidence of normal variants of the anatomy of the vascular pedicle when compared to other free flaps that are commonly used for anterior skull base reconstruction, and anterolateral thigh flaps offer a poor match for resected facial skin color, thickness, and hair growth patterns.

Rectus Free Flap

The rectus abdominus muscle free flap offers a large amount of soft tissue bulk for reconstruction of high volume defects. Historically, the rectus abdominus flap is the most commonly used flap in anterior skull base reconstruction (Figs 8.9A and B). However, in recent years it has been used less frequently, as anterolateral thigh flaps often offer similar flap characteristics with decreased potential for flap donor site morbidity. Rectus flaps can be harvested as a muscle flap, a myofascial flap, or a myocutaneous flap. Rectus flaps have been used to obliterate large volume defects, including orbital and palatal defects that occur in conjunction with anterior skull base defects. Vascularized anterior rectus sheath can be harvested for repair of dural defects. The skin component of rectus abdominus flaps offers a poor match for resected facial skin with regards to skin color, skin texture, and hair growth patterns. Potential donor site complications include abdominal wall hernia formation, and abdominal wall laxity is relatively common even if a hernia does not occur.

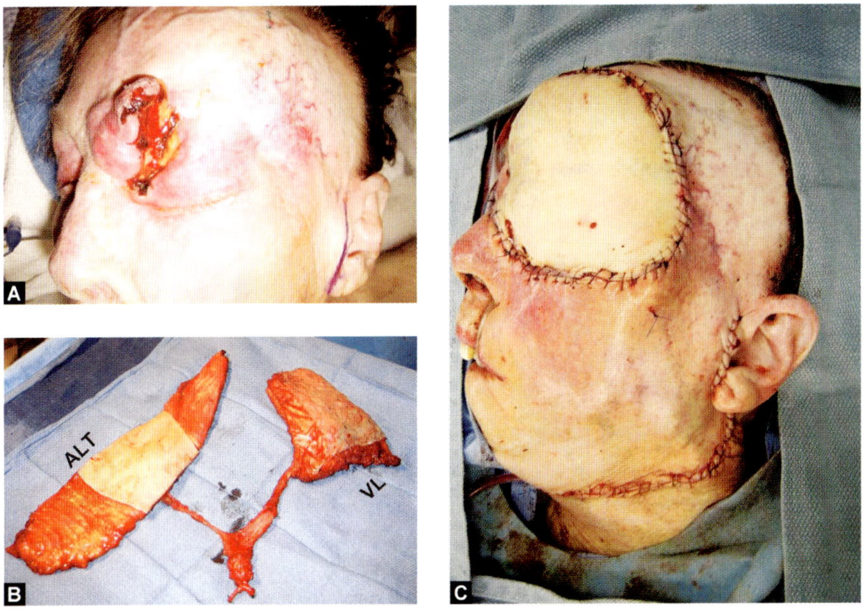

Figs 8.8A to C: (A) An advanced recurrent squamous carcinoma of the orbit and eyebrow requiring craniofacial resection and orbital exenteration; (B) An anterolateral thigh-vastus lateralis flap that has separate fasciocutaneous and myofascial components that are both perfused by the lateral circumflex femoral vessels is useful for reconstruction of complex or high-volume skull base defects; (C) The defect has been obliterated and the intracranial space has been separated from the orbit and paranasal sinuses using a bulky anterolateral thigh flap. Unfortunately, the flap skin provides a poor match for the color, texture and contour of the resected facial skin.

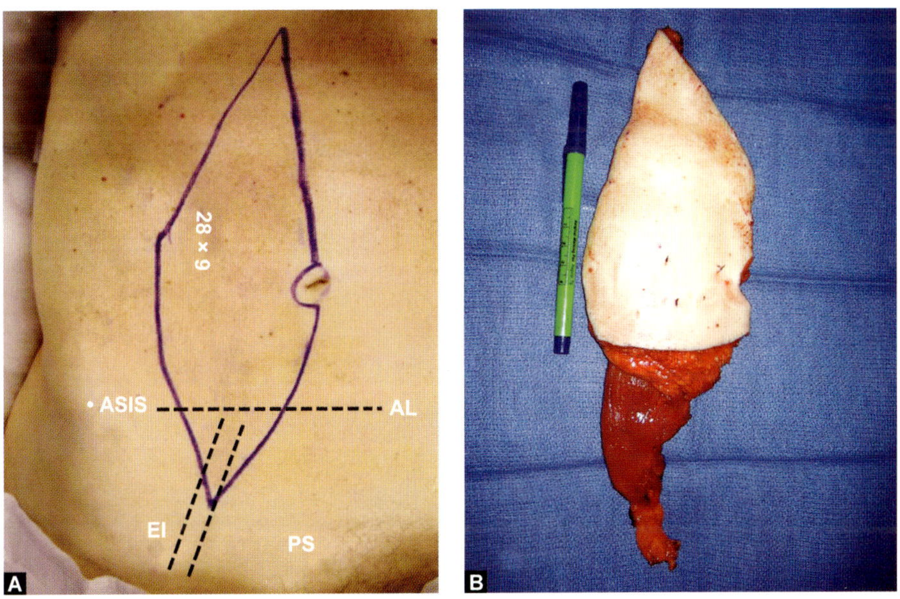

Figs 8.9A and B: (A) A vertical rectus abdominus myocutaneous flap is designed on the right abdominal wall; (B) The rectus abdominus myocutaneous flap is a bulky flap that contains more subcutaneous fat than other flaps commonly used for anterior skull base reconstruction. It should be considered for reconstruction of high-volume defects.

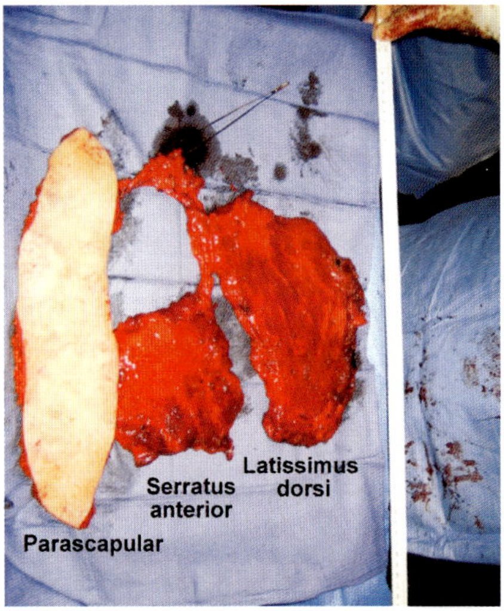

Fig. 8.10: A so-called "megaflap" contains a latissimus dorsi myofascial component, a serratus anterior myofascial component and a parascapular fasciocutaneous component that are all perfused by the subscapular vascular pedicle. This flap offers sufficient surface area to reconstruct the entire scalp and forehead, and each soft tissue component can be inset independently, allowing for reconstruction of complex three-dimensional anatomy.

Latissimus Dorsi Free Flap

The latissimus dorsi free flap was initially described by Olivari in 1979.[15] It offers a high volume flap that has lower donor site morbidity in comparison to the rectus abdominus muscle free flap.[16] Multiple flaps components that are perfused by a single subscapular vascular pedicle can be included in addition to the latissimus dorsi muscle, including a scapular fasciocutaneous component, a parascapular fasciocutaneous component, a serratus anterior muscle component, and vascularized scapular and rib bone components. This allows for reconstruction of very large and complex defects using a single free flap (Fig. 8.10). Latissimus dorsi myofascial flaps are often used in conjunction with a split thickness skin graft to reconstruct large surface areas of the scalp and forehead, and aesthetic outcomes are often very acceptable with regard to the resulting scalp and forehead contour and color (Fig. 8.11). In cases of skull base reconstruction where there is a defect of the dura or use of an alloplastic cranioplasty, myocutaneous flaps are often preferred over myofascial flaps, as use of a flap with a thick myocutaneous skin paddle facilitates creation of a water-tight soft tissue closure to reduce the risk of cerebrospinal fluid leak and reduces the risk of cranioplasty extrusion (Figs 8.12 and 8.13).

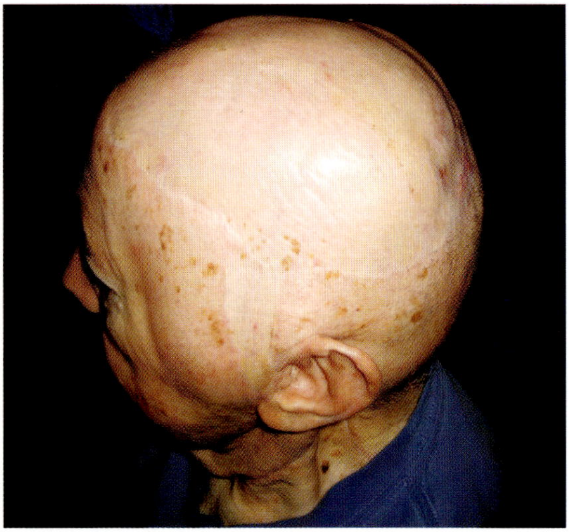

Fig. 8.11: Scalp reconstruction using a latissimus dorsi myofascial flap and a split thickness skin graft offers a very reasonable long-term esthetic outcome, with an acceptable scalp contour, skin color and skin texture.

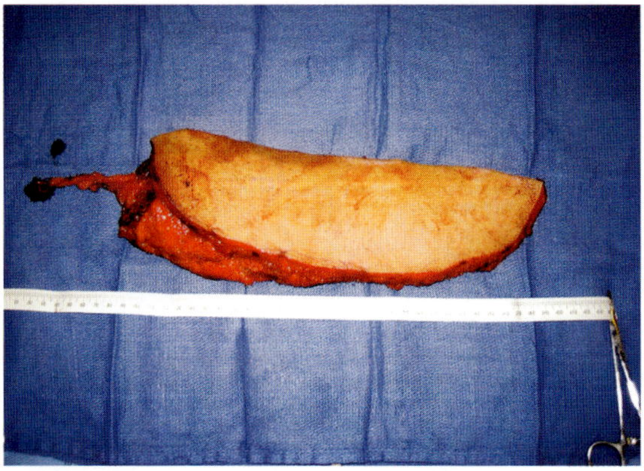

Fig. 8.12: A latissimus dorsi myocutaneous flap offers a moderately thick flap and a skin paddle that facilitates creation of a water-tight wound closure. This is often the flap of choice for forehead and scalp reconstruction when there is an alloplastic cranioplasty or a high-risk of cerebrospinal fluid leak.

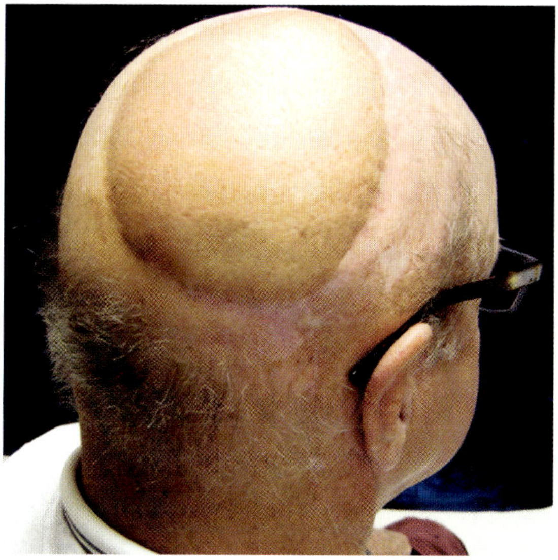

Fig. 8.13: Scalp reconstruction using a latissimus dorsi myocutaneous flap in a patient with a duraplasty and titanium mesh cranioplasty. There was no cerebrospinal fluid leak or cranioplasty extrusion, but the esthetics of the reconstruction is compromised when compared to using a myofascial flap with a skin graft.

Special Considerations

Anterior skull base defects do not always require bone replacement; however, it should be considered if the defect measures greater than 3 square centimeters.[17] Bony reconstruction is also recommended if greater than one-third of the orbital roof is lost; otherwise the patient may experience pulsatile enophthalmos. In addition, loss of the supraorbital bar, frontal bone, and malar eminence necessitates bone replacement in order to achieve optimal esthetic results.

Patients who have had radiation therapy, or will undergo radiotherapy postoperatively are at a higher risk of developing significant fibrosis and decreased vascularization. As a result, non-vascularized grafts may reabsorb over time. In addition, alloplastic agents should be used with caution in an irradiated field due to an increased risk of extrusion and wound complications.

CONCLUSION: MICROVASCULAR FREE FLAPS

Open reconstruction of anterior skull base defects can usually be accomplished with local flaps. Free tissue transfer may be necessary for large volume defects, defects that involve a significant amount of forehead, scalp, or orbital skin, or in cases when prior surgery and/or radiation therapy makes local flaps unreliable. A thorough understanding of the reconstructive options, including free tissue transfer, will provide optimal results after skull base surgery.

REFERENCES

1. Wolfe SA. The utility of pericranial flaps. Ann Plast Surg. 1978;1(2):147-53.
2. Smith JE, Ducic Y. The versatile extended pericranial flap for closure of skull base defects. Otolaryngol Head Neck Surg. 2004;130(6):704-11.
3. Snyderman CH, Janecka IP, Sekhar LN, et al. Anterior cranial base reconstruction: role of galeal and pericranial flaps. Laryngoscope. 1990;100(6): 607-14.
4. Neligan PC, Mulholland S, Irish J, et al. Flap selection in cranial base reconstruction. Plast. Reconstr. Surg. 1996;98(7):1159-66; discussion 1167-8.
5. Georgantopoulou A, Hodgkinson PD, Gerber CJ. Cranial-base surgery: a reconstructive algorithm. Br J Plast Surg. 2003;56(1):10-3.
6. Fu C, Hao S, Hsu Y. Use of a galeopericranial flap for the reconstruction of anterior cranial base defects. Chang Gung Med J. 2005;28(5):341-8.
7. Brown WJ. Extraordinary case of horse bite: the external ear completely bitten off and successfully replaced. Lancet. 1898;1:1533.
8. Monks GH. The restoration of a lower lid by a new method. N Eng J Med. 1898.
9. Fortes FSG, Carrau RL, Snyderman CH, et al. Transpterygoid transposition of a temporoparietal fascia flap: a new method for skull base reconstruction after endoscopic expanded endonasal approaches. Laryngoscope. 2007;117(6):970-6.
10. Speculand B. The origin of the temporalis muscle flap. Br J Oral Maxillofac Surg. 1992;30(6):390-2.

11. Estellés Ferriol JE, Carrasco Llatas M, Ferrer Ramírez MJ, et al. Temporalis myofascial flap: technique description and results in our patients. Acta Otorrinolaringol Esp. 2005;56(6):257-60.
12. Suh JD, Sercarz JA, Abemayor E, et al. Analysis of outcome and complications in 400 cases of microvascular head and neck reconstruction. Arch. Otolaryngol. Head Neck Surg. 2004;130(8):962-6.
13. Chiu ES, Kraus D, Bui DT, et al. Anterior and middle cranial fossa skull base reconstruction using microvascular free tissue techniques: surgical complications and functional outcomes. Ann Plast Surg. 2008;60(5):514-20.
14. Gil Z, Abergel A, Leider-Trejo L, et al. A comprehensive algorithm for anterior skull base reconstruction after oncological resections. Skull Base. 2007;17(1):25-37.
15. Olivari N. Use of thirty latissimus dorsi flaps. Plast. Reconstr. Surg. 1979;64(5):654-61.
16. Bootz F, Gawlowski J. Free latissimus dorsi flap for reconstruction of the anterior base of the skull. Skull Base Surg. 1995;5(4):207-12.
17. Schmalbach CE, Webb DE, Weitzel EK. Anterior skull base reconstruction: a review of current techniques. Curr Opin Otolaryngol Head Neck Surg. 2010;18(4):238-43.

9

Skull Base Reconstruction: Endoscopic

Darshni Vira, MD; Jeffrey D Suh, MD

INTRODUCTION

For the last two decades, skull base surgeons have been employing endoscopic approaches to the skull base to resect a variety of both benign and malignant tumors. These techniques evolved from experience accumulated treating benign sinonasal inflammatory conditions, repairing meningoencephaloceles, closing small cerebrospinal fluid (CSF) fistulas and treating pituitary adenomas. To close larger defects after skull base surgery, a variety of techniques have been developed with the same goal of creating a watertight seal separating the cranial cavity from the nasal cavity. This chapter will discuss endoscopic approaches to skull base reconstruction, while open skull base reconstruction is covered in chapter 8.

Skull base defects reconstructed with purely endoscopic techniques spare patients an external incision and the morbidity associated with a craniotomy. Results, in a number of large series, show comparable to superior success to open reconstructive techniques. In a meta-analysis of endoscopic CSF leak repair, Hegazy et al.[1] reported a 90% closure rate for primary surgery and a 96% rate of success for revision attempts. Lanza et al.[2] in 1996 and Zweig et al.[3] in 2000 reported similar excellent success rates approaching 95% after initial endoscopic repair. Endoscopic repairs are also successful in long-term prevention of intracranial infective complications such as meningitis, pneumocephalus and abscess. Harvey et al.[4] reported only a 0.9% risk of subsequent intracranial complications after endoscopic skull base reconstruction in 106 endoscopic skull base repairs over a 5-year period. As will be described in this chapter, dural defects after open or endoscopic surgery can be sealed using a combination of bone, fat, fascia, synthetic dural substitutes, and mucosal grafts.

BACKGROUND

Dandy first described the use of fascia lata in the repair of dural tears for pneumocephalus after traumatic frontal sinus injury in 1926.[5] In time, a success rate of 60–80% was achieved, and the frontal craniotomy approach soon became the standard of care. Improved instrumentation for sinus surgery led to the endoscopic repair of CSF leaks by Wigand in 1981.[6] Many techniques have subsequently been described further improve success rates of endoscopic repair, including the use of fat packing, pedicled flaps, gaskets, and sutures. Arguably the greatest advancement in cranial base defect repairs has been the Hadad flap, which is a vascularized pedicled nasoseptal flap based on the sphenopalatine artery.[7] Currently, many of the methods of skull base reconstruction are often supported by the vascularized nasoseptal pedicle flap.

Numerous sources have reported on the inciting factors for CSF leaks with accidental trauma being the most frequent cause (44%), followed by surgical trauma (29%) and tumors (22%).[8] Most commonly, the CSF leaks are found at a cribiform plate (35%), followed by sphenoid sinus (26%), anterior ethmoid (18%), frontal sinus (10%), posterior ethmoid (9%) and inferior clivus (2%).[9] The leak site often determines the choice of reconstruction.

DESCRIPTIONS OF VARIOUS ENDOSCOPIC METHODS OF CSF LEAK REPAIR

Nasoseptal Flap

The most commonly used flap to cover large dural defects is the nasoseptal flap. Originally described by Hirsch in 1952, this flap is harvested as a mucoperichondrial flap with its pedicle originating near the sphenopalatine foramen.[10] The blood supply of this rotational flap is derived from the nasoseptal artery, a branch of the posterior septal artery from the sphenopalatine artery. The pedicle of mucosa extends from the nasal septum back to the sphenopalatine foramen. Two incisions are made following the plane of the septum sagittally. The superior incision is made 2 cm below the superior aspect of the septum, and the inferior incision is made on the maxillary crest or the nasal floor depending on the required width. The incisions are connected anteriorly and posteriorly are extended laterally to allow for a large arc of rotation. This flap can be used to reach the frontal recess anteriorly and can extend to the clivus posteriorly. Typically, a layer of collagen matrix, fibrin sealant and a fat graft are placed in the defect prior to laying down the nasoseptal flap. Figures 9.1A to F illustrates a left skull base defect repaired with a multilayer closure including bone and a nasoseptal flap. The flap is generally harvested prior to tumor resection and stored in the nasopharynx or maxillary sinus for use after the cranial resection. Therefore, the surgeon must be cognizant in designing a flap appropriate to cover the resultant defect prior to reconstruction. In addition, this flap cannot be used in patients who have had a posterior septectomy, unless patency of the vessel can be confirmed with intraoperative Doppler ultrasonography. In the author's initial description of 44 patients with skull base defects repaired with the nasoseptal flap for a variety of pathologies, only two patients (5%) had postoperative CSF leaks requiring subsequent surgery.[7]

Nasoseptal Flap for High-flow CSF Leaks

The group at the University of Pittsburgh also evaluated the nasoseptal flap to repair high-flow CSF leaks.[11] In this technique, a dural substitute such as DuraGen (Integra, Plainsboro, NJ) is used first to cover the exposed intracranial structures as an inlay graft. The nasoseptal flap is then rotated over the defect and overlaps the bony boundaries of the defect. A layer of surgical (Ethicon, Cornelia, GA) is then placed around the edges of the flap. Then DuraSeal (Confluent Surgical, Waltham, MA) is sprayed over the entire surface of the flap. Then, Gelfoam (Pfizer, New York, NY) is placed over the entire surface after which a Foley balloon or sponge is used to support the repair. For these high-flow leaks, lumbar drains were used in 65/70 patients in this study for three days at 10 mL/hour. The postoperative CSF leak rate using this method was 5.7% (4/70). Occult high intracranial pressure is cited as a risk factor for repair failure.

Turbinate Flaps

An alternative to the nasoseptal flap for small defects is the inferior or middle turbinate flap (Figs 9.2A to D). These pedicled flaps were originally described for use of septal perforation repairs.[12] For skull base repairs, it is more common to use the turbinate tissue as a free mucosal graft. Fortes and the group at the University of Pittsburgh evaluated the use of the posterior pedicled inferior turbinate flap

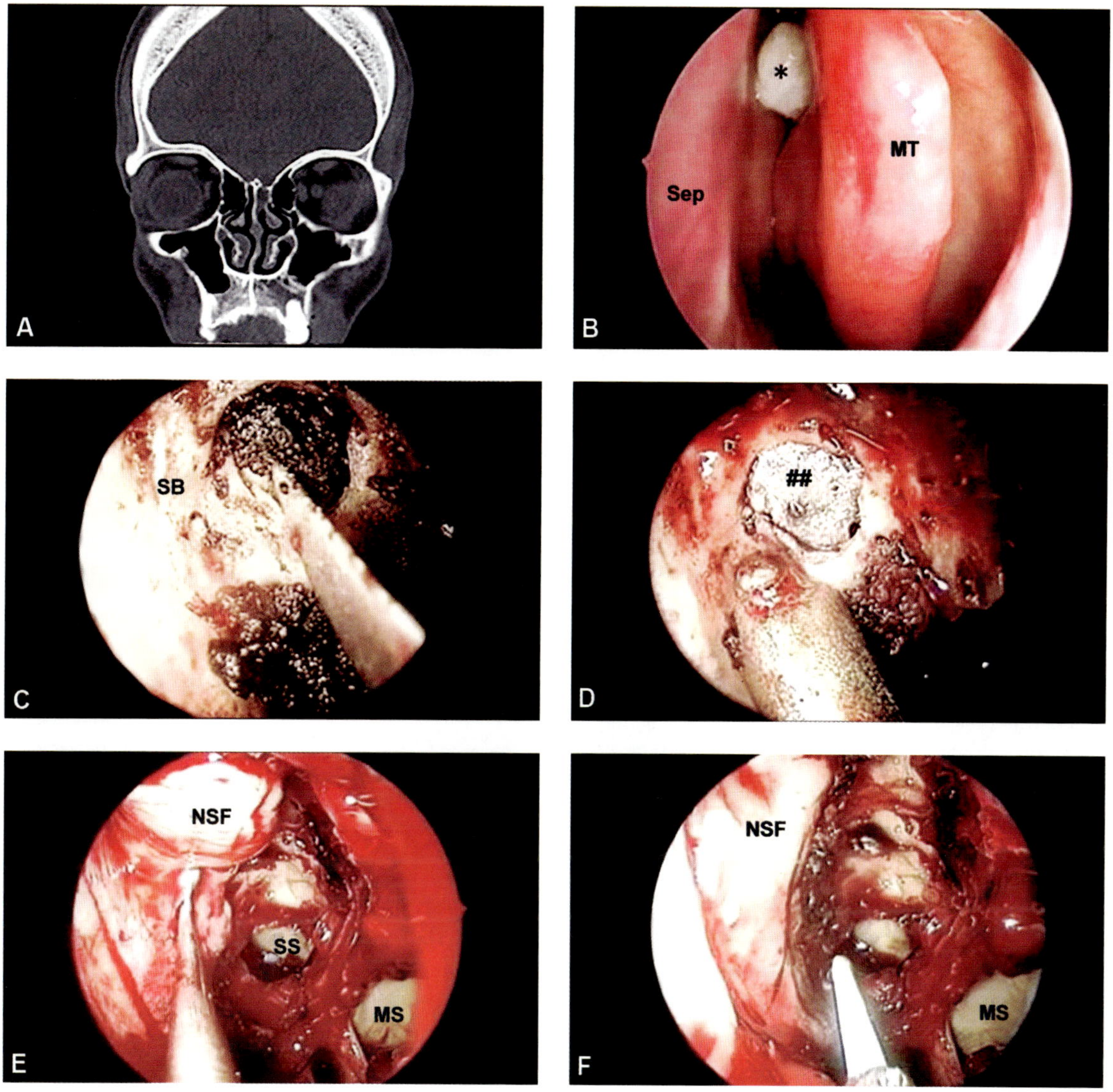

Figs 9.1A to F: Left cribriform plate encephalocele repair. Repair was done with intracranial bone inlay graft followed by nasoseptal flap.

Sep: Nasal septum; MT: Middle turbinate; *: Encephalocele; SB: Skull base; ##: Medial bone graft; NSF: Nasoseptal flap; SS: Sphenoid sinus; MS: Maxillary sinus.

in a small study of four patients after endoscopic skull base surgery.[13] The flap was used in two cases to close CSF leaks and was successful. The authors suggest that the flap is a viable option for patients with small skull base defects when the Hadad flap is not available.

The middle turbinate has been evaluated as a pedicled flap for skull base repair in one cadaver study.[14] The authors concluded that the flap is "technically demanding" and requires precise endoscopic dissection to be successful. The mean length of the flap was 4 cm, with an average width of

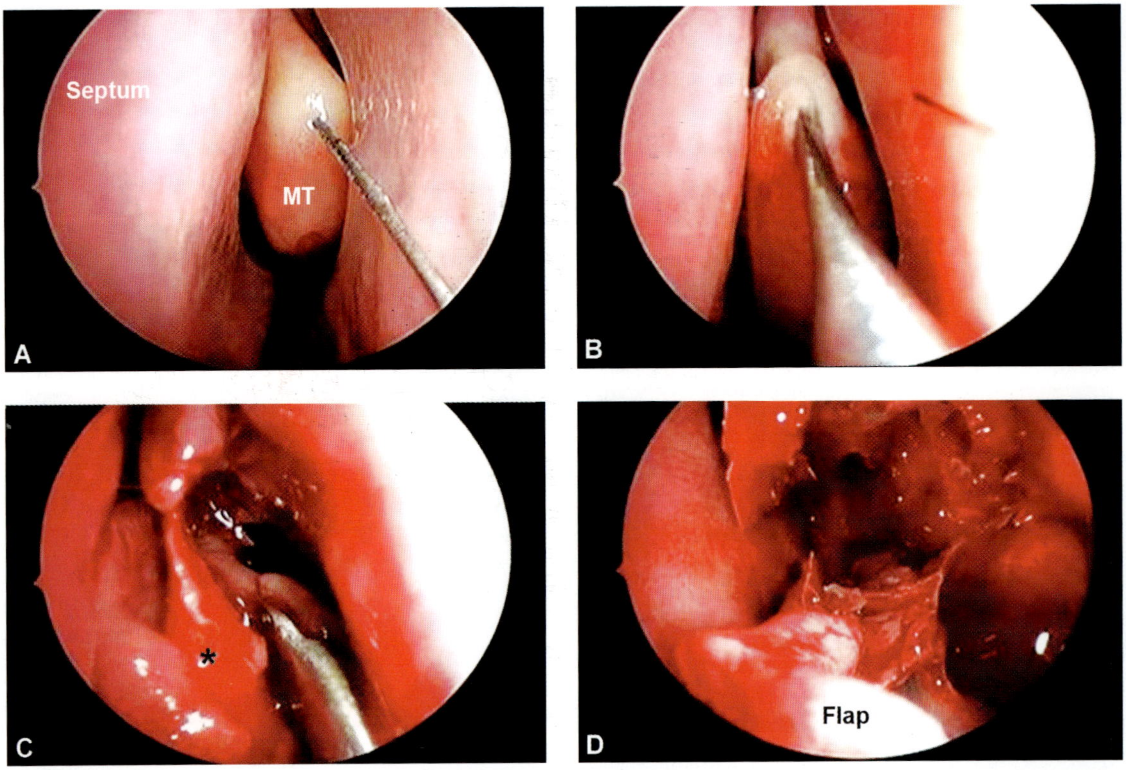

Figs 9.2A to D: Left middle turbinate flap. (A) Injection of left middle turbinate; (B) Vertical incision; (C) Dissection of flap away from turbinate bone; (D) Flap based posteriorly with intact blood supply.

MT: Middle turbinate; *: Turbinate bone.

2.8 cm. The flap was considered to be large enough in 10/12 sides to cover a sellar defect. The authors concluded that the flap would be more suitable for covering defects of the planum and fovea ethmoidalis.

Bilayer Button

This technique, recently described by the group at Jefferson University in Philadelphia in 2010, appears to be useful in the closure of high-flow leaks.[15] In this technique, a button is made with two separate pieces of fascia lata (Fig. 9.3). The inlay graft, which eventually sits on the inside of the dural defect is 25–30% larger than the defect. The onlay graft is made to be only 5–10% larger than the opening. Two 4-0 nylon sutures are used to secure the two pieces of fascia lata together. In this study, using this technique to repair skull base defects, the authors showed a statistically significant decrease in CSF leaks ($P< 0.03$) compared to their traditional repair methods. The 16/20 patients in this study

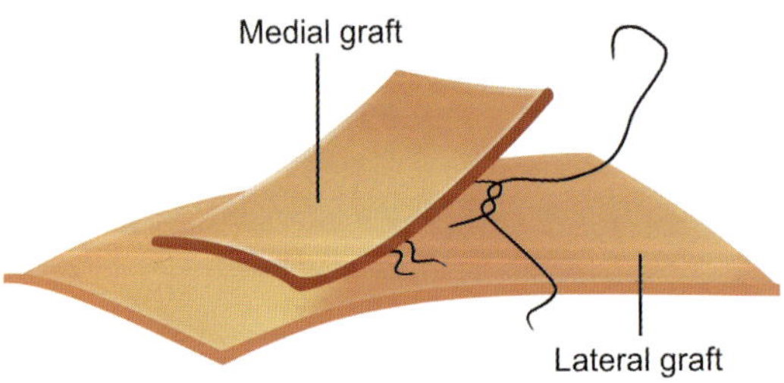

Fig. 9.3: Bilayer button technique with fascia lata. Medial graft is placed intracranially while the lateral graft lies over the skull base defect[15].

Source: Luginbuhl AJ, Campbell PG, Evans J, et al. Endoscopic repair of high-flow cranial base defects using a bilayer button. Laryngoscope. 2010;120(5):876-80.

also had a nasoseptal flap over the button repair. Lumbar drains were used in 40% (8/20) of patients in this study. One benefit of this technique is that it theoretically reduces the incidence of graft migration and subsequent failure due to the medial graft being placed intracranially.

Gasket Seal

This technique described by the group at Cornell in 2008, consists of a soft-tissue graft (generally fascia lata or Alloderm) centered over the defect with the edges of the graft exceeding the bony defect circumferentially.[16] Next, a piece of bone (such as from the vomer) is fashioned to be roughly the size of the bony defect. The bone is centered over the soft-tissue graft so that there was excess soft-tissue graft circumferentially around the rigid graft. The rigid graft is placed into the bony defect forming a watertight gasket seal around the bone. In this pilot study, they reported a 0% leak rate. When the defect is large, the group also describes using a nasoseptal flap as the final layer of closure.[17]

Bath-Plug Closure

Wormald offered a novel technique in 2003 for maintaining the watertight seal for prevention of CSF leaks in the anterior skull base.[18] Initially, a lumbar drain is placed and 10 mL of CSF is mixed with 0.2–0.25 mL of 5% fluorescein. Once identified, the bony defect is measured and a similar sized piece of fat is harvested from the ear lobe or abdomen, depending on the size of the defect. A 4-0 Vicryl (Ethicon Inc., Somerville, NJ) suture is secured through one end of the fat plug and gently the fat is pushed through the bony defect intracranially using a blunt probe. Once the fat is inserted, the suture is gently pulled to allow the fat plug to expand on the intracranial surface, filling the dural defect. The seal is then tested using the fluorescein-stained CSF for confirmation. A free mucosal graft, fibrin glue and Gelfoam are then laid over the plug. Of the 33 patients who underwent this procedure, 31 patients had no recurrence of the CSF leak yielding a 94% success rate for primary closures. The two patients who did recur had repeat bath-plug closures and subsequently did not recur.

Free Mucosal Grafts

One of the simplest methods of closing a CSF leak is with a free mucosal graft. Mucosa can be harvested from a number of sites, including the nasal floor, turbinates or septum. This method of repair is usually used in conjunction with another medial layer of repair, including bone, fat or fascia. Areas of common fascial harvest are outlined in Table 9.1. Tissue glue is used to secure the graft in place. Figures 9.4A to D and 9.5A to D demonstrates a large skull base encephalocele repaired with a medial bone graft harvested from the nasal septum and a lateral free mucosal graft. The graft is usually then supported by packing material or balloon to prevent postoperative migration.

Adjuvant Therapies

Acetazolamide is a diuretic that can decrease CSF production up to 48%.[19] Acetazolamide can be considered in cases of elevated intracranial pressure (ICP), such as in benign intracranial hypertension, as an adjuvant therapy after CSF leak repair. The authors recommend either dosing two times a day with the 500 mg sustained-release form or providing only an evening dose. Theoretically, this approach will maximize the effects of the drug during rapid eye movement (REM) sleep when ICPs peak. The optimal timing, dosing and long-term benefits of this approach have not been proven, but it may reduce the risk of developing subsequent skull-base defects in patients with elevated CSF pressures.

Table 9.1 Types of Free fascia grafts

Types of free-fascia grafts
• Alloderm (synthetic)
• Temporalis fascia
• Pericranial fascia
• Fascia lata
• Anterior rectus sheath

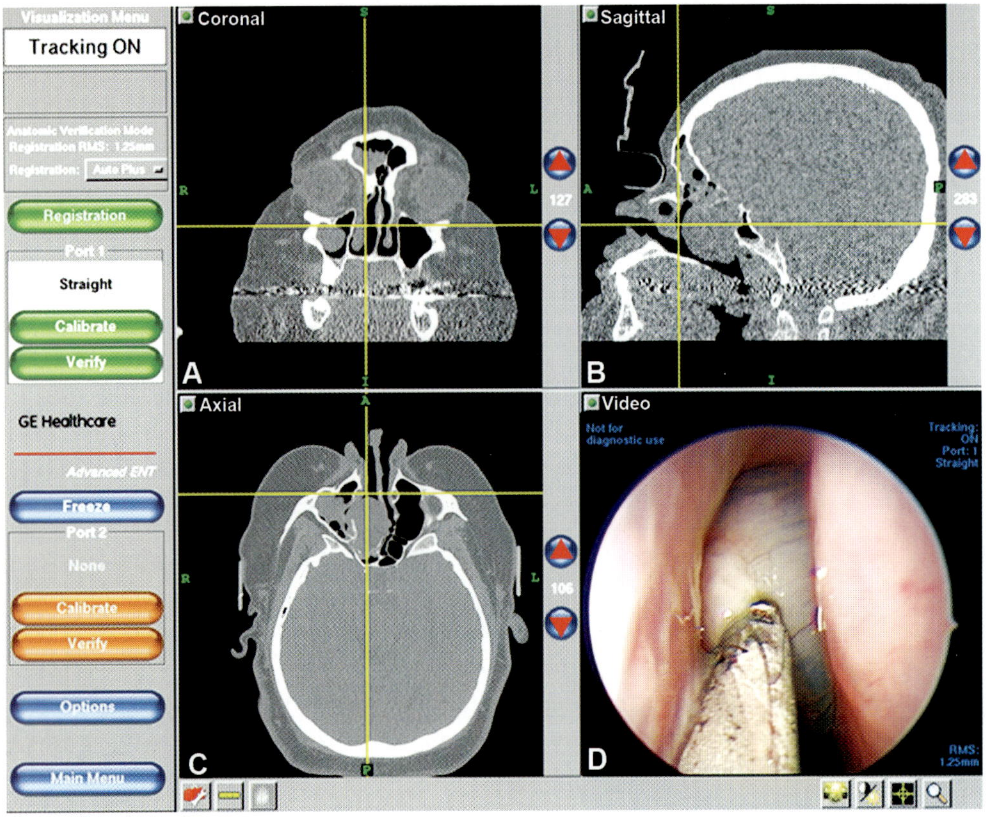

Figs 9.4A to D: Endoscopic views of right nasal cavity encephalocele.

Lumbar drains may be used postoperatively with drainage set at 5–10 mL/hour. Risks and side effects of lumbar drain placement are well described. Their use in the postoperative setting may help graft take during the first 48–72 hours. Many groups prefer to reoperate in the setting of a postoperative CSF leak, where adjustment of graft placement or focused supplementation with abdominal fat may resolve the leak.

Ventriculoperitoneal drains are typically reserved for patients with spontaneous leaks who have recurrences post closure or very high ICP or those who do not respond to acetazolamide.

Endoscopic Skull Base Repair Failure

Endoscopic skull base repair is generally very successful in closing CSF fistulas, but failures do occur. In a 10 year review of 72 endoscopic CSF leak repairs, Mirza et al.[20] reported a 90% success rate with the first repair and 97% with the second. Six (75%) of the eight failures occurred in the spontaneous CSF leak group and seven (88%) occurred in those cases with evidence of raised ICP. Lindstrom et al.[9] identified four factors related to failure of the repair: (1) spontaneous CSF leak, (2) elevated BMI, (3) the location of the leak in the lateral sphenoid where access is difficult and (4) a massive skull base defect.

In a review of long-term outcomes of endoscopic repair, Zuckerman et al.[21] focused on the timing of recurrent CSF leaks. The average time for recurrence in their series was seven months, ranging from 1–25 months. Another study from the group at the University of Pennsylvania[22] found a

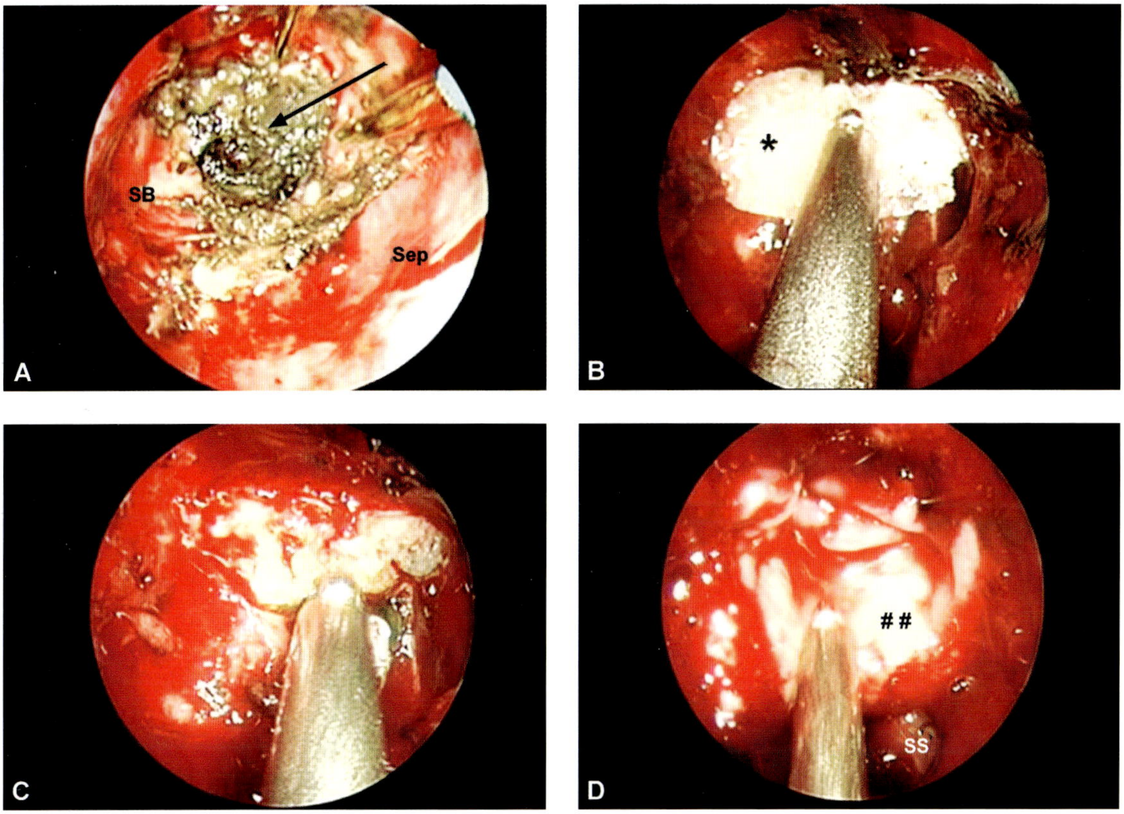

Figs 9.5A to D: Same patient after encephalocele removal. (A) The skull base defect is clearly defined; (B) Placement of bone harvested from nasal septum; (C) Bone graft is placed medial to skull base; (D) Free mucosal graft from septum over skull base defect.

SB: Skull base; Sep: Left nasal septum; Arrow: Skull base defect; *: Bone graft; ##: Free mucosal graft; SS: Sphenoid sinus.

similar time frame for repair failure, with spontaneous leaks recurring in an average of seven months, ranging from 4 days to 24 months, and traumatic leaks recurring in an average of four months, ranging from 4 days to 29 months. With an average followup of 23 months, the overall rate of failure was 9% (17 of 193).

CONCLUSION

Local pedicled flaps, free tissue transfer and endoscopic techniques are currently the mainstay of skull base reconstruction. As endoscopic resections of skull base tumors have gained popularity, reconstructive efforts using endoscopic techniques have kept pace and proven to be effective. As these and new methods of endoscopic skull base reconstruction become further refined and developed, skull base surgeons will have even more methods to successfully repair large defects without the morbidity of open approaches.

REFERENCES

1. Hegazy HM, Carrau RL, Snyderman CH, et al. Transnasal endoscopic repair of cerebrospinal fluid rhinorrhea: a meta-analysis. Laryngoscope. 2000;110:1166-72.
2. Lanza DC, O'Brien DA, Kennedy DW. Endoscopic repair of cerebrospinal fluid fistulae and encephaloceles. Laryngoscope. 1996;106:1119-25.

3. Zweig JL, Carrau RL, Celin SE, et al. Endoscopic repair of cerebrospinal fluid leaks to the sinonasal tract: predictors of success. Otolaryngol Head Neck Surg. 2000;123(3):195-201.
4. Harvey RJ, Smith JE, Wise SK, et al. Intracranial complications before and after endoscopic skull base reconstruction. Am J Rhinol. 2008;22(5):516-21.
5. Dandy W. Pneumocephalus (intracranial pneumatocele or aerocele). Arch Surg. 1926;12:959-82.
6. Wigand ME. Transnasal, endoscopical sinus surgery for chronic sinusitis. IA biomechanical concept of the endonasal mucosa surgery (author's transl). HNO. 1981;29(7):215-21.
7. Hadad G, Bassagasteguy L, Carrau RL, et al. A novel reconstructive technique after endoscopic expanded endonasal approaches: vascular pedicle nasoseptal flap. Laryngoscope. 2006;116(10): 1882-6.
8. Martin TJ, Loehrl TA. Endoscopic CSF leak repair. Curr Opin Otolaryngol Head Neck Surg. 2007;15(1):35-9.
9. Lindstrom DR, Toohill RJ, Loehrl TA, et al. Management of cerebrospinal fluid rhinorrhea: the Medical College of Wisconsin Experience. Laryngoscope. 2004;114:969-74.
10. Hirsch O. Successful closure of cerebrospinal fluid rhinorrhea by endonasal surgery. AMA Arch Otolaryngol. 1952;56(1):1-12.
11 Zanation AM, Carrau RL, Snyderman CH, et al. Nasoseptal flap reconstruction of high flow intraoperative cerebral spinal fluid leaks during endoscopic skull base surgery. Am J Rhinol Allergy. 2009;23(5):518-21.
12. El-Banhawy OA, Halaka AN, Altuwaijri MA, et al. Long-term outcome of endonasal endoscopic skull base reconstruction with nasal turbinate graft. Skull Base. 2008;18(5):297-308.
13. Fortes FSG, Carrau RL, Snyderman CH, et al. Transpterygoid transposition of a temporoparietal fascia flap: a new method for skull base reconstruction after endoscopic expanded endonasal approaches. Laryngoscope. 2007;117(6):970-6.
14. Prevedello DM, Barges-Coll J, Fernandez-Miranda JC, et al. Middle turbinate flap for skull base reconstruction: cadaveric feasibility study. Laryngoscope. 2009;119(11):2094-8.
15. Luginbuhl AJ, Campbell PG, Evans J, et al. Endoscopic repair of high-flow cranial base defects using a bilayer button. Laryngoscope. 2010;120(5):876-80.
16. Leng LZ, Brown S, Anand VK, et al. "Gasket-seal" watertight closure in minimal-access endoscopic cranial base surgery. Neurosurgery. 2008;62(5 Suppl 2):ONSE342-3;discussion ONSE343.
17. Nyquist GG, Anand VK, Mehra S, et al. Endoscopic endonasal repair of anterior skull base non-traumatic cerebrospinal fluid leaks, meningoceles, and encephaloceles. J. Neurosurg. 2010;113(5):961-6.
18. Wormald PJ, McDonogh M. The bath-plug closure of anterior skull base cerebrospinal fluid leaks. Am J Rhinol. 2003;17(5):299-305.
19. Schlosser RJ, Bolger WE. Nasal cerebrospinal fluid leaks: critical review and surgical considerations. Laryngoscope. 2004;114(2):255-65.
20. Mirza S, Thaper A, McClelland L, et al. Sinonasal cerebrospinal fluid leaks: management of 97 patients over 10 years. Laryngoscope. 2005;115(10):1774-7.
21. Zuckerman J, Stankiewicz JA, Chow JM. Long-term outcomes of endoscopic repair of cerebrospinal fluid leaks and meningoencephaloceles. Am J Rhinol. 2005;19(6):582-7.
22. Banks CA, Palmer JN, Chiu AG, et al. Endoscopic closure of CSF rhinorrhea: 193 cases over 21 years. Otolaryngol Head Neck Surg. 2009; 140(6):826-33.

10

Surgical Complications Associated with Sinonasal Tumor Resection

Sharon Morong, MD, MSc; Allan Vescan, MD, FRCSC; John Lee, MD, FRCSC

INTRODUCTION

Endoscopic skull base surgery is a field within otolaryngology and neurosurgery that is still in its infancy and is rapidly progressing. With the advent of new techniques and instrumentation, the boundaries of the endoscopic approach continue to be expanded. However, as we continue to further define the role of endoscopic skull base surgery in the treatment of sinonasal tumors, we must remain objective in our assessment of the risks and benefits of these newer approaches. Currently, there is limited literature regarding the complications associated with these endoscopic techniques. Many of the complications associated with endoscopic skull base surgery are akin to those we are currently familiar with from our experience with functional endoscopic sinus surgery. There are, however, unique differences that require a thorough working knowledge of skull base anatomy, multidisciplinary involvement and early recognition of concerning signs and symptoms to avoid potential morbidity and mortality. In this chapter, we will review the current literature on complications associated with endoscopic skull base surgery and also highlight diagnostic and management pearls to minimize these risks.

CEREBROSPINAL FLUID LEAKS

Cerebrospinal fluid leakage is the most reported complication when examining endoscopic skull base surgery, with a published rate as high as 20%.[1] These rates were initially based on the learning curve associated with endonasal repair following skull base and dural entry. As a comparison, open skull base approaches have CSF leak rates ranging from 5–15%. The low rate of 5% is attributed to repair with a free tissue transfer. However, the morbidity of having to harvest tissue from a secondary donor site is clearly a disadvantage of this option.[2] With respect to endoscopic skull base repair, various autologous materials have been used for reconstructive purposes to prevent postoperative CSF leaks. Some of these materials have included muscle, cartilage, fat, muopericondrium and mucoperiostium.[3-6] Synthetic materials have also been used but host-tissue reactions and magnetic resonance imaging (MRI) interference are some of their disadvantages.[7-10] The earlier higher rates of CSF leak following endoscopic skull base surgery were primarily based on repairs using inlay fascia and fat grafts alone.[1] However, with the introduction of the nasoseptal flap described by Hadad et al, reported rates of CSF leak have been reduced to less than 5%.[3] This flap is a vascular pedicled flap based on the posterior septal artery. It can be designed to incorporate the mucosa of the nasal cavity floor and also extend to the nasal sill, thus providing a large surface area and tremendous versatility for an onlay repair. For large dural defects, a composite repair is employed using an inlay fascia graft that is combined with the nasoseptal flap to provide a well-vascularized skull base closure. Within our institution, the routine use of the nasoseptal flap in 69 patients undergoing endoscopic skull base surgery resulted in a CSF leak rate of only 4%.

Cerebrospinal fluid leaks that occur despite the use of a nasoseptal flap often occur in skull base defects that involve the ethmoid roof and pituitary sella. In these cases, high volume CSF leaks associated with the suprasellar cistern require a bulky graft in order to withstand the pressures of the high volume leak. In addition, repair of the length of the skull base from pituitary sella to along the ethmoid roof often causes parts of the length of the flap to fall away from the skull base. This is due to the three turns the flap has to make: from the floor of the sphenoid to the clival recess, the clival recess to the pituitary sella, and then finally the sella to the planum sphenoidale. The senior textbook editor has addressed this by using fat graft in 2 fashions: first, to fill the clival recess prior to placement of the flap so that there is a less acute angle from the floor of sphenoid to pituitary sella and second, by using fat as an onlay around the edges of the flap as it makes the turn from the sphenoid floor to the pituitary sella. In the senior editor's experience, this is the location in which nasoseptal flaps for large skull base defects involving the pituitary sella and extending to the ethmoid roof are most likely to fail.

Various studies have attempted to identify risk factors for CSF leaks following endoscopic skull base surgery. From a purely anatomical stand point, the commonest locations for CSF leak include the roof of the ethmoid sinus, cribriform plate and the sphenoid sinus.[11,12] Additional risk factors include prior irradiation or surgery to the skull base, surgical communication with the ventricles, opening into the suprasellar cistern, large dural defects, non compliance with postoperative instructions, and obesity.[1] With regards to the endoscopic approach, patients undergoing a transplanum-tuberculum approach appear to be most vulnerable to postoperative CSF leaks. Anatomically, this approach opens into the suprasellar cistern that houses a large volume of CSF. In comparison, other approaches such as the transcribriform technique open into the subarachnoid space underneath the frontal lobes which contains a relatively low volume of CSF. Also, taking the reconstructive repair into consideration, transcribriform reconstruction is aided by the weight of the frontal lobes, providing a natural water-tight seal against any inlay dural repair. The region of the sella however, offers no such support. As such, postoperative packing in these patients is extremely important in counteracting the effects of gravity.[13]

Patients with CSF leak are also susceptible to pneumocephalus. All patients undergoing skull base surgery may have a small trapping of air secondary to opening of the skull base. This however, can expand, leading to pneumocephalus and in even rarer cases, tension pneumocephalus (Fig. 10.1).[13] Tension pneumocephalus can lead to

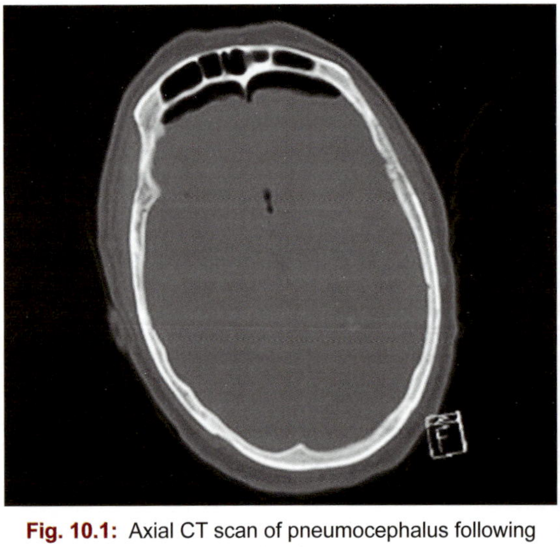

Fig. 10.1: Axial CT scan of pneumocephalus following endoscopic skull base surgery.

compression of intracranial structures, restriction of blood flow and possible herniation. The computed tomography (CT) characteristic features for this event is the Mount Fuji sign.[14] It is so called because of the compression of the frontal lobes and widening of the interhemispheric space between the frontal lobes, resembling the silhouette of Mount Fuji.

A retrospective review looked at ten cases of pneumocephalus after either endoscopic sinus or microscopic skull base surgery. These patients all had associated CSF leaks. They found that lumbar drainage worsened the pneumocephalus and that although six out of eight patients who underwent endoscopic sinus surgery had spontaneous resolution of their CSF leak and pneumocephalus, endoscopic exploration in these patients revealed quite thin or incompletely regenerated mucosa that needed to be repaired with mucosal grafting. Based on these findings, recommendations were made from this group to consider endoscopic exploration for patients with pneumocephalus, even if there is spontaneous resolution. The rationale for this being the possibility of ascending infection through incompletely healed mucosa.[15] To reduce the risk of this complication, tracheotomies were performed during open craniofacial resections to enable airflow diversion from the nose and pharynx. Currently, postoperative packing with materials such as epistaxis balloons, urinary catheters, nasopharyngeal airways and topical hemostatic agents are used to support skull base reconstructive efforts and serve as a less morbid method of preventing pneumocephalus.[13]

INFECTIOUS COMPLICATIONS

Another complication associated with endoscopic skull base surgery is infection. These infections may be either sinonasal or intracranial in nature. Two reports in the literature cited the occurrence of sinusitis in 7.5 and 29% of their patients after undergoing endoscopic skull base surgery.[16,17] Culture under endoscopic guidance is recommended for these patients before the initiation of broad-spectrum antibiotics. Patients within this population suffering sinusitis should be treated rapidly to avoid infection ascending intracranially. Intracranial infections can occur as sequelae of sinusitis or from contamination via surgical instruments. Intracranial infections can include meningitis, epidural, subdural or intracranial abscesses. Patients with these infections typically grow Methicillin-resistant Staphylococcus aureus (MRSA), gram-negative rods and polybacterial organisms.

In open skull base procedures, a standardized regimen of triple antibiotics is used with an associated low incidence of postoperative infections.[18] An endoscopic approach, however, has different considerations and potential risks which may not make this regimen applicable. Surgical access is through the sinonasal cavity to an otherwise sterile intracranial region. One study looked at the use of cefazolin (vancomycin or clindamycin in patients with a penicillin allergy) for 24–48 hours for prophylaxis of CNS infections in patients undergoing endoscopic skull base surgery. Their choice of antibiotic was based on a study which looked at patients suffering acute sinusitis following endoscopic sinus surgery, with the majority of culture positive infections being Staphylococcus aureus.[19] Their first dose was administered upon induction of general anesthesia and continued at timely intervals until nasal packs were removed on postoperative day 1 or 2. The duration of antibiotics used in this study was based on Carrau et al's work looking at antibiotic prophylaxis in open cranial base surgery, where they found that patients taking antibiotics for 24 hours had a decreased incidence in infectious complications with no added benefit of extending the duration beyond 48 hours.[20] Patients were then placed on gentamycin nasal spray 2 weeks after surgery until the sinonasal cavity was considered well healed. Patients who were diagnosed with sinusitis on follow-up were given additional antibiotic therapy. No cases of intracranial infections or meningitis were reported in this study.[21] It is important to note however that there was no control group for comparison. Additionally, the risk of developing resistant organisms when using prophylactic antibiotics must be considered. One study looking at the use of prophylactic antibiotics in neurosurgery found that while this proved effective for reducing incision related infections, it failed to prevent meningitis and tended to select for resistant organisms.[22]

SINONASAL COMPLICATIONS

Epistaxis is one of the most common sinonasal complications following endoscopic skull base surgery. While the majority can typically be controlled with packing or cautery, it is prudent to bear in mind that possibility of a major vascular or intracranial bleed. Epistaxis in these patients should be carefully explored endoscopically. If no source can be localized, one should consider an angiogram to rule out the possibility of a major vascular bleed.

Other sinonasal complications include synechiae, atrophic rhinitis and nasal airflow obstruction. The most common location for synechiae to form within the nasal cavity is between the turbinate and the septum. Special care during the operation to avoid overt trauma to these locations can help prevent this complication. In addition, the use of silastic stents during the postoperative period may prevent adhesions from forming between opposing traumatized surfaces.

Atrophic rhinitis can also occur from iatrogenic trauma to the nasal cavity. It is typically defined as inflammation of the nasal cavity following removal of large mucosal surfaces and can be classified as primary or secondary. Secondary atrophic rhinitis typically occurs after inferior turbinectomies, but may also occur during endoscopic skull base surgery, middle turbinectomies or aggressive septectomies. Approximately one-third of patients undergoing endoscopic skull base surgery experience this, with symptoms of chronic crusting, and foul smell (Fig. 10.2).[13] Currently, there is no universally accepted cure for atrophic rhinitis. Management for this condition has been mostly conservative with the use of humidification, irrigation and topical antibiotics. Topical antibiotics, such as bacitracin, are used with the thought that patients who develop atrophic rhinitis may suffer from superimposed bacterial infections from Klebsiella, which has been shown to be cultured in patients with primary atrophic rhinitis.[23] Case reports have looked at surgical interventions for "closing the nose" as a means of alleviating atrophic rhinitis.[24,25] This method is based on the theory that a more open sinonasal cavity allows for turbulent airflow, which can ultimately lead to atrophic rhinitis. This has yet to be tried, however, in patients following endoscopic skull base surgery.

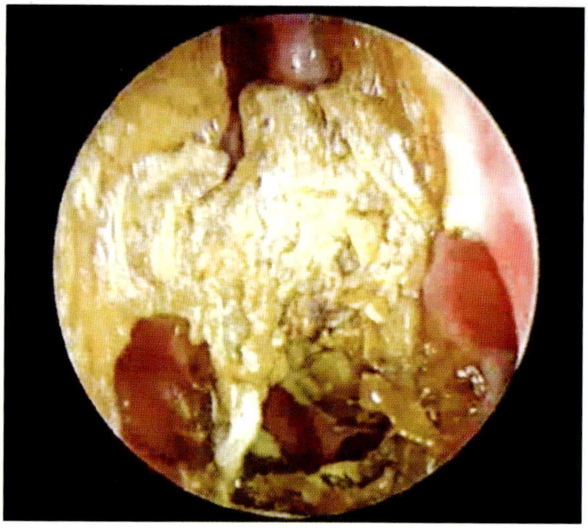

Fig. 10.2: Sinonasal crusting in a patient three months s/p endoscopic craniofacial resection for a mucosal melanoma.

The senior textbook editor has had the most success in managing post-resection crusting with a combination of mupirocin and surfactant irrigations along with frequent in-office debridements. Postoperative crusting is nearly always seen after irradiation and will persist until mucociliary function returns, classically seen anywhere from 6–12 months following end of therapy. During this period, patients are instructed to irrigate with a mixture of bactroban and Sinusurf™ (NeilMed Pharmaceuticals) twice a day and are seen in the office every 2–3 weeks for debridements.

Hyposmia and anosmia are another subset of sinonasal complications that can be found in patients who have undergone endoscopic skull base surgery. Typically, patients have some element of decreased smell in the immediate postoperative period secondary to nasal packing, old blood and debris. Hyposmia or anosmia can only truly be elicited once all packing has been removed and the nasal cavity has fully healed. It is important to note however that patients undergoing an endoscopic craniofacial resection are also more likely to be susceptible to this complication. This is secondary to the surgical resection of the superior septum, middle turbinate and cribriform plate that would be carried out with this approach. More importantly, surgical resection of esthesioneuroblastomas often incorporate removal of the olfactory bulb irregardless of tumor involvement.[26] Anosmia would be an expected outcome in these patients, and thus an important topic in preoperative counseling.

VASCULAR COMPLICATIONS

One of the major challenges in endoscopic skull base surgery is the ability to control bleeding in the surgical field. While sinonasal bleeding can be easily managed with standard endoscopic bipolar or monopolar devices, skull base surgery opens new possibilities of serious vascular complications. One of the most feared neurovascular injuries in endoscopic skull base approaches is internal carotid artery injury. To date, very little skull base literature exists on this specific topic. Wormald et al developed an animal model for vascular injuries whereby 42 endoscopic carotid artery injuries and 25 endoscopic venous injuries were created. They found that the two-surgeon technique, proper selection of the appropriate nostril for endoscope positioning and the use of a large bore suction to clear the bleeding field in order to identify and control the source were useful techniques to control the surgical field while addressing the injury.[27] For localization of the internal carotid artery, transsphenoidal intraoperative ultrasound and pulse Doppler ultrasonography can also be employed as additional adjuncts. This is especially useful in the intracavernous portion of the carotid artery.[28,29]

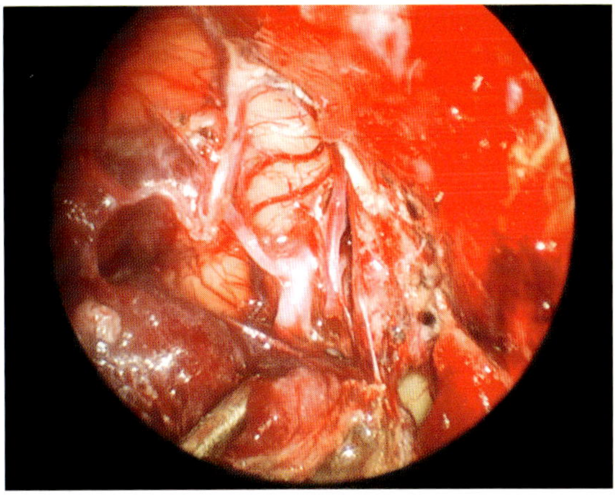

Fig. 10.3: Endoscopic view of the branches of the anterior communicating artery.

Other vascular structures that may be injured include the circle of Willis, with potentially disastrous neurologic sequelae. The arteries that are most likely injured are the anterior cerebral and anterior communicating arteries, particularly during the trans-tuberculum approach (Fig. 10.3). In order to reduce the risk of vascular complications, basic endoscopic principles should be maintained. This includes meticulous dissection, careful use of cautery, image guidance, hemostatic agents and the use of the 2 nostril- 4 hand technique to ensure adequate visualization and stabilization.[13]

ENDOCRINE COMPLICATIONS

Endocrine complications following endoscopic skull base surgery can occur as a result of manipulation to the pituitary gland or its vasculature. This is more commonly seen in open procedures. Severe injury can lead to panhypopituitarism, for which patients need lifelong hormone supplementation. Isolated dysfunction is more common, typically manifesting as diabetes insipidus (DI) or syndrome of inappropriate diuretic hormone (SIADH). Diabetes insipidus occurs as a result of lack of secretion of the antidiuretic hormone. This results in the production of copious amounts of dilute urine and a subsequent low serum sodium concentration. Symptoms may include mental status changes, and cardiovascular collapse. These patients are typically treated with IV hypotonic fluid and desmopressin (DDAVP) if needed. DI is typically transient but can be permanent. SIADH is particularly seen in patients with pituitary adenoma removal. These patients secrete inappropriate amounts of antidiuretic hormone, despite drop in serum sodium concentration. Their renal excretion of sodium remains constant, resulting in the production of concentrated urine. Their low serum sodium may manifest with symptoms of nausea, vomiting , confusion, coma and even death. Patients with SIADH typically require fluid restriction. In more severe cases IV furosemide and urea can be given. SIADH may often be difficult to differentiate from cerebral salt wasting syndrome (CSWS). CSWS is caused as a result of abnormalities within the renal sodium transport system in response to trauma, brain injury or tumors within or surrounding the brain. These patients also have low serum sodium concentration because of excessive renal excretion of sodium. These patients, unlike those with SIADH, are hypovolemic and require fluid resuscitation. The best indicators to differentiate between SIADH and CSWS are ADH levels and fluid status.[30]

Some patients can also present with combined DI and hyponatremia. This presentation is not as frequent, with a quoted incidence range of 4.5–20%.[31] These patients typically present with DI and through overaggressive ADH replacement, subsequently show symptoms of hyponatremia.[32] Studies looking at patients with DI and hyponatremia have found that they typically present with symptoms around postoperative day 2 and 9, and should therefore be monitored closely during this time period. Patients that are discharged home should be educated on the signs and symptoms of these endocrine disturbances to reduce the risk of serious morbidity at home.[32]

ORBITAL COMPLICATIONS

Currently, the incidence of orbital complications following endoscopic skull base surgery is unknown. However, we can extrapolate from what is known in the literature from endoscopic sinus surgery. Overall, the most feared complication is orbital hematoma, with a reported incidence of less than 1%. Patients typically present with signs and symptoms of proptosis, chemosis, diplopia, vision loss (red being the first color to be lost) and elevated intraocular pressure leading to ischemia of the optic nerve. Intraocular pressures in these situations are typically more than 40 mm Hg. Orbital hematomas can be either venous or arterial in nature. Venous hematomas more commonly occur as a result of an inadvertent puncture of the lamina papyracea, with disruption of the veins within the orbital fat. These hematomas are typically slow and progressive in nature. Arterial hematomas arise from either anterior or posterior ethmoidal artery injury and can develop very rapidly (Fig. 10.4).[33]

While the incidence of this event is unknown in endoscopic skull base surgery, it can theoretically be expected to be less for various reasons. During endoscopic sinus surgery, the lamina papyracea is preserved. As such, a breach in the lamina papyracea is likely to be inadvertent in nature, causing traumatic bleeding. A bleed within a closed orbital cavity in situations such as this, will lead to increased intraocular pressure and hematoma formation. With endoscopic skull base surgery,

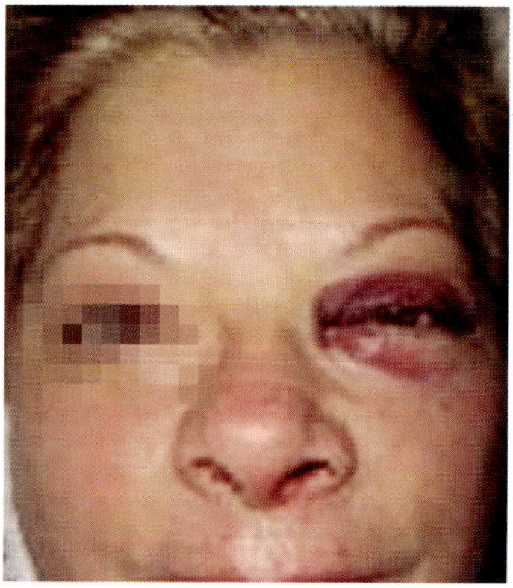

Fig. 10.4: Orbital hematoma following endoscopic sinus surgery.

however, the lamina papyracea is likely taken down if orbital work is being carried out. Bleeding is therefore much more readily visualized and controlled. Also, as a result of the lamina papyracea being removed, hematoma formation within the orbit will likely spill out into the nasal cavity instead of accumulating within a closed space. Without the intraocular pressure buildup, compression and subsequent ischemia of the optic nerve is less likely to occur. Another reason why hematoma formation is less likely to occur in endoscopic skull base surgery is secondary to primary control of the anterior or posterior ethmoid arteries during the skull base approach. With the use of surgical clips or endoscopic cautery devices, the risk of bleeding from these vessels is minimized during the surgical procedure.[13]

Management of orbital and optic nerve complications comprise both conservative and ultimately surgical management. Conservative management consists of orbital massage, IV mannitol with or without IV steroids, while surgical intervention comprises of a lateral canthotomy with cantholysis, orbital decompression and lateral orbitotomy if needed. The difference in management of a venous versus arterial hematoma lies in the timeline for conservative management. Patients with venous hematomas are estimated to have a timeline of 60–90 minutes before vision impairment, thereby giving the surgeon more time to administer conservative treatment before initiating surgical intervention. Arterial hematomas, however, almost always require surgical intervention.[33]

There is a theoretical risk of optic nerve injury during endoscopic skull base surgery. To date, no cases have been reported. Direct injury can occur as a result of accidental instrumentation or manipulation. Currently there are no options for visual restoration after complete nerve trans-section. Preoperative imaging is essential to assess for anatomical variants that may predispose an individual to greater risk of optic nerve injury. These includes the presence of Onodi cells as well as a dehiscent optic nerve within the sphenoid sinus.

Medial rectus injury has been shown to occur in less than 0.5% of endoscopic sinus surgery cases.[13] There are no reports, however, of this type of injury occurring in endoscopic skull base surgery. Risk factors for medial rectus injury include a dehiscent lamina papyracea and the use of powered instrumentation. These types of injuries are difficult to repair, and patients complain of diplopia and ophthalmoplegia. Oculoplastic techniques to repair the medial rectus muscle with subsequent Botox injection into the lateral rectus have been tried, but the results of these procedures have been quite poor.[34,35]

LUMBAR DRAIN PLACEMENT

Over the last several years, the routine use of perioperative lumbar drain placement in endoscopic skull base cases has decreased. This has largely been due to the refinements in endoscopic skull base repair but also because of the associated potential morbidity associated with lumbar drains. Catheter infections, overdrainage with possible herniation and persistent lumbar leak requiring a blood patch for subsequent spinal headaches are some of the complications that may occur. Sciarretta et al. argue that lumbar drains should only be used when there is high pressure hydrocephalus or a direct communication between the surgical cavity and the third ventricle to avoid reconstruction failure.[36] Additionally, a lumbar drain may be useful in cases where there are large dural defects or in transplanum and trans-tuberculum approaches given their proximity to the suprasellar cistern. Ultimately, prophylactic use of a lumbar drain to minimize the risk of CSF leak should be weighed against the risk of complications associated with the drain itself.

CONCLUSION

Endoscopic skull base surgery is a continually advancing field in research, technology, patient care and management. As we move forward, however, it is important to remain cognizant of complications that can occur with this type of surgery, to ensure that safety is maintained. Having a high index of suspicion, recognizing complications early and intervening in a timely manner all serve to reduce potential morbidity and mortality. Further studies are needed, not only to better report complication rates as it pertains to various approaches within endoscopic skull base surgery, but to also define the effect of endoscopic resection and its associated reconstructive techniques, on emotional well-being and physical function.

REFERENCES

1. Snyderman CH, Kassam AB, Carrau R, et al. Endoscopic reconstruction of cranial base defects following endonasal skull base surgery. Skull Base. 2007;17(1):73-8.
2. Neligan PC, Mulholland S, Irish J, et al. Flap selection in cranial base reconstruction. Plast Reconstr Surg. 1996;98(7):1159-66; discussion 67-8.
3. Hadad G, Bassagasteguy L, Carrau RL, et al. A novel reconstructive technique after endoscopic expanded endonasal approaches: vascular pedicle nasoseptal flap. Laryngoscope. 2006;116(10):1882-6.
4. Locatelli D, Rampa F, Acchiardi I, et al. Endoscopic endonasal approaches for repair of cerebrospinal fluid leaks: nine-year experience. Neurosurgery. 2006;58(4 Suppl 2):ONS-246-56; discussion ONS-56-7.
5. McMains KC, Gross CW, Kountakis SE. Endoscopic management of cerebrospinal fluid rhinorrhea. Laryngoscope. 2004;114(10):1833-7.
6. Zweig JL, Carrau RL, Celin SE, et al. Endoscopic repair of cerebrospinal fluid leaks to the sinonasal tract: predictors of success. Otolaryngol Head Neck Surg. 2000;123(3):195-201.
7. Kaptain GJ, Vincent DA, Laws ER, Jr. Cranial base reconstruction after transsphenoidal surgery with bioabsorbable implants. Neurosurgery. 2001;48(1):232-3; discussion 3-4.
8. Dusick JR, Mattozo CA, Esposito F, et al. BioGlue for prevention of postoperative cerebrospinal fluid leaks in transsphenoidal surgery: A case series. Surg Neurol. 2006;66(4):371-6; discussion 6.
9. Arita K, Kurisu K, Tominaga A, et al. Size-adjustable titanium plate for reconstruction of the sella turcica. Technical note. J Neurosurg. 1999;91(6):1055-7.
10. Cavallo LM, Messina A, Esposito F, et al. Skull base reconstruction in the extended endoscopic transsphenoidal approach for suprasellar lesions. J Neurosurg. 2007;107(4):713-20.
11. Lindstrom DR, Toohill RJ, Loehrl TA, et al. Management of cerebrospinal fluid rhinorrhea: the Medical College of Wisconsin experience. Laryngoscope. 2004;114(6):969-74.
12. Lee TJ, Huang CC, Chuang CC, et al. Transnasal endoscopic repair of cerebrospinal fluid rhinorrhea and skull base defect: ten-year experience. Laryngoscope. 2004;114(8):1475-81.
13. Ransom ER, Chiu AG. Prevention and management of complications in intracranial endoscopic skull base surgery. Otolaryngol Clin North Am. 2010;43(4):875-95.
14. Sadeghian H. Mount Fuji sign in tension pneumocephalus. Arch Neurol. 2000;57:1366.
15. DelGaudio JM, Ingley AP. Treatment of pneumocephalus after endoscopic sinus and microscopic skull base surgery. Am J Otolaryngol. 2010;31(4):226-30.
16. Unger F, Haselsberger K, Walch C, et al. Combined endoscopic surgery and radiosurgery as treatment modality for olfactory neuroblastoma (esthesioneuroblastoma). Acta Neurochir (Wien). 2005;147(6):595-601; discussion -2.
17. Batra PS, Citardi MJ, Lanza DC. Isolated sphenoid sinusitis after transsphenoidal hypophysectomy. Am J Rhinol. 2005;19(2):185-9.
18. Kraus DH, Gonen M, Mener D, et al. A standardized regimen of antibiotics prevents infectious complications in skull base surgery. Laryngoscope. 2005;115(8):1347-57.
19. Bhattacharyya N, Gopal HV, Lee KH. Bacterial infection after endoscopic sinus surgery: a controlled prospective study. Laryngoscope. 2004;114(4):765-7.
20. Carrau RL, Snyderman C, Janecka IP, et al. Antibiotic prophylaxis in cranial base surgery. Head Neck. 1991;13:311-7.
21. Brown SM, Anand VK, Tabaee A, et al. Role of perioperative antibiotics in endoscopic skull base surgery. Laryngoscope. 2007;117(9):1528-32.
22. Morong S, Goetz P, Ooi EH, et al. The nasoseptal flap for skull base defects: an institutional experience. Manuscript in Preparation.
23. Zohar Y, Talmi YP, Strauss M, et al. Ozena revisited. J Otolaryngol. 1990;19(5):345-9.

24. Shehata MA. Atrophic rhinitis. Am J Otolaryngol. 1996;17(2):81-6.
25. Shehata M, Dogheim Y. Surgical treatment of primary chronic atrophic rhinitis (an evaluation of silastic implants). J Laryngol Otol. 1986;100(7): 803-7.
26. Har-El G, Casiano RR. Endoscopic management of anterior skull base tumors. Otolaryngol Clin North Am. 2005;38:133-44, ix.
27. Valentine R, Wormald PJ. Controlling the surgical field during a large endoscopic vascular injury. Laryngoscope; 2010.
28. Yamasaki T, Moritake K, Hatta J, et al. Intraoperative monitoring with pulse Doppler ultrasonography in transsphenoidal surgery: technique application. Neurosurgery. 1996;38(1):95-7; discussion 97-8.
29. Ram Z, Bruck B, Hadani M. Ultrasound in pituitary tumor surgery. Pituitary. 1999;2(2):133-8.
30. Deslarzes T, Turini P, Friolet R, et al. Cerbral salt wasting syndrome versus SIADH. Rev Med Suisse. 2009;5(225):2281-4.
31. Hensen J, Henig A, Fahlbusch R, et al. Prevalence, predictors and patterns of postoperative polyuria and hyponatraemia in the immediate course after transsphenoidal surgery for pituitary adenomas. Clin Endocrinol (Oxf). 1999;50(4):431-9.
32. Kristof RA, Rother M, Neuloh G, et al. Incidence, clinical manifestations, and course of water and electrolyte metabolism disturbances following transsphenoidal pituitary adenoma surgery: a prospective observational study. J Neurosurg. 2009;111(3):555-62.
33. Bhatti MT, Stankiewicz JA. Ophthalmic complications of endoscopic sinus surgery. Surv Ophthalmol. 2003;48(4):389-402.
34. Huang CM, Meyer DR, Patrinely JR, et al. Medial rectus muscle injuries associated with functional endoscopic sinus surgery: characterization and management. Ophthal Plast Reconstr Surg. 2003; 19(1):25-37.
35. Penne RB, Flanagan JC, Stefanyszyn MA, et al. Ocular motility disorders secondary to sinus surgery. Ophthal Plast Reconstr Surg. 1993;9(1):53-61.
36. Sciarretta V, Mazzatenta D, Ciarpaglini R, et al. Surgical repair of persisting CSF leaks following standard or extended endoscopic transsphenoidal surgery for pituitary tumor. Minim Invasive Neurosurg. 2010;53(2):55-9.

11

Surgical Debate: Open Versus Endoscopic

Jeffrey D Suh, MD

BACKGROUND

The treatment of skull base and paranasal sinus tumors is a challenging frontier that is constantly evolving. In 1941, Dandy first described the craniofacial approach for resection of orbital tumors with central nervous system extension.[1] In 1954, Smith reported a case in which the craniofacial concept was applied for the first time. A neurosurgeon and a second surgeon worked in conjunction to resect, *en bloc*, an ethmoid-orbital tumor.[2] Only in 1963, when Ketcham published his paramount paper reporting a series of 17 anterior craniofacial resections (CFR), did this surgical procedure become the standard treatment of malignant tumors of the skull base.[3] Similarly, VanBuren et al. in 1968, Terz et al in 1969, Shah and Galicich in 1977, and others[4-7] all reported good results with CFRs. Since Ketcham's series, complication rates of open anterior skull base surgery have steadily fallen, and the craniofacial approach has become the gold standard for tumors in this area.

The first reports of endoscopic skull base surgery emerged in the late 1990s. Endoscopic resection of the sinonasal tumors has become a reality because of a better understanding of the anatomy from an endoscopic perspective, improved surgical experience, advances in skull base reconstruction, and concomitant technological advances. However, just as importantly, head and neck surgeons have accepted that an oncologic resection of sinonasal malignancies can be achieved by piecemeal resection. Large experiences with transoral robotic surgery (TORS) and transoral laser microsurgery have helped show that piecemeal resection can have results that are at least equal to traditional approaches where *en bloc* resections can be achieved. Sinonasal inverted papilloma and juvenile nasopharyngeal angiofibroma (JNA) were some of the first tumors that fueled controversy on the need for open resection. Since then, multiple reports have demonstrated its feasibility, safety, and efficacy of the endoscopic approach to treat both benign and malignant sinonasal tumors. This chapter will outline the advantages and disadvantages of the open and endoscopic approaches to treat sinonasal pathology.

CONVENTIONAL TREATMENT OF SINONASAL CANCER: OPEN APPROACHES TO THE NASAL CAVITY, PARANASAL SINUSES AND SKULL BASE

The lateral rhinotomy and midface degloving incisions are the most commonly used traditional approaches to access tumors within the paranasal sinuses and nasal cavity. These techniques are also used as a part of the CFR for skull base neoplasms. Other more limited approaches include the Caldwell-Luc, external ethmoidectomy via a Lynch incision, or non-endoscopic transnasal surgery.

Mid-Facial Degloving Approach

This technique was first described by Casson in 1974.[8] This approach consists of lifting the soft tissue from the mid portion of the face by means of a sublabial incision. Four incisions are required in this approach to facilitate exposure of the pyriform aperture, lateral nasal wall, and medial orbital wall: (i) Bilateral intercartilaginous incisions (ii) Complete septocolumellar transfixion incision (iii) Sublabial incision (iv) Bilateral pyriform aperture incisions extending to the vestibule. It offers excellent bilateral exposure of the nasal cavities, middle third of the face and central skull base. Limitations of this technique include access and visualization of the nasal bones, lacrimal pathway, frontal sinus, premaxillary soft tissues, and orbit.

Lateral Rhinotomy Approach

This technique was first described by Moure in 1902.[9] This approach provides excellent exposure of the nasal cavity, the paranasal sinuses, and the nasopharynx with minimal postoperative deformity when meticulously closed. A representative incision is displayed in Figure 11.1. It is most often employed to perform a medial maxillectomy. To achieve *en bloc* resection, osteotomies are performed through the inferior and anterior aspects of the medial wall of the maxilla, through the medial wall of the orbit just inferior to the frontoethmoid suture line, and through the inferior orbital rim and orbital floor. One potential complication is the development of scar tissue or narrowing of the nasal vestibule. However, Lueg et al. demonstrated that both the lateral rhinotomy and midface degloving approaches do not negatively affect the nasal airway.[10]

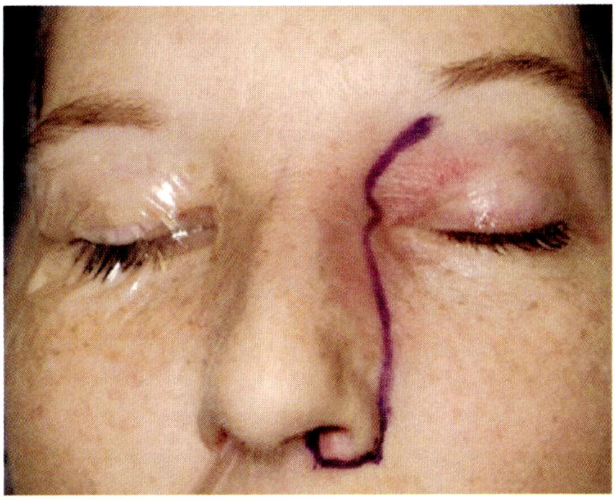

Fig. 11.1: Lateral rhinotomy incision.

Craniofacial resection is typically regarded as the treatment of choice for paranasal malignant tumors invading the anterior skull base (Fig. 11.2). The general technique includes a bicoronal incision, bifrontal craniotomy to the orbital rims, gentle elevation of the frontal lobes extradurally, and entry into the paramedian structures beneath the floor of the anterior cranial fossa. The frontal sinus is cranialized, and the frontal recess plugged. During posterior dissection, the olfactory fibers are cauterized. The tumor is then approached from the inferior aspect via one of several transfacial approaches, usually the lateral rhinotomy or midfacial degloving to remove the intranasal portions (Fig. 11.3). Contraindications to this approach include

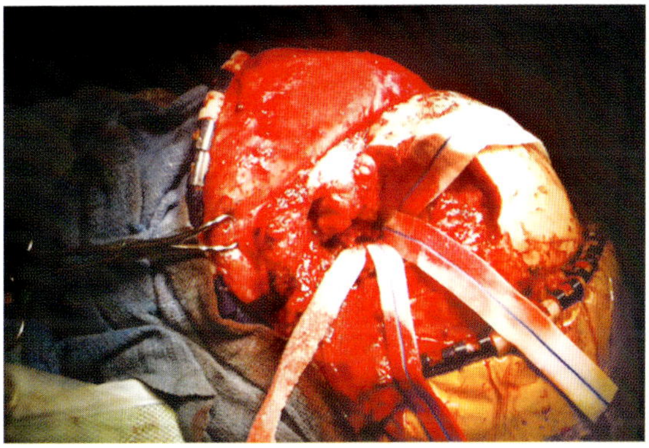

Fig. 11.2: Bicoronal approach for frontal sinus tumor.

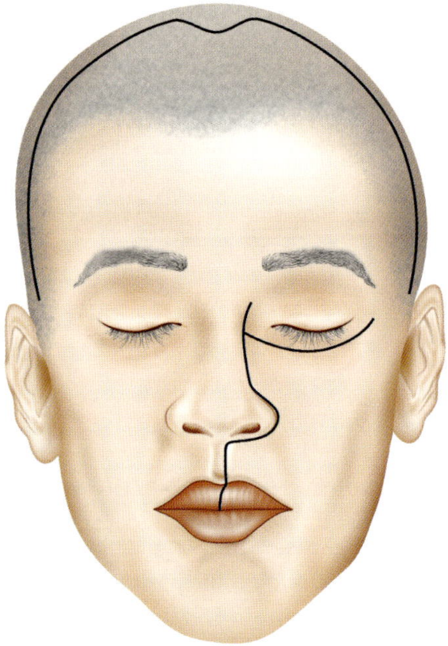

Fig. 11.3: A transfacial approach, where usually the lateral rhinotomy or midfacial degloving is done to remove the intranasal portions.

gross massive invasion of the brain; invasion of the optic chiasm; invasion of both orbits; gross invasion of the internal carotid artery (relative); and elderly patients physiologically and psychosocially unsuitable for a major operation. There are various modifications of the craniofacial resection that have been described to afford adequate exposure. Theoretically, this approach does allow for *en bloc* tumor resection.

Complications of Standard Craniofacial Resection

The traditional CFR has several limitations. The approach has been associated with significant perioperative morbidity with major complications being reported in 30–40% of the cases and mortality from the surgery has been reported in 0–13% of cases.[11-13] Another factor includes significant frontal lobe retraction which leads to permanent anosmia. In addition, the use of facial incisions can be a source of significant patient morbidity in traditional CFRs. Deschler et al. looked at their complications associated with anterior skull base surgery in 49 patients treated between 1986 and 1993.[14] The authors noted a 40% complication rate, with one postoperative death. Infectious complications occurred in 19% of cases, with one case of meningitis. Seven CSF leaks occurred (13%), with two cases requiring reoperation. A recent, international, multicenter study by Ganly et al. reported 334 patients who underwent CFR for paranasal sinus malignancies. Postoperative complications occurred in 110 patients (32.9%). Postoperative mortality was 4.5%. The 5-year overall, disease-specific, and recurrence free survival rates were 48.3%, 53.3%, and 45.8%, respectively.[12] In another series, Batra et al. described 16 patients who were treated with traditional open approaches. Major complications occurred in 44% of cases, and overall mortality was 27% over a 2.6 year medial follow-up period. Major complications included pneumocephalus (4), seizures (2), CSF leak (1), hemorrhage (1), meningitis (1), frontal lobe infarct (1), and aspiration pneumonia (1).[15]

Special Considerations of Open Craniofacial Resection

With the trend toward more minimally invasive surgeries, an obvious criticism to the craniofacial approach is the need for a facial and scalp incision. The fully endoscopic endonasal approach obviously eliminates the use of facial incisions. However, to date, there has been no literature describing patient dissatisfaction with the cosmetic result from the lateral rhinotomy approach versus a completely endoscopic approach. In a series from UCLA by Nabili et al. looking at a transnasal, transfacial modification of the craniofacial resection, no patient discomfort or subjective complaints were noted in the postoperative course as it pertained to the external incision.[16] When properly done, the lateral rhinotomy scar typically can be well-camouflaged, as demonstrated in the short- and long-term follow-ups in this study.

Loss of olfactory function after craniofacial resection is a common sequela of the approach. However, variations of the approach have been described which can limit total anosmia by modifying the resection specimen.[17] Also, olfaction can be preserved when the lesion is unilateral and effort is made to spare the contralateral olfactory nerves.[18]

Lastly, most surgeons agree that a complete *en bloc* resection is difficult to achieve despite the wide exposure afforded by the approach. Theoretically, a piecemeal resection could result in intraoperative tumor seeding and increase the risk of local recurrence. However, in practice, *en bloc* versus piecemeal resection does not appear to change prognosis. McCutcheon reported that given the anatomic confines of this region, "... the oncological ideal of a wide, *en bloc* resection was rarely achieved...."[19] Cantu wrote of the difficulty of obtaining *en bloc* resection "as the deep margins may be better overlooked and resected after the removal of the vegetating component of the tumor."[20] Ultimately the *most* important prognostic factor is the presence of a positive margin, thus the choice of approach must be adequate for complete tumor resection.

ENDOSCOPIC SKULL BASE SURGERY

Over the last decade, surgeons have expanded the boundaries of what is accessible using the endonasal approach. Pathology of almost all parts of the ventral skull base has been treated using endoscopic techniques. The current limitations of endoscopic skull base surgery are yet to be determined, and the indications seem to be increasing as more and more experience is accumulated. Surgeons must take into consideration experience of the skull base team, availability of necessary equipment, and the ability to control hemorrhage.

Advantages of Endoscopic Skull Base Surgery

The most apparent advantage of endoscopic skull base surgery is that it avoids the facial incisions. Other benefits include a wide and clear surgical view which is difficult to achieve otherwise within the sphenoid sinus, clivus, posterior skull base, and nasopharynx. Endoscopic approaches also eliminate the need for craniofacial soft-tissue dissection, skeletal disassembly, and brain retraction. Development of angled endoscopes, drills, and instruments has also kept pace with surgeon needs to access tumors and perform resections. Most benign tumors are treated now with endoscopic resections at most tertiary medical centers. Review of the recent literature suggests that endoscopic skull base surgery for malignant tumors can have equal overall and disease free survival compared to CFR.

Batra et al. in 2005 compared 16 patients with CFR with nine cases of minimally invasive endoscopic resection (MIER). In this small study, MIER of anterior skull base tumors did not differ significantly from CFR in operative time, estimated blood loss, hospital stay, or complication rate. Survival and recurrence rates were similar also. Most common tumor types were esthesioneuroblastoma, squamous cell carcinoma, and adenocarcinoma.[15] In 2007, Nicolai et al. reviewed their 10-year experience on exclusive endoscopic approach (EEA) or cranioendoscopic approach (CEA) for malignant tumors of the sinuses and skull base. One hundred and thirty four patients underwent a purely endoscopic approach, while fifty underwent a cranioendoscopic approach. Most common histologic types were adenocarcinoma (37%) and SCCA (14%). The patients were followed up for a mean of 34.1 months (range, 2–123 months). The 5-year disease-specific survival was 91.4% and 58.86% ($p<0.01$) for the EEA and CEA group, respectively, however the CEA group tended to have tumors of higher T stage compared the EEA group.[21]

A more recent study by Eloy et al. in 2009 compared transnasal endoscopic (n=18) and open CFR (=48) for malignant tumors of the skull base and concluded that hospital stays were shorter (3.8 versus 8.1 days). There was no significant difference in survival, metastatic, or complications rates (28% vs 25%), however most of the tumors that were resected endoscopically were esthesioneuroblastomas compared to squamous cell carcinoma in the CFR group.[22] Hanna et al in 2009 published one of the largest series to date comparing endoscopic resection of sinonasal cancers with and without craniotomy. The study evaluated 120 total patients and divided them into two groups, one with exclusively endoscopic approach (n=93), and another group that included a craniotomy (n=27). Of note, most tumors that were removed without craniotomy were of lower T stage (T1 or T2) while 95% of patients treated with the cranioendoscopic approach were T3 or T4. Postoperative complications were low, and the rate of CSF leak was 3% and not statistically different between the two groups. Five and ten-year survival were 87% and 80%, respectively, and did not differ between the two groups. This study suggests that endoscopic surgery (alone or combined with adjuvant treatment), when properly planned and performed by experienced surgeons, may be an effective alternative to standard approaches in the management of malignancies of the sinonasal tract.[23]

Contraindications, Precautions, and Limitations of the Endoscopic Approach

Contraindications to exclusive endoscopic approaches for cure include extensive tumors that involve the facial soft tissues. One relative contraindication is a large dural involvement. Gaining a wide margin of dura may preclude a purely endoscopic approach. Another relative contraindication is a highly vascular tumor, or tumors that involve major vascular structures that hemostasis would be difficult to achieve. In these situations, a combined open and endoscopic approach may be utilized to obtain clear margins.

Precautions

Surgeons performing endoscopic skull base surgery should be concerned about approaching critical areas such as the orbit and optic nerve, brain, surrounding dura, and the internal carotid artery. Endoscopic surgeons also need to be aware of complications such as bleeding, which can be difficult to control quickly, as well as the potential for blindness, brain injury, and spinal fluid leakage. The most important innovation in ESB surgery for the prevention of complications has been the introduction of multidisciplinary teams. Close review of all pertinent radiology and discussion with relevant consultants is essential for complicated skull base pathology.

Complications of Endoscopic Skull Base Resection

Many of the complications of open skull base surgery can also occur in the endoscopic approach as well. Some of the more common sequela of endoscopic skull base surgery include nasal blockage from crusting, impaired olfaction, and altered sensation. Some of the surgical morbidity can be predicted if there is significant drilling leaving with exposed bone, dissection near the olfactory cleft, and resection or manipulation of the neurovascular structures in the pterygopalatine fossa. In most cases, these symptoms are temporarily, and resolve with time and careful postoperative management. A study by the group at the University of Pittsburgh looking at morbidity after endoscopic skull base surgery found that nasal crusting was present for an average of 101 days, and was slightly longer for complex compared to simple approaches. Remucosalization of the nasal septum after nasoseptal flap usually took place by 89 days.[24]

Despite non-sterile conditions in the nasal cavity and sinuses, infectious complications are rare with ESB surgery. The incidence of meningitis after traditional transsphenoidal surgery ranges from 0.7% to 3.1% and for open craniotomy it ranges from 0.9% to 2.5%. A review of 1,000 endoscopic skull base cases, 1.8% developed meningitis, which is comparable to open approaches.[25] Postoperative CSF leak, another potential complication and cause of morbidity after endoscopic skull base surgery, is usually below 10%.[15,21,23] Most CSF fistulas can often be successfully managed clinically with a lumbar drainage or with endoscopic surgical repair. In almost all cases, the repair can be augmented with a small fascial or fat graft or with repositioning of the mucosal flap.

Pneumocephalus also represents a rare, but potentially catastrophic complication of endoscopic skull base surgery. Expanding pneumocephalus can present with a spectrum of symptoms or findings, including headache, mental status changes, coma, or death. Several large series report that the incidence of clinically significant pneumocephalus in patients undergoing anterior skull base procedures is 0–12%.[26] Management symptomatic pneumocephalus usually includes decompression and aspiration of the air, and closure of the skull base defect.

One of the most devastating complications is ICA injury. ICA injury during endoscopic pituitary surgery is an infrequent event, with an incidence of 0.5–1.1%. However, more extended endoscopic skull base resections have a reported incidence between 4–9%.[27] In general, these types of injury are treated with packing and coiling of the ICA by neurointerventional radiology. In an animal model, Valentine and Wormald suggest that the ICA could be repaired at the time of injury with a 4-handed approach employing multiple suctions and vascular clips.[27]

THE FUTURE

Experience and technological advances suggest that the future of endoscopic skull base is very bright. Surgeons are assessing the possibility of robotic surgery to treat skull base pathology,[28] and using 3D technology to improve visualization.[29] Also, improvements in skull base reconstruction will allow for larger tumors to be resected, while simultaneously reducing many postoperative complications such as CSF leaks and infection.

SUMMARY

Despite an exponential increase of recent literature describing the different applications of endoscopic skull base surgery, more long-term data will be necessary to prove its effectiveness compared to traditional open approaches. However, early results suggest that endoscopic tumor resections as at least equal to CFR, with the potential of less morbidity when cases are chosen correctly.

REFERENCES

1. Dandy WE. Orbital tumors: Results following the transcranial attack. New York: Oskar Priest; 1941. p. 1154.
2. Smith RR, Klopp CT, Williams JM. Surgical treatment of cancer of the frontal sinus and adjacent areas. Cancer. 1954;7(5):991-4.
3. Ketcham AS, Wilkins RH, Van Buren JM, et al. A combined intracranial facial approach to the paranasal sinuses. Am J Surg. 1963;106:698-703.
4. Van Buren JM, Ommaya AK, Ketcham AS. Ten years' experience with radical combined craniofacial resection of malignant tumors of the paranasal sinuses. J Neurosurg. 1968; 28:341-50.
5. Terz JJ, Alksne JF, Lawrence W. Craniofacial resection for tumors invading the pterygoid fossa. Am J Surg. 1969;118:732-40.
6. Shah JP, Galicich JH. Craniofacial resection for malignant tumors of ethmoid and anterior skull base. Arch Otolaryngol. 1977;103:514-7.
7. Schramm VL, Myers EN, Maroon JC. Anterior skull base surgery for benign and malignant disease. Laryngoscope. 1979;89:1077-91.
8. Casson PR, Bonnano PC, Converse JM, et al. The midface degloving procedure. Plast Reconstr Surg. 1974;53(1):102-3.
9. Moure EJ. Traitement des tumors malignes primitives de l'ethmoide. Rev Laryngol Otol Rhinol (Bord). 1902;23:401-12
10. Lueg EA, Irish JC, Roth Y, et al. An objective analysis of the impact of lateral rhinotomy and medial maxillectomy on nasal airway function. Laryngoscope. 1998;108(9):1320-4.
11. Lund VJ, Harrison DF. Craniofacial resection for tumors of the nasal cavity and paranasal sinuses. Am J Surg. 1988;156:187-90.
12. Ganly I, Patel SG, Singh B, et al. Craniofacial resection for malignant paranasal sinus tumors: Report of an International Collaborative Study. Head Neck. 2005;27(7):575-84.

13. Sakashita T, Oridate N, Homma A, et al. Complications of skull base surgery: an analysis of 30 cases. Skull Base. 2009;19(2):127-32.
14. Deschler DG, Gutin PH, Mamelak AN, et al. Complications of anterior skull base surgery. Skull Base Surg. 1996;6(2):113-8.
15. Batra PS, Citardi MJ, Worley S, et al. Resection of anterior skull base tumors: comparison of combined traditional and endoscopic techniques. Am J Rhinol. 2005;19(5):521-8.
16. Nabili V, Kelly DF, Fatemi N, et al. Transnasal, transfacial, anterior skull base resection of olfactory neuroblastoma. Am J Otolaryngol; 2010.
17. Feiz-Erfan I, Han PP, Spetzler RF, et al. Preserving olfactory function in anterior craniofacial surgery through cribriform plate osteotomy applied in selected patients. Neurosurgery. 2005;57(1 Suppl):86-93.
18. Browne JD, Mims JW. Preservation of olfaction in anterior skull base surgery. Laryngoscope. 2000;110(8):1317-22.
19. McCutcheon IE, Blacklock JB, Weber RS, et al. Anterior transcranial (craniofacial) resection of tumors of the paranasal sinuses: Surgical technique and results. Neurosurgery. 1996;38:471-80.
20. Cantù G, Riccio S, Bimbi G, et al. Craniofacial resection for malignant tumours involving the anterior skull base. Eur Arch Otorhinolaryngol. 2006;263(7):647-52.
21. Nicolai P, Battaglia P, Bignami M, et al. Endoscopic surgery for malignant tumors of the sinonasal tract and adjacent skull base: a 10-year experience. Am J Rhinol. 2008;22(3):308-16.
22. Eloy JA, Vivero RJ, Hoang K, et al. Comparison of transnasal endoscopic and open craniofacial resection for malignant tumors of the anterior skull base. Laryngoscope. 2009;119(5):834-40.
23. Hanna E, DeMonte F, Ibrahim S, et al. Endoscopic resection of sinonasal cancers with and without craniotomy: oncologic results. Arch Otolaryngol Head Neck Surg. 2009;135(12):1219-24.
24. de Almeida JR, Snyderman CH, Gardner PA, et al. Nasal morbidity following endoscopic skull base surgery: A prospective cohort study. Head Neck; 2010.
25. Horiguchi K, Murai H, Hasegawa Y, et al. Endoscopic endonasal skull base reconstruction using a nasal septal flap: surgical results and comparison with previous reconstructions. Neurosurg Rev. 2010;33(2):235-41.
26. Clark DW, Citardi MJ, Fakhri S. Endoscopic management of skull base defects associated with persistent pneumocephalus following previous open repair: a preliminary report. Otolaryngol Head Neck Surg. 2010;142(6):820-6.
27. Valentine R, Wormald PJ. Controlling the surgical field during a large endoscopic vascular injury. Laryngoscope; 2010. [Epub ahead of print].
28. Lee JY, O'Malley BW Jr, Newman JG, et al. Transoral robotic surgery of the skull base: a cadaver and feasibility study. ORL J Otorhinolaryngol Relat Spec. 2010;72(4):181-7. Epub 2010.
29. Brown SM, Tabaee A, Singh A, et al. Three-dimensional endoscopic sinus surgery: feasibility and technical aspects. Otolaryngol Head Neck Surg. 2008;138(3):400-2.

12

Surgical Debate: Orbital Exenteration

Benjamin S Bleier, MD; Derrick T Lin, MD, FACS

INTRODUCTION

Since the first successful radical resection of a maxillary sinus cancer in 1828,[1] trends in the treatment of sinonasal malignancy have reflected the shift towards organ preservation and multimodality therapy seen in head and neck cancer as a whole. Optimizing management of the orbit has been a subject of intense study given the obvious functional and cosmetic deficits associated with the radical exenteration procedures popularized in the 1950s.[2] Despite profound advances in surgical instrumentation, preoperative imaging modalities, and delivery of radiotherapy, there remains a lack of consensus over the utility and indications for orbital exenteration. While no level 1 evidence exists to aid in the development of a formal therapeutic algorithm, analysis of multiple prior retrospective studies may be used to frame the discussion and identify critical areas for future investigation.

HISTORICAL APPROACH TO ORBITAL MANAGEMENT

Because of their generally late presentation, malignant sinonasal tumors are typically diagnosed at an advanced stage. Involvement of the orbit may be seen in 60–80% of maxillary and ethmoid sinus malignancies[3-5] of whom 30–50% demonstrate periorbital involvement.[4,6] Patients may complain of ocular symptoms in up to 62% of ethmoidal tumors which is consistent with their high rate of orbital invasion. These symptoms tend to correlate with tumor site and include motility disturbance (31%), afferent system dysfunction (29%), proptosis (29%), eyelid abnormalities (19%), dystopia (17%), and lacrimal outflow obstruction in 5%.[7] Perineural involvement may also occur resulting in numbness or less frequently pain in the trigeminal distribution.[8]

As the tumor spreads towards the orbit, the bone and periorbita function as effective barriers against further invasion. However once these anatomic boundaries have been transgressed, there are no natural extra or intraconal limits to continued spread throughout the orbit. With further growth, lesions may gain intracranial access through a variety of anatomic pathways including skull base foramina, neurovascular structures, or directly through bone.[9]

Surgical extirpation remains the primary mode of treatment but its value relative to other adjunctive therapies is controversial. Though first described by Bartisch in 1583,[10] orbital exenteration was not routinely performed in the setting of sinonasal malignancy until the late 1950s.[2] It was soon recognized that many of the pathologic specimens were free of disease and thus a rational approach to orbital sparing techniques began to evolve. With the introduction of computed tomography (CT) in the 1970s, surgeons were able to visualize the tumor preoperatively and evaluate the degree of bony orbital involvement to the extent afforded by the resolution of the early scans. Although imaging modalities continue to improve, their sensitivity in detecting orbital invasion remains limited. While magnetic resonance imaging (MRI) is superior to both positron emission tomography (PET) and CT in the determination of periorbital violation, it has yet to approach the sensitivity of intraoperative evaluation.[11,12]

As the use of CT gained widespread acceptance, the value of concurrent chemoradiotherapy also began to be recognized. These advances led to the proliferation and implementation of multiple orbital sparing surgical protocols.[2] While these protocols have led to a progressive diminution in the indications for exenteration there is still considerable disagreement over how to optimize management of orbital involvement.[9]

Difficulty in Interpretation of the Literature

The etiology of this debate arises from the inherent limitations of current data on orbital sparing approaches. Given the low incidence of sinonasal malignancy each study varies widely incohort size, tumor histology, site of lesion, extent of orbital involvement, surgical technique, and use of adjunctive therapies.[13] Consequently, deriving meaningful comparisons within and across studies is difficult. The data is further confounded by the lack of randomized, prospective trials. As a result while most studies compare recurrence and survival data between orbital sparing and orbital sacrificing groups, an inherent selection bias exists as the latter group will typically represent more advanced lesions whose prognosis is known to be worse a priori.[13]

Despite this uncertainty, there is some agreement with regards to management of the orbit with extensive involvement. Tumor infiltration of the extraocular musculature, involvement of bulbar conjunctiva or sclera, and full thickness retrobulbar fat invasion all represent reasonable indications for orbital sacrifice. Similarly, most authors agree that contraindications to exenteration include extensive involvement of brain parenchyma, cavernous sinus, carotid artery, bilateral optic nerves, and optic chiasm.[10]

Thus, the focus of the debate centers on the management of the orbit with only minimal bony or soft tissue involvement. Meaningful data with respect to this scenario must be gleaned from studies reporting not only oncologic results but functional outcomes as well.

Impact of Tumor and Extent of Invasion on Prognosis

A key factor influencing the argument for aggressive surgical management is data from multiple studies identifying orbital invasion as a strong and independent predictor of poor outcome. Ianetti et al.[14] established three stages of orbital invasion where Grade I represents erosion/destruction of the medial orbital wall, Grade II indicates extraconal invasion of periorbital fat, and Grade III is infiltration of the medial rectus muscle, optic nerve, ocular bulb, or the skin overlying the lid where increasing grade suggests a poorer prognosis (Figs 12.1A to D).

In a multi-institutional study of 334 patients who underwent craniofacial resection for ethmoid tumors, lack of involvement of the orbital contents was found to predict recurrence free, disease-specific, and overall survival. Disease specific survival was 41% as compared to 75% without orbital involvement.[4] Similarly, McCaffrey et al. reported that tumor grade and presence of orbital invasion were the only two independent variables adversely affecting survival in their series.[15]

In another review of 100 patients with ethmoid tumors, multivariate analysis demonstrated that involvement of orbital soft tissue was an independent

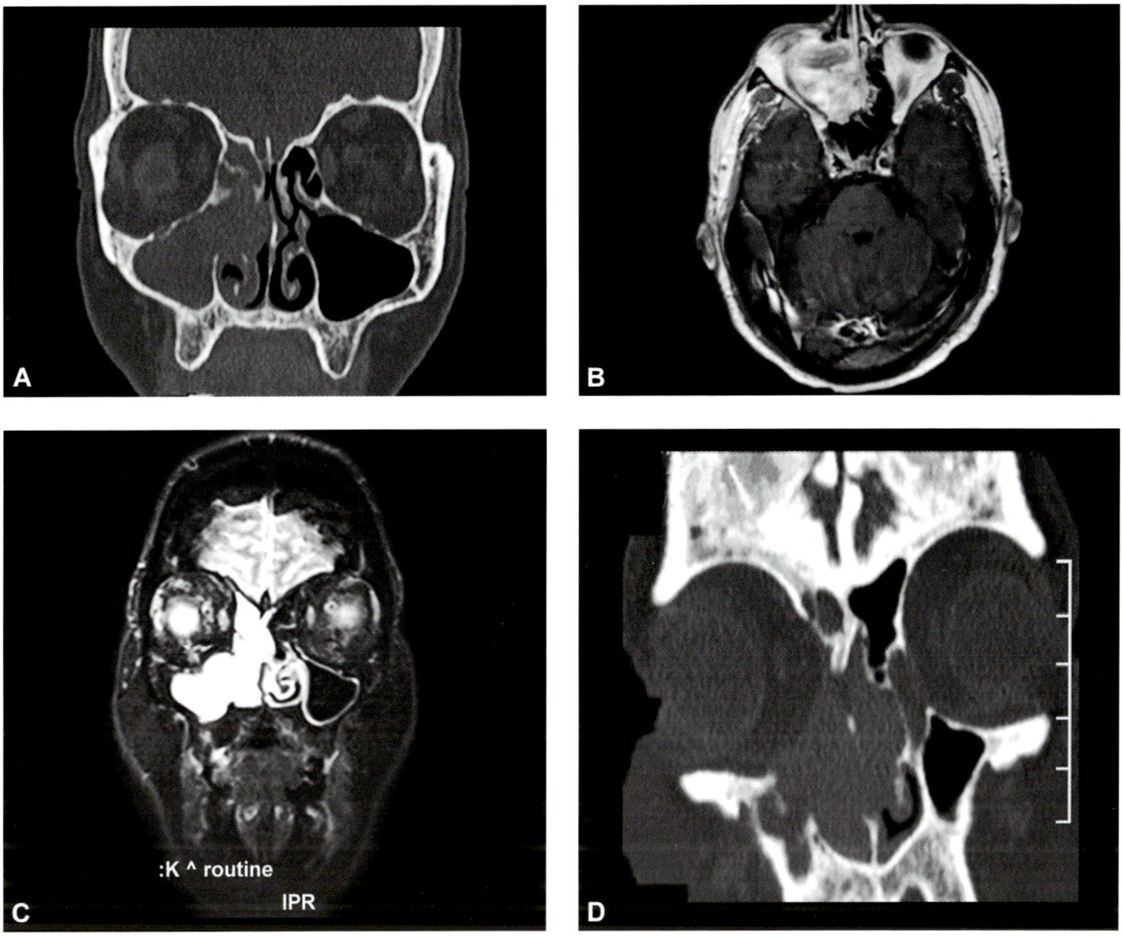

Figs 12.1A to D: Sinonasal tumors present with varying degrees of orbital involvement. (A) Poorly differentiated carcinoma adjacent to orbit with preservation of the medial and inferior bony walls; (B) High grade fibroblastic sarcoma with gross intraconal and orbital apex invasion; (C) T2-weighted MRI of invasive Squamous Cell Carcinoma Arising (SCCA) from an inverting papilloma; (D) CT of the same patient in panel C demonstrating gross bony orbital erosion. Management of orbit with this type of lesion depends on the status of the periorbita as determined at the time of surgery.

factor influencing survival however when invasion was limited to the orbital periosteum (Ianetti Grade I), survival was unchanged.[6]

Most authors have found that orbital invasion has a deleterious impact on the outcome of maxillary sinus tumors as well.[16-18] In a series of 95 tumors, Carrillo et al. reported that T4 maxillary sinus tumors with orbital involvement had a worse prognosis than other T4 tumors again establishing orbital involvement as an independent poor prognostic factor.[17] In a review of 57 patients who underwent maxillectomy, multivariate analysis confirmed that only skull base and orbital involvement were factors significantly associated with disease specific survival. Involvement of the orbit was associated with a 5-year survival of 17% as opposed to 49% in patients without invasion. Interestingly, this study also suggested that no survival benefit was achieved by orbital clearance and only 11 patients with orbital involvement remained alive after 5 years despite complete extirpation of the orbit.[18]

In a series of 259 sinonasal malignancies undergoing anterior craniofacial resection, Howard et al.[19] reported that 53 required orbital clearance while 50 underwent resection of the orbital periosteum with preservation of the eye. Five of those went on to subsequently require orbital clearance between 5 months and 4 years later. In their multivariate analysis the three most important prognostic factors were brain involvement, type of malignancy, and orbital involvement. In contrast to the prior reports, this study suggested that the decision to resect orbital periosteum alone did impact patient outcome.

Impact of Tumor Histology on Prognosis

The impact of histology on orbital invasion related survival has also been separately studied with varying results. Nishino et al.[20] reported a series of 26 patients with orbital invasion who underwent simultaneous chemoradiotherapy with preservation of orbital contents. His group found a significant differences between the 5-year overall survival rate for patients with squamous cell carcinoma (SCCA) (74%) versus patients with other histologic subtypes (40%).

Imola et al.[21] also looked at oncologic outcomes among SCCA, adenomatous carcinomas, and undifferentiated carcinoma. In contrast to Nishino, none of these groups demonstrated a significant survival difference regardless of whether they were managed by orbital preservation or orbital sacrifice.

SURGICAL RATIONALE FOR ORBITAL PRESERVATION

While these prognostic studies suggest that orbital invasion and potentially histology represent independent risk factors for poor outcome, the benefit of surgical resection is far less clear. At present, there is no consensus on the degree of orbital invasion which is safe when considering sparing of the orbital contents.[9]

Early reports called for orbital clearance in all cases with any bony orbital invasion. In a retrospective review of 111 patients with maxillary sinus tumors involving the orbital floor, 5-year survival and local recurrence rates were reported at 27.3% and 12.5% following orbital exenteration. In the orbital preservation arm, the corresponding rates were 34.8% and 8.6% with no significant differences between groups.[22]

In a less conservative approach, Carrau et al.[5] compared survival in patients with SCCA in whom orbital clearance was performed only in the setting of periorbital involvement. At 3-year follow-up 50% of patients whose orbits were cleared were alive and disease free as compared to 56% in patients whose orbital contents were preserved. The difference in rate of local recurrence (40% vs 18%) was not statistically significant. This approach is supported by another study in 53 patients with maxillary sinus SCCA in which clearance was performed in 25 patients for gross involvement of the periorbita whereas the other 28 patients were treated with orbital preservation. Again, in this study the results did not demonstrate any difference in local recurrence or actuarial survival between the orbital preservation or the orbital clearance groups.[23]

Imola et al.[21] allowed for even further invasion in their study of 66 patients in which orbital preservation was performed in all patients with tumor extension up to and including resectable periorbital involvement. Within the orbital preservation group local recurrence occurred in 30% compared to 33% in patients treated by orbital clearance. Nazar et al.[18] utilized similar criteria and reported local recurrence in 13% of patients with orbital preservation while 15% of patients who underwent orbital clearance recurred in the orbit. This study supported Imola et al. showing that preservation of the orbit does not adversely affect outcome.

Of note, these findings are contrasted by a separate retrospective study by Dulguerov et al.[24] in which 220 patients with a range of tumor stages and histologic subtypes did demonstrate improved survival when undergoing orbital clearance.

The addition and timing of adjunctive therapies has also been explored with respect to the role of orbital exenteration. Itami et al.[25] looked at local control in patients with SCCA undergoing piecemeal debulking followed by conventional fractionated XRT and found a local recurrence free survival rate at 5 years of 59%. Orbital clearance was only performed in one patient. For patients with macroscopic residual disease, at least 58 Gy was needed to improve local control. Jansen et al.[26] performed a similar study examining local control and survival in a variety of histologic subtypes. They found that 5-year local control and overall survival with combined treatment were 65% and 60% respectively compared to 47% and 9% with XRT alone. Of note the groups were not fully comparable as patients with more advanced disease tended to choose XRT alone.

While the data derived from these studies is at times conflicting, they reflect an overall trend towards orbital sparing approaches for more advanced degrees of periorbital involvement with no obvious decrement in 5-year actuarial survival or local control rates (Table 12.1).

Histologic Rationale for Orbital Preservation

Histologic studies of exenteration specimens also support the evolving role of orbital preservation. In one study of 25 cases with radiologic evidence of orbital invasion, 6 were found to require exenteration at the time of surgery. Subsequent pathologic analysis of those specimens revealed that only one demonstrated actual invasion into the orbital fat. This study also noted the presence of an additional periocular fascial layer. This plane is distinct from the periorbita and while it cannot be distinguished radiologically, it is capable of preventing further tumor spread into the eye.[27] Similarly in a retrospective review of 139 surgical specimens, it was found that the orbit could have been spared in 95% of cases using only limited periorbital dissection.[20]

Functional Outcomes in the Setting of Orbital Invasion

As organ preservation protocols have evolved for management of lesions throughout the head and neck, functional outcomes have also been recognized as a critical metric in the assessment of therapeutic success. Thus an analysis of the role of orbital sparing protocols must include an evaluation of post-treatment ocular function. An eye that is preserved anatomically may not be functionally intact secondary to a variety of factors including loss of bony support, radiation induced cataract or optic neuropathy, and exposure keratitis due to loss of eyelid or lacrimal system dysfunction.

In their study, Imola et al.[21] reported an overall functional preservation in 54% with impairment in 37% and a nonfunctional eye in 9%. The most common abnormality was globe malposition in 63% and this was associated with a lack of adequate rigid reconstruction of complete orbital floor defects. Of note, the use of adjunctive radiotherapy was associated with increased risk of ocular complications including optic atrophy, cataracts, excessive dryness, and extropion. Nishino at al.[20] reported more favorable outcomes with 73% of patients demonstrating adequate ocular function as defined by the study.

Reconstruction of the orbital floor with an intact orbit is among the most difficult challenges faced by the reconstructive surgeon. Without appropriate reconstruction of the bony floor, the orbital contents can migrate inferiorly leading to dystopia, diplopia, and an essentially nonfunctional eye.[28-30] Cordiero et al.[31] has recommended reconstruction with nonvascularized bony grafts along with vascularized locoregional flaps or free tissue transfer such as the temporalis muscle or rectus abdominis muscle, respectively. Still others have advocated the use of composite flaps including fibula, scapula, osteocutaneous forearm, and iliac crest.[32]

Anderson et al.[33] reported a 32% incidence of developing a nonfunctional eye in their series of 58 consecutive patients who underwent anterior craniofacial resection with orbital preservation and postoperative radiotherapy. Based on these relatively high impairment rates, some authors[23] have recommended strong consideration for orbital exenteration purely based on anticipated functional outcome with tumors requiring significant floor

Table 12.1 Different studies reflecting an overall trend towards orbital sparing approaches with no obvious decrement in 5-year actuarial survival or local control rates

Author	*Year*	*LOE*	*Histology*	*N(OS)*	*N(OE)*	*Adjuvent therapy*	*Surviv-al OS*	*Survivial OE*	*Local control OS*	*Local control OE*	*Comments*
Nazar et al.[18]	2004	2b	Multiple	30	16	Postoperative XRT	49%	17% ($p<0.05$)	87%	85% (NS)	Required cuff of periorbital fat for preservation
Nishino et al.[20]	2003	2b	Multiple	26		Postoperative XRT, regional 5FU	68%		66%		Required cuff of periorbital fat for preservation
Imola et al.[21]	2002	2b	Multiple	54	12	Postoperative XRT	53%	46% (NS)	70%	67% (NS)	Required cuff of periorbital fat for preservation
Carrau et al.[5]	1999	2b	SCCA	37	21	Postoperative XRT	56%	50% (NS)	60%	82% (NS)	Exentered for any perioribital involvement
Itami et al.[25]	1998	2b	SCCA	36	1	Preoperative XRT, regional 5FU			59%		Left residual gross disease in orbit
Wu et al.[22]	1995	2b	SCCA	23	88	Preoperative XRT	35%	27% (NS)	91%	87% (NS)	Exenterated for any bony invasion
Perry et al.[2]	1988	2b	Multiple	2	4	Not listed	50%	50% (NS)	50%	75% (NS)	Exentered for significant periorbital involvement

OS - Orbital Sparing, OE - Orbital Exenteration
LOE - Level of Evidence

resection or radiation fields that included the globe and optic apparatus. In the setting of exenteration, reconstruction to obliterate the orbit is essential as the defect may be quite extensive with a large volume requirement. Free tissue flaps with a muscular component such as the rectus abdominis, anterolateral thigh, or latissimus dorsi are usually used in this setting.[31]

FUTURE DIRECTIONS

In the studies available for evaluating orbital function, almost half of the ophthalmologic complications could be attributed to radiation. Consequently, evolving techniques in radiotherapy may help to further expand the role of orbital preservation.[13] In a long-term study of clinical outcomes in patients with sinonasal neoplasms treated with XRT, Chen et al.[34] found a progressive improvement in Grade III and IV toxicity in patients treated since the late 1960s. Further reductions in complications were seen with the use of three-dimensional conformal radiotherapy and intensity modulated radiotherapy.

Newer radiotherapy modalities promise to further decrease radiation-related orbital dysfunction in the setting of multi-modality orbital sparing protocols. In a retrospective review of 16 patients undergoing cyberknife image guided radiosurgery for lesions immediately adjacent to the optic nerve, 12 demonstrated either stabilization or a decrease in tumor size without sacrifice of visual acuity.[35] Similarly, Kim et al. studied 15 patients with orbital tumors treated with gamma knife and found tumor control in 12 of 15. Of these, six patients showed improvement in visual acuity while three showed deterioration.[36]

Novel chemotherapeutic regimens are also being explored which may further reduce the need for orbital exenteration. Kanoto et al.[37] described a superselective transarterial infusion with high dose cisplatin and concomitant radiotherapy in a prospective study of 15 patients with orbital invasion in the setting of maxillary sinus cancer. The study reported a pathologic complete response rate of 93.3% and 87.5% disease free survival with preservation of all orbits and local recurrence in only one patient.

Finally as endoscopic techniques progress, transnasal orbital surgery may offer alternative approaches for the management of these lesions (Figs 12.2A to C). Yoshimura et al.[38] describe an endoscopic approach to an orbital apex cavernous hemangioma in an effort to improve upon classical lateral orbitotomy, transconjunctival, and frontotemporal approaches. These methods may eventually allow for less invasive methods of periorbital and soft tissue sampling in order to clear the orbit of infiltrating tumor.

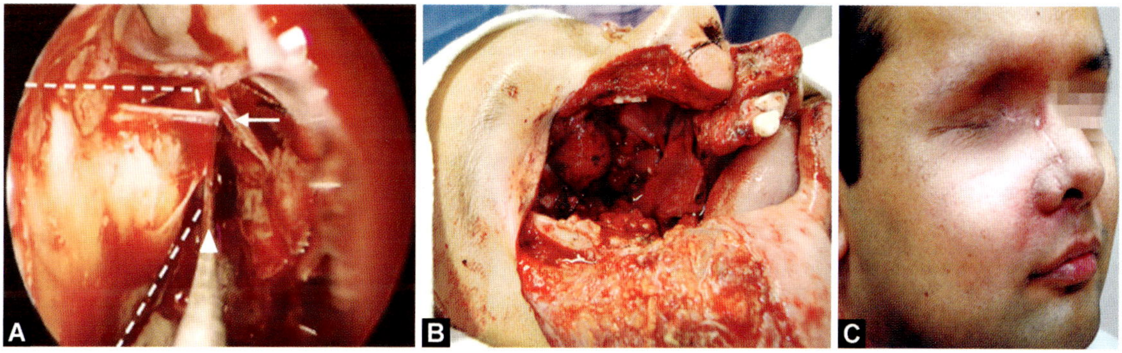

Figs 12.2A to C: (A) Endoscopic approach to the orbit (outlined in white dashed line) with controlled resection of the periorbita (white arrow); (B) Intraoperative image of an orbital exenteration in a patient with high-grade fibroblastic sarcoma; (C) Postoperative appearance of patient in panel B demonstrating a well-healed lateral rhinotomy incision.

CONCLUSION

Advances in our understanding of multimodality therapy in the treatment of sinonasal cancer has led to a shift towards organ sparing protocols in the setting of orbital invasion. However, the lack of level 1 evidence and considerable variability in management paradigms between studies have fostered continued debate with regards to the degree of invasion which may be safely managed using conservative methods. Analysis of currently available data suggests that resection of involved periorbita with negative margins on frozen section may be oncologically sound with respect to 5-year survival and local control rates. As oncologic and functional outcomes of evolving adjunctive chemoradiotherapeutic regimens improve, the indications for orbital exenteration may continue to diminish.

REFERENCES

1. Sisson GA. Symposium: 3. Treatment of malignancies of paranasal sinuses. Discussion and summary. Laryngoscope. 1970;80(6):945-53.
2. Perry C, Levine PA, Williamson BR, et al. Preservation of the eye in paranasal sinus cancer surgery. Arch Otolaryngol Head Neck Surg. 1988;114(6): 632-4.
3. Iannetti G, Valentini V, Rinna C, et al. Ethmoido-orbital tumors: our experience. J Craniofac Surg. 2005;16(6):1085-91.
4. Ganly I, Patel SG, Singh B, et al. Craniofacial resection for malignant paranasal sinus tumors: Report of an International Collaborative Study. Head Neck. 2005;27(7):575-84.
5. Carrau RL, Segas J, Nuss DW, et al. Squamous cell carcinoma of the sinonasal tract invading the orbit. Laryngoscope. 1999;109(2 Pt 1):230-5.
6. Suárez C, Llorente JL, Fernandez De Leon R, et al. Prognostic factors in sinonasal tumors involving the anterior skull base. Head Neck. 2004;26(2):136-44.
7. Stamm A, Nogueira JF. Orbital cavernous hemangioma: transnasal endoscopic management. Otolaryngol Head Neck Surg. 2009;141(6):794-5.
8. Tyers AG. Orbital exenteration for invasive skin tumours. Eye (Lond). 2006;20(10):1165-70.
9. Suárez C, Ferlito A, Lund VJ, et al. Management of the orbit in malignant sinonasal tumors. Head Neck. 2008;30(2):242-50.
10. Copcu E, Sivrioglu N, Baytekin C, et al. How can we decide on orbital exenteration for second eye in a patient with basal cell carcinoma? Plast Reconstr Surg. 2006;117(7):2512-4.
11. Kim HJ, Lee TH, Lee HS, et al. Periorbita: computed tomography and magnetic resonance imaging findings. Am J Rhinol. 2006;20(4):371-4.
12. Lane KA, Bilyk JR. Preliminary study of positron emission tomography in the detection and management of orbital malignancy. Ophthal Plast Reconstr Surg. 2006;22(5):361-5.
13. Essig GF, Newman SA, Levine PA. Sparing the eye in craniofacial surgery for superior nasal vault malignant neoplasms: analysis of benefit. Arch Facial Plast Surg. 2007;9(6):406-11.
14. Iannetti G, Valentini V, Rinna C, et al. Ethmoido-orbital tumors: our experience. J Craniofac Surg. 2005;16(6):1085-91.
15. McCaffrey TV, Olsen KD, Yohanan JM, et al. Factors affecting survival of patients with tumors of the anterior skull base. Laryngoscope. 1994;104(8 Pt 1):940-5.
16. Gullane PJ, Conley J. Carcinoma of the maxillary sinus. A correlation of the clinical course with orbital involvement, pterygoid erosion or pterygopalatine invasion and cervical metastases. J Otolaryngol. 1983;12(3):141-5.
17. Carrillo JF, Güemes A, Ramírez-Ortega MC, et al. Prognostic factors in maxillary sinus and nasal cavity carcinoma. Eur J Surg Oncol. 2005;31(10):1206-12. Epub 2005 May 31.
18. Nazar G, Rodrigo JP, Llorente JL, et al. Prognostic factors of maxillary sinus malignancies. Am J Rhinol. 2004;18(4):233-8.
19. Howard DJ, Lund VJ, Wei WI. Craniofacial resection for tumors of the nasal cavity and paranasal sinuses: a 25-year experience. Head Neck. 2006;28(10):867-73.
20. Nishino H, Ichimura K, Tanaka H, et al. Results of orbital preservation for advanced malignant maxillary sinus tumors. Laryngoscope. 2003;113(6): 1064-9.
21. Imola MJ, Schramm VL Jr. Orbital preservation in surgical management of sinonasal malignancy. Laryngoscope. 2002;112(8 Pt 1):1357-65.

22. Wu X, Tang P, Qi Y. Management of the orbital contents in radical surgery for squamous cell carcinoma of the maxillary sinus. Chin Med J (Engl). 1995;108(2):123-5.
23. Stern SJ, Goepfert H, Clayman G, et al. Orbital preservation in maxillectomy. Otolaryngol Head Neck Surg. 1993;109(1):111-5.
24. Dulguerov P, Jacobsen MS, Allal AS, et al. Nasal and paranasal sinus carcinoma: are we making progress? A series of 220 patients and a systematic review. Cancer. 2001;92(12):3012-29.
25. Itami J, Uno T, Aruga M, et al. Squamous cell carcinoma of the maxillary sinus treated with radiation therapy and conservative surgery. Cancer. 1998;82(1):104-7.
26. Jansen EP, Keus RB, Hilgers FJ, et al. Does the combination of radiotherapy and debulking surgery favor survival in paranasal sinus carcinoma? Int J Radiat Oncol Biol Phys. 2000;48(1):27-35.
27. Tiwari R, van der Wal J, van der Waal I, et al. Studies of the anatomy and pathology of the orbit in carcinoma of the maxillary sinus and their impact on preservation of the eye in maxillectomy. Head Neck. 1998;20(3):193-6.
28. Swartz WM, Banis JC. Orbital Maxillary Reconstruction. In WM Schwartz and JC Banis (Eds). Head and Neck Microsurgery. Baltimore: Williams & Wilkins; 1990. p. 225.
29. Cordiero PG, Santamaria E, Kraus D, et al. Reconstruction of Total Maxillary Defects with Preservation of Orbital Contents. Plast Reconstr Surg. 1998;102:1874.
30. Shusterman MA. Reconstruction of Total Maxillectomy Defects with Preservation of Orbital Contents (Discussion). Plast Reconstr Surg. 1998;102: 1885.
31. Cordiero PG, Santamaria E. A Classification System and Algorithm for Reconstruction of Maxillectomy and Midfacial Defects. Plast Reconstr Surg. 2000;105:2331-46.
32. Brown J, Shaw R. Reconstruction of the Maxilla and Midface: Introducing a New Classification. Lancet Oncol. 2010;11:1001-8.
33. Anderson PE, Kraus DH, Arbit E, et al. Management of the orbit during anterior fossa craniofacial resection. Arch Otolaryngol Head Neck Surg. 1996;122(12):1305-7.
34. Chen AM, Daly ME, Bucci MK, et al. Carcinomas of the paranasal sinuses and nasal cavity treated with radiotherapy at a single institution over five decades: are we making improvement? Int J Radiat Oncol Biol Phys. 2007;69(1):141-7. Epub 2007 Apr 24.
35. Hirschbein MJ, Collins S, Jean WC, et al. Treatment of intraorbital lesions using the Accuray Cyberknife system. Orbit. 2008;27(2):97-105.
36. Kim MS, Park K, Kim JH, et al. Gamma knife radiosurgery for orbital tumors. Clin Neurol Neurosurg. 2008;110(10):1003-7.
37. Kanoto M, Oda A, Hosoya T, et al. Impact of superselective transarterial infusion therapy of high-dose cisplatin on maxillary cancer with orbital invasion. AJNR Am J Neuroradiol. 2010;31(8): 1390-4.
38. Yoshimura K. Removal of a cavernous hemangioma in the orbital apex via the endoscopic transnasal approach: a case report. Minim Invasive Neurosurg. 2010;53(2):77-9.

13

Management of the Neck in Sinonasal Malignancy

Lindsay S Reder, MD; Niels Kokot, MD

INTRODUCTION

Cancer of the nose and paranasal sinuses is rare, accounting for approximately 3–6% of all head and neck cancers. Types of malignancy that occur in this site are most commonly squamous cell carcinoma (SCC), with significantly less adenocarcinoma, minor salivary gland malignancies, and non-epithelial carcinomas such as sarcomas, lymphomas, neuroendocrine malignancies and melanoma. Treatment modalities vary depending on tumor type, location, and extent of disease and include surgery, radiation, chemotherapy and a combination of two or more modalities.

Discussion of cancer of the sinonasal cavity and its management is complicated by several factors. For example, the rarity of cancer in this location limits large, prospective, multicenter trials. Therefore, many of the published reports both in the Otolaryngology as well as the Radiation and Medical Oncology literatures are retrospective, single center reviews, often with a small sample size. Additionally, the diversity of tumor types limits comparison, as inherent tumor characteristics and metastatic features vary between types of malignancies. This can be demonstrated by the American Joint Committee on Cancer (AJCC) staging for cancer of the paranasal sinuses (Table 13.1). The AJCC stages sinonasal tumors by location of primary site, separating site into maxillary sinus or in the nasal cavity/ethmoid sinuses. Of note, these include only epithelial tumor types, so malignant processes such as lymphoma, mesenchymal tumors and melanoma are not included in this staging system. Other tumor subtypes have staging systems of their own, however none are universally accepted. The 7th edition of the AJCC Cancer staging handbook, however, does propose a staging system for mucosal melanoma of the head and neck, which may become more universally accepted (Table 13.2). Olfactory neuroblastoma (also referred to as esthesioneuroblastoma), over the years, has had several staging systems proposed, the most well known are the Kadish system and the Dulguerov Classification (Table 13.3). The Kadish staging system was originally based solely on clinical presentation and tumor location, whereas the Dulguerov Classification relies on examination as well as radiographic findings, and also takes regional disease into consideration. Several groups who have published institutional data of this subset of patients over the last decade have suggested there should be a standardized staging system, and assert that the Dulguerov Classification is the most inclusive and has solid

Table 13.1 TNM staging for epithelial tumors of the nasal cavity and paranasal sinuses

Primary Tumor (T)

TX	Primary tumor cannot be assessed
T0	No evidence of primary tumor
Tis	Carcinoma *in situ*
Maxillary Sinus	
T1	Tumor limited to maxillary sinus mucosa with no erosion or destruction of bone
T2	Tumor causing bone erosion or destruction including extension into the hard palate and/or middle nasal meatus, except extension to posterior wall of maxillary sinus and pterygoid plates
T3	Tumor invades any of the following: bone of the posterior wall of maxillary sinus, subcutaneous tissues, floor or medial wall of orbit, pterygoid fossa, ethmoid sinuses
T4a	Tumor invades anterior orbital contents, skin of cheek, pterygoid plates, infratemporal fossa, cribriform plate, sphenoid or frontal sinuses
T4b	Tumor invades any of the following: orbital apex, dura, brain, middle cranial fossa, cranial nerves other than maxillary division of trigeminal nerve (V2), nasopharynx, or clivus
Nasal Cavity and Ethmoid Sinus	
T1	Tumor restricted to any one subsite, with or without bony invasion
T2	Tumor invading two subsites in a single region or extending to involve an adjacent region within the nasoethmoidal complex, with or without bony invasion
T3	Tumor extends to invade the medial wall or floor of the orbit, maxillary sinus, palate, or cribriform plate
T4a	Tumor invades any of the following: anterior orbital contents, skin of nose or cheek, minimal extension to anterior cranial fossa, pterygoid plates, sphenoid or frontal sinuses
T4b	Tumor invades any of the following: orbital apex, dura, brain, middle cranial fossa, cranial nerves other than (V2), nasopharynx, or clivus
Regional Lymph Nodes (N)	
NX	Regional lymph nodes cannot be assessed
N0	No regional lymph node metastasis
N1	Metastasis in a single ipsilateral lymph node, 3 cm or less in greatest dimension
N2	Metastasis in a single ipsilateral lymph node, more than 3 cm but not more than 6 cm in greatest dimension, or in multiple ipsilateral lymph nodes, none more than 6 cm in greatest dimension, or in bilateral or contralateral lymph nodes, none more than 6 cm in greatest dimension
N2a	Metastasis in a single ipsilateral lymph node, more than 3 cm but not more than 6 cm in greatest dimension
N2b	Metastasis in multiple ipsilateral lymph nodes, none more than 6 cm in greatest dimension
N2c	Metastasis in bilateral or contralateral lymph nodes, none more than 6 cm in greatest dimension
N3	Metastasis in a lymph node, more than 6 cm in greatest dimension
Distant Metastasis (M)	
M0	No distant metastasis
M1	Distant metastasis

ANATOMIC STAGE/PROGNOSTIC GROUPS

Stage 0	Tis	N0	M0
Stage I	T1	N0	M0
Stage II	T2	N0	M0
Stage III	T3	N0	M0
	T1–T3	N1	M0
Stage IVA	T4a	Any N	M0
	T1–T3	N2	M0
Stage IVB	T4b	Any N	M0
	Any T	N3	M0
Stage IVC	Any T	Any N	M1

Source: AJCC. The AJCC Cancer Staging Manual, 7th edition. In: Edge SB, Byrd DR, Compton CC, et al. (Eds). New York: Spinger; 2010. pp. 93-102.

Table 13.2 AJCC Staging for mucosal melanoma of the head and neck

Primary Tumor

T3	Mucosal disease
T4a	Moderately advanced disease Tumor involving deep soft tissue, cartilage, bone, or overlying skin
T4b	Very advanced disease Tumor involving brain, dura, skull base, lower cranial nerves (IX, X, XI, XII), masticator space, carotid artery, prevertebral space, or mediastinal structures

Regional Lymph Nodes

NX	Regional lymph nodes cannot be assessed
N0	No regional lymph node metastases
N1	Regional lymph node metastases present

Distant Metastasis

M0	No distant metastasis
M1	Distant metastasis present

ANATOMIC STAGE/PROGNOSTIC GROUPS

Stage III	T3	N0	M0
Stage IVA	T4a	N0	M0
	T3–T4a	N1	M0
Stage IVB	T4b	Any N	M0
Stage IVC	Any T	Any N	M1

Source: AJCC. The AJCC Cancer Staging Manual, 7th edition. In: Edge SB, Byrd DR, Compton CC, et al. (Eds). New York: Spinger; 2010. pp. 123-6.

Table 13.3 Olfactory neuroblastoma staging systems

Kadish Staging System

A	Tumor limited to the nasal cavity
B	Tumor involving the nasal and paranasal cavities
C	Tumor extends beyond the nasal and paranasal cavities (Kadish SM, Goodman, Wang CC, et al. Olfactory neuroblastoma. A clinical analysis of 17 cases. Cancer. 1976;37(3):1571-6)

Dulguerov Classification

T1	Tumor involving the nasal cavity and/or paranasal sinuses (excluding sphenoid), sparing the most superior ethmoidal cells
T2	Tumor involving the nasal cavity and/or paranasal sinuses (including the sphenoid) with extension to or erosion of the cribriform plate
T3	Tumor extending into the orbit or protruding into the anterior cranial fossa, without dural invasion
T4	Tumor involving the brain
N1	Any form of cervical lymph-node metastasis
M0	No metastases
M1	Distant metastasis (Dulguerov P, Calcaterra T. "Esthesioneuroblastoma: the UCLA experience 1970-1990." Laryngoscope. 1992;102(8):843-9)

prognostic value.[1,2] Staging of the neck has been included in most staging systems, however unlike other head and neck malignancies, staging of the neck in sinonasal tumors has not necessarily brought about a standardized treatment regimen for cervical lymph nodes.

Recurrence of malignancies in the head and neck, including those in the nose and paranasal sinuses, is usually related to local failure; however recurrence can also occur due to regional and distant metastasis. There has been little consensus on treatment of the cervical lymph nodes in malignancies of the sinonasal cavity, largely due to the low incidence of these diseases and subsequent difficulty conducting large research protocols to evaluate treatment modalities. Nevertheless, management of the cervical lymphatics is a critical aspect of treatment in individuals with nasal/paranasal sinus tumors.

This chapter will discuss the anatomy of the cervical lymphatics and surgical landmarks for lymph node levels and neck dissection. This will be followed by an overview of treatment of both the node-negative (N0) and node-positive (N+) neck for epithelial and non-epithelial tumors that occur in the nose and paranasal sinuses. Finally nasopharyngeal carcinoma will be discussed separately since it occurs more commonly, and it is treated somewhat differently than many sinonasal tumors.

ANATOMY: LYMPHATICS OF HEAD AND NECK

The lymphatic drainage of the face is extensive and redundant; however malignant spread via lymphatics has been well characterized over time. The network of lymphatics of the head and neck first drain into the superficial nodes at various locations where the head and neck convene. These first echelon nodes are named for their location (occipital, retroauricular, parotid, submandibular, submental, and retropharyngeal), and they continue to drain into the deeper jugulodigastric lymph nodes.[3]

Over the last 20 years, the classification of cervical lymph node levels has been described and updated based on reports of metastasis of various head and neck malignancies. In conjunction with the American Academy of Otolaryngology – Head and Neck Surgery's Committee for Head and Neck Surgery and Oncology, Robbins et al. initially published a statement article in 1991 to standardize neck dissection terminology, and it was followed up with an update in 2002 that further subdivided the neck levels. This standardization incorporates surgical and radiological anatomical landmarks to allow surgeons, oncologists and radiologists to communicate clearly, and allows for treatment protocols to be standardized based on disease extent. Table 13.4 and Figures 13.1 and 13.2 describes the lymphatic levels and the head and neck primary sites that commonly drain to each level, as described in the updated report published in 2002.[4,5] Briefly, level I is composed of the submental and submandibular lymph nodes, levels II–IV are the jugulodigastric nodes, and level V includes the posterior triangle nodes.

The retropharyngeal lymph nodes are not included in the conventional classification of cervical lymph nodes. However, an understanding of their anatomy and the drainage patterns is essential during this discussion, as there appears

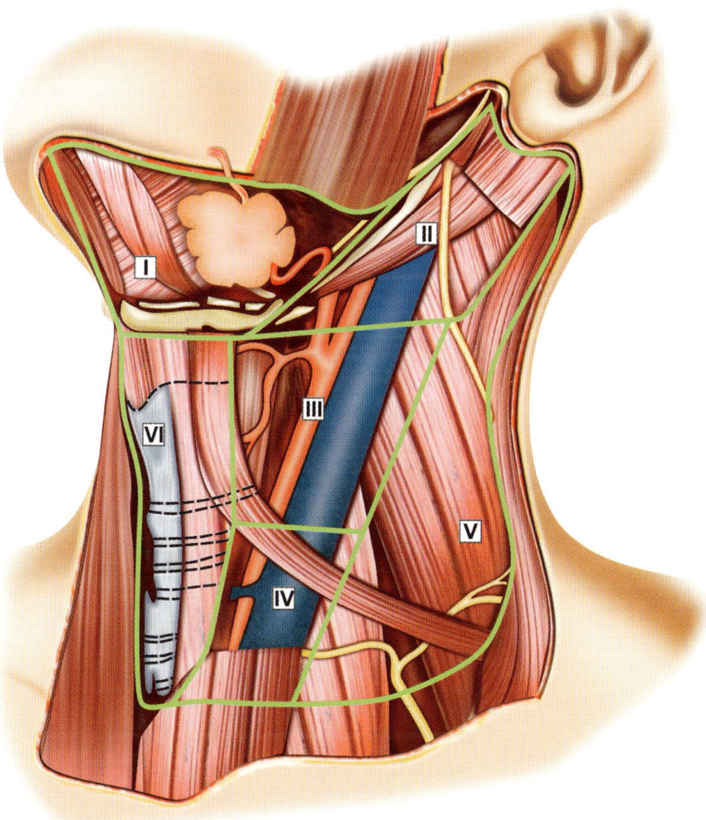

Fig. 13.1: The six levels of the neck.

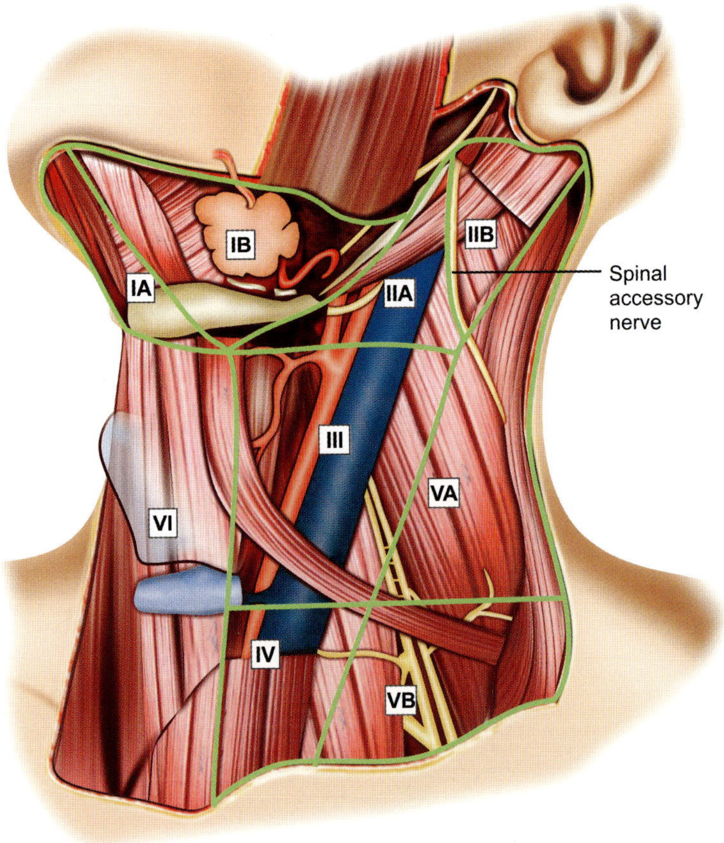

Fig. 13.2: The six sublevels of the neck.

to be a consensus that this group of nodes is likely the first drainage basin for the lymphatics of the sinonasal tract.[6,7] Classically the retropharyngeal lymph nodes have been described as consisting of six nodes in two columns (a medial and a lateral column) on each side of the retropharynx.[8] Over the last 50 years, little work has been published looking specifically at this area. In order to improve our understanding of the lymphatic channels of the nose and paranasal sinuses, and as a result of availability of improved technology, Pan et al. performed an anatomical study to examine the lymphatic drainage of the nasal fossae and nasopharynx. Using human cadaver heads, their study described the lymphatic drainage of the nasal cavity as follows: Lymphatic channels begin in the mucous membranes at various sites within the nasal cavity (atrium, three turbinates, nasal floor), form a network and drain into a precollector system that further drains into lymph basins in the lateral wall of the nasopharynx. These channels then form two lymph collectors that pass along the lateral pharyngeal wall into the parapharyngeal fat tissue. From this point the channels converge, then divide into a lateral and a medial vessel. The lateral vessel drains into the lateral pharyngeal lymph node, which is found on the lateral side of the external carotid artery at the origin of the facial artery. The medial vessel eventually divides again into two vessels, one enters the lateral pharyngeal lymph node, and the other divides again into an anterior branch and a posterior branch. The anterior branch again enters the lateral pharyngeal lymph node, and the posterior branch drains into a retropharyngeal lymph

Table 13.4 The lymphatic levels, and the head and neck primary sites that commonly drain into the levels

Lymph node level	*Anatomical boundaries*	*Metastastic risk*	
IA, Submental	Symphysis of Mandible Body of Hyoid Anterior bellies of bilateral Digastric muscles	Floor of mouth Anterior oral tongue Lower lip	Anterior mandibular alveolar ridge
IB, Submandibular	Body of Mandible Anterior and posterior bellies of ipsilateral Digastric Stylohyoid muscle Submandibular gland included in specimen	Oral cavity Anterior nasal cavity Midfacial soft tissues Submandibular gland	
IIA, Upper jugular (anterior)	Skull base Horizontal line defined by inferior border of Hyoid body Styloid muscle (anterior border) * Vertical line defined by CN XI (posterior border)	Oral cavity Nasal cavity Nasopharynx Hypopharynx	Larynx Parotid gland
IIB, Upper jugular (posterior)	Skull base Horizontal line defined by inferior border of Hyoid body Vertical line defined by CN XI (anterior border) Lateral border of SCM	Oral cavity Nasal cavity Nasopharynx Hypopharynx	Larynx Parotid gland
III, Middle jugular	Horizontal line defined by inferior border of Hyoid body Horizontal line defined by inferior border Cricoid cartilage Lateral border of Sternohyoid muscle Lateral border of SCM/sensory branches of cervical plexus	Oral cavity Nasopharynx Oropharynx Hypopharynx	Larynx
IV, Lower jugular	Horizontal line defined by inferior border Cricoid cartilage Clavicle Lateral border of Sternohyoid muscle Lateral border of SCM/sensory branches of cervical plexus	Hypopharynx Thyroid Cervical esophagus Larynx	
VA, Posterior triangle (superior) (Spinal accessory nodes)	Apex of convergence of SCM and Trapezius muscles Horizontal line defined by inferior border Cricoid cartilage Lateral border of SCM/sensory branches of cervical plexus Anterior border of Trapezius muscle	Nasopharynx Orophyarynx Posterior scalp/neck skin	
VB, Posterior triangle (inferior) (TCA and supra-clavicular nodes)	Horizontal line defined by inferior border Cricoid cartilage Clavicle Lateral border of SCM/sensory branches of cervical plexus Anterior border of Trapezius muscle	Nasopharynx Oropharynx Posterior scalp/neck skin	
VI, Anterior compartment	Hyoid bone Sternal notch Bilateral Common Carotid arteries	Thyroid Larynx (glottic and supraglottic)	Pyriform sinus apex Cervical esophagus

CN, Cranial Nerve; SCM, Sternocleidomastoid muscle; TCA, transverse cervical artery

** Radiological border defined by vertical line at posterior border of Submandibular gland*

Adapted from (Robbins, Clayman, Levine, et al. 2002)

Robbins KT, Clayman G, Levine PA, et al. Neck dissection classification update: revisions proposed by the American Head and Neck Society and the American Academy of Otolaryngology-Head and Neck Surgery. Arch Otolaryngol Head Neck Surg. 2002;128(7):751-8.

node. The study continued to describe the pattern of the lymphatics in the nasopharynx, which first drains into a retropharyngeal lymph node.[9]

The lymphatics of the anterior nasal cavity drain along the pathway of the skin of the nose and end in the area of the submandibular gland (anterior drainage pathway). The lymphatic drainage of the middle and posterior nasal cavity as well as the paranasal sinuses drain both through the nasopharynx to the retropharyngeal group of lymph nodes as well as to the superior jugulodigastric nodal group (posterior drainage pathway).

Rates of Cervical Lymph Node Metastasis

Paranasal sinus tumors of the epithelial type include SCC, adenocarcinoma, and minor salivary gland malignancies (most commonly adenoid cystic and mucoepidermoid carcinomas). Of these, the most common type is SCC, and the most common site is in the maxillary sinus. The literature varies in reports of histologic types and location, with quotes of 44–92% of tumors being of the SCC type. The range is attributed to geographical location of the patient population as well as sample size. The most common site of occurrence is the maxillary sinus, making up 46–62% of paranasal tumors. Rates of cervical metastasis from SCC have been reported in the 8–12% range at initial presentation and up to 33% at recurrence.[10-17]

There are few studies that look at other epithelial subtypes and their specific rates of regional metastasis. Adenocarcinoma is rarer; most centers report less than 12% incidence in their populations, however two centers in Europe found 46% and 24% of patients in their cohorts.[10,11] Le et al. reported 25% risk of nodal involvement (inclusive of N+ and recurrence), however most other authors report 2–20% risk of lymph node metastasis.[11,14,16,17] Salivary gland malignancies of the nose/paranasal sinuses are even rarer. Minor salivary gland malignancies, such as adenoid cystic and mucoepidermoid carcinomas, comprise less than 10% of tumors in most studies. However, Cantu et al. found salivary gland tumors in 20% of their set.[11] There are few studies that isolate lymph node involvement specifically for minor salivary gland histology types, but the few that do report no more than 5% of patients with salivary gland histologies have nodal involvement upon presentation and up to 10% experience lymph node metastasis at some point during the disease.[11,14,16]

Several tumor types deserve mention that do not fall into the more common epithelial subtypes mentioned above: neuroendocrine tumors, mucosal melanoma, and sarcomas. Sinonasal neuroendocrine tumors represent a spectrum of carcinoma, which includes olfactory neuroblastoma, neuroendocrine carcinoma, and according to some sources, sinonasal undifferentiated carcinoma.[18] These tumors arise from the cells of the neuroepithelium, and develop exclusively from the nasal cavity and ethmoid sinuses. These neuroendocrine tumors are responsible for 3–5% of sinonasal malignancies, although some propose that they may be under diagnosed due to confusion with other subtypes.[19] Sinonasal undifferentiated carcinoma comprises 5–20% of tumor types and has been shown in several studies to have up to 50% rate of cervical lymph node involvement. Olfactory neuroblastoma has been shown to have cervical lymph node metastasis at presentation or recurrence in 5–33% of patients. In their meta-analysis that included 390 patients, Dulguerov et al. found 5% cervical node involvement at presentation and 16% of subjects recurred in the neck. However, individual studies have quoted up to 33% of lymph node involvement at some point during the disease.[1,2,19,20] Mucosal melanoma is responsible for less than 10% of all head and neck melanomas and less than 1% of all melanomas reported in Western countries. Several large series (N= 42–160) out of the United States and Europe all report the most common location of mucosal melanomas of the head and neck is in the sinonasal cavity with 54–90% of patients presenting with lesions in this area.[21-26] Until the most recent AJCC Cancer Staging Manual update,[27] staging of mucosal melanoma was most commonly categorized using the

Ballantyne clinical staging system. The Ballantyne classification[28] includes all melanoma of the head and neck (cutaneous, ocular and mucosal) and is dependent on site of disease, with Stage I being confined to the primary site, Stage II with cervical lymph node metastasis and Stage III with distant metastasis. The most recent AJCC staging system attempts to stage this entity like other tumors in the TNM classification. Given its aggressive nature, the lowest stage is Stage III, and involvement of regional lymph nodes is seen in Stage IV disease (see Table 13.2). The rate of cervical lymph node metastasis (based on the conventional Ballantyne system, i.e. Stage II) has been reported as 1–8% at presentation and up to 20% at recurrence.[22,24,29] Most authorities agree that mucosal melanoma, like its cutaneous counterpart, is more likely to metastasize hematogenously, but cervical lymph node involvement should not be dismissed.

Sarcomas of the head and neck are also rare, comprising approximately 5–15% of all sarcomas, but only 1% of all head and neck malignancies.[30,31] The incidence of sarcomas of the nose and paranasal sinus has been reported in up to 28% of all head and neck sarcomas. However, the large retrospective analysis that had this high percentage included esthesioneuroblastoma in their analysis, an entity that currently is classified separately. Other reports quote the frequency of sarcomas arising in the nose and paranasal sinuses at 7–25%.[31,32] Sinonasal sarcomas are most commonly derived from bone (chondrosarcoma, osteosarcoma) and fibroblasts (fibrosarcoma, malignant fibrous histiocytoma), and in pediatric populations rhabdomyosarcoma is frequently seen. Additionally, there are reports of various vascular sarcomas, neural-derived sarcomas, Ewing's sarcoma and post-irradiation sarcomas arising in the sinonasal tract. Cervical lymph node metastasis from all sarcomas of the head and neck has been seen in up to 8% of subjects. There are few published reports looking exclusively at sinonasal sarcomas; Koka et al. retrospectively looked at their institution's population of patients with osteosarcoma, chondrosarcoma or fibrosarcoma of the nose/paranasal sinuses and found that no patients presented with cervical lymph node involvement, and 4.7% of their cohort had recurrence in the neck.[33] Rhabdomyosarcoma is noted to be the most common malignancy of the sinonasal tract in the pediatric population, but can be seen in adults as well.[34,35] Several authorities note a relatively high rate of regional metastasis in rhabdomyosarcomas of the head and neck, and studies examining rhabdomyosarcoma in the nose and paranasal sinuses, cervical lymph node metastasis has been seen in 15–38% of patients.[31,35,36]

Treatment of the Node-Negative (N0) Neck

Head and neck oncologists have established a treatment paradigm to address the cervical lymphatics when the risk of cervical lymph node metastasis is equal to or greater than 20%.[37] This includes the risk upon presentation in addition to the risk of recurrent disease involving lymph node metastasis. The reasoning for this model, in short, is that there has been well documented evidence that cervical lymph node involvement, either on presentation or recurrence, leads to poorer outcomes and should therefore be treated aggressively.[11,14-16,38] Although most of the studies that established this model were based on oral and oropharyngeal cancers, the data have been extrapolated to become the standard for most head and neck malignancies.

Consensus has not been established for treatment of the clinically negative (N0) neck. Overall, the rate of cervical metastasis from sinonasal tumors has been quoted as 8–14%, but as described above, the numbers vary widely depending on histological type.[39-41] The dilemma in decision-making for treatment of the neck is largely due to the rarity of cancers in the sinonasal cavity and therefore the lack of randomized controlled studies comparing various treatments and no treatment. Historically, most centers did not recommend elective treatment of the neck for sinonasal tumors due to reportedly low rate of lymph node metastasis in multiple studies. Between 1991 and 2000 however, three multidisciplinary groups in the United States published retrospective data of patients with maxillary sinus malignancies and evaluated each tumor type, lymph node involvement, and survival data. Jiang and his collaborators showed that while only 8% of all patients initially presented with nodal involvement, 22% of patients that were initially staged N0 and were not electively treated recurred in the neck. This was further broken down into tumor type, and in their population 33% of patients that were initially N0 with SCC and 50% of patients with SNUC had recurrence in the neck. The rates of lymph node metastasis from other tumor types such as adenocarcinoma and salivary gland malignancies remained low. They concluded, therefore, that patients with SCC or SNUC histologies should have elective neck treatment of at least the ipsilateral neck for T2-4 maxillary sinus carcinomas.[16] Similarly, Paulino and colleagues reported nearly 30% of patients with SCC of the maxillary sinus had regional lymph node recurrence. Furthermore, the patients with T1 and T2 tumors actually had a higher propensity to develop lymph node metastasis than T3-4 tumors (although the numbers of T1-2 tumors was small), so they concluded that all patients with SCC of the maxillary sinus should have elective treatment of the ipsilateral neck.[15] Finally, Le et al. found an overall risk at diagnosis or recurrence of lymph node metastasis in the cohort with SCC of 28%. All patients with cervical lymph node involvement had T3 or T4 tumors. Additionally, for those who presented with an N0 neck, the 5-year risk of recurrence in the neck for those that did not receive treatment was 20%, versus 0% of patients who had elective treatment of the neck.[14] All three studies also show significantly decreased survival for those that relapse in the neck, further supporting the role of elective neck treatment. Since then, several Head and Neck surgeons and multidisciplinary groups have published institutional studies and have evaluated both tumor type and tumor site and risk of metastasis to cervical lymphatics. Elective irradiation of the neck is generally given at a dose of 45–50 Gy.[42]

Although not including sinonasal or nasopharyngeal tumors in their cohorts, there are various reports that involvement or recurrence in the retropharyngeal nodes in patients with head and neck cancer may lead to worse results. Several groups have proposed addressing the retropharyngeal nodes either during resection of the primary site or with radiotherapy for other head and neck malignancies based on significant findings or trends toward poorer outcomes.[43,44]

To summarize, there appears to be a role for elective neck treatment for SCC and SNUC originating in the maxillary sinus, and there is some evidence for treatment of the N0 neck for SNUC at any site. The treatment modality can be determined by the treatment modality for the primary site. In other words, if surgery is most appropriate for managing the primary site or a free flap reconstruction will be required, a neck dissection (possibly also addressing the retropharyngeal nodes) should be planned. If radiation or chemoradiotherapy is the primary treatment, or will be given in the adjuvant setting, then at least the ipsilateral neck and retropharyngeal nodes should be included in the radiation field. In this situation, if there is no reason to open the neck (i.e. to isolate vessels for micorvascular reconstruction), then the neck will be addressed with non-surgical therapy. On the other hand, other histologic types such as adenocarcinoma and adenoid cystic carcinoma originating from the ethmoid sinuses, seldom (up to 5%) present with lymph node metastasis either at presentation or as a recurrence so few advocate for elective treatment of the neck. As mentioned above, risk of metastasis varies based on tumor type and histology and each case should be considered individually considering tumor type, location and stage. The decision-making process to manage the N0 neck should be made in a multi-disciplinary manner.

Treatment of the Node-Positive Neck

There is little doubt that positive cervical lymph node metastasis found on presentation should be treated, as there is copious evidence that cervical node involvement or failure in the regional lymph nodes portends a worse prognosis. Management options of cervical metastasis include surgery, usually at the time of the primary site resection, as well as definitive or adjuvant irradiation. Additionally, if the cervical lymph nodes show high-risk features, the addition of chemotherapy may also be considered. Surgical management generally includes neck dissection of levels I–III or levels I–IV, as the first echelon of lateral cervical lymph nodes will be levels I and II. However, more complete modified radical or radical neck dissections should be performed if there are clinically positive nodes in other anatomical levels, or if disease is extensive. The standard selective or modified radical neck dissection does not address the retropharyngeal lymph nodes. Since, lymph drainage of the nasal cavity and paranasal sinuses is known to drain into the retropharyngeal nodes, there may be an argument for extended dissection, either during resection of the primary site or neck dissection to investigate the retropharyngeal nodes. Several authors have described retropharyngeal lymph node dissection in recent literature. Briefly, the retropharyngeal space can be accessed via the standard neck dissection incision with or without a mandibulectomy or mandibulotomy. With a mandibulotomy, the space is entered above the posterior belly of the digastric and styloid muscle group; without mandibular incision these muscles require division to access the retropharyngeal space. The nodes are found in the fascia between the pharyngeal wall medially and internal carotid artery laterally; the dissection begins from inferiorly at the level of the tongue base and proceeds superiorly toward the skull base.[43,45] Depending on the tumor type and stage, irradiation of the cervical lymph nodes can be a definitive treatment, but more commonly is given adjuvantly in the postoperative setting. There is a role, however, for definitive radiotherapy especially if the primary site will also be definitively treated with radiation therapy. Radiotherapy usually entails around 70 Gy to bilateral neck regions in the case of definitive treatment, and the retropharyngeal lymph nodes can be included in the radiation fields.[42] Indications for postoperative radiotherapy follow suit with other head and neck malignancies. Relative indications for postoperative radiotherapy to the neck include one lymph node positive, while two or more positive lymph nodes is generally considered an absolute indication for postoperative radiotherapy. Level I evidence was published by two large groups in 2004 in an effort to standardize treatment of cervical metastasis in head and neck cancer. The United States Radiation Therapy Oncology Group (RTOG) and the European Organization Research and Treatment of Cancer (EORTC) separately performed randomized trials to compare postoperative treatment of cervical lymph nodes using radiation alone or concomitant chemoradiotherapy. Although these trials looked at patients with SCC, most of whom had primary disease in the oral cavity, oropharynx, hypopharynx and larynx, the evidence for postoperative treatment has been extrapolated to include most head and neck malignancies. In regards to regional lymphatic involvement, the ROTG trial included histologic evidence of invasion of two or more regional lymph nodes and extracapsular extension of nodal disease as high-risk characteristics.[46,47] Patients who received chemoradiation had improved locoregional control and disease-free survival. EORTC considered patients with high-risk neck disease to have level IV or V lymph nodes (oral cavity and oropharyngeal primary tumors) or extracapsular extension. When the data was pooled, the combined analysis showed that only extracapsular extension is an indication for postoperative chemoradiation.[48]

Nasopharyngeal Carcinoma

Nasopharyngeal carcinoma (NPC) is included in this discussion as disease in the neck is common and requires treatment. Early stage NPC is usually treated with radiation therapy alone to the primary tumor and the neck. The standard of care treatment for advanced NPC in the United States was established based on results of Intergroup-0099

(INT-0099) phase III trial, which found benefit from the addition of chemotherapy to radiation with respect to rates of recurrence, distant metastasis and overall survival. The treatment regimen consists of concurrent chemoradiotherapy (CCRT) consisting of fractionated radiotherapy to a total of 70 Gy with concurrent cisplatin and postoperative cisplatin plus 5-fluorouracil for three cycles.[49] There has been controversy in carrying out this management in Asia, where NPC is much more prevalent, however, recent studies appear to confirm the findings of INT-0099 and uphold the use of CCRT in endemic areas.[50,51]

Cervical node metastasis occurs in up to 75% of patients with NPC and a large proportion present with the initial complaint of a neck mass.[52] The first echelon of lymph nodes that drain the nasopharynx are the retropharyngeal lymph nodes, however these are usually not detectable upon initial physical examination. Lymphatic drainage of the nasopharynx then continues both via the retropharyngeal path and also via direct channels to the jugulodigastric level II and level V lymph nodes, and can then continue to involve the lower jugulodigastric nodes. There are several different staging classifications of nodal involvement in NPC, all based on clinical exam and therefore do not take the retropharyngeal group into consideration. Table 13.5 summarizes several staging systems of nodal disease in NPC. The AJCC/UICC systems highlight laterality and size of nodes. Similarly, the Huang system emphasizes size and laterally of lymph nodes. The Ho staging system stresses the level of node(s) only whereas the Changsha system encompasses size, location and fixation of nodes. The prognostic value of nodal stage has been debated. Node size, laterality and neck level are addressed in the various staging systems, and most agree that nodal disease may be an indicator for distant metastasis. Additionally, most agree that the level of disease in the neck is also a significant prognostic factor, with lower nodal level carrying a worse prognosis. However, there continues to be controversy regarding the other factors. Laterality has been debated, as some authors feel that since the nasopharynx is a midline structure, the existence of contralateral disease should not change prognosis or management. On the other hand, the supporters of the Huang and UICC/AJCC systems have shown that bilateral neck disease is an independent indicator of outcome. Of note, the reports that support this

Table 13.5 Nasopharyngeal staging systems

AJCC/UICC	
Nx	Regional lymph nodes cannot be assessed
N0	No regional lymph node metastases
N1	Unilateral metastasis in lymph node(s), 6 cm or less in greatest dimension, above the supraclavicular fossa
N2	Bilateral metastases in lymph node(s), 6 cm or less in greatest dimension, above the supraclavicular fossa
N3a	Metastasis in a lymph node(s) greater than 6 cm in dimension
N3b	Metastasis in a lymph node(s) greater than 6 cm in dimension in the supraclavicular fossa
HUANG	
N0	No clinically positive nodes
N1	Unilateral (ipsilateral) node ≤ 5 cm
N2	Bilateral or contralateral node(s) >5 cm
HO	
N0	No palpable nodes
N1	Node(s) entirely in the upper cervical level, limited below by the neck crease extending laterally and posteriorly from just below thyroid notch
N2	Palpable nodes between the crease and supraclavicular fossa, upper limit being a line joining the upper margins of the sternal end of the clavicle and the apex of an angle formed by the lateral surface of the neck and the superior margin of the trapezius
N3	Palpable nodes in supraclavicular fossa and/or skin involvement in the form of carcinoma en cuirasse or satellite nodules above clavicle
CHANGSHA	
N0	No palpable nodes
N1	Mobile and/or <3 cm above supraclavicular fossa
N2	Fixed and/or (3–8 cm) above supraclavicular fossa
N3	Supraclavicular and/or >8 cm

(Adapted from Brown JJ, Fee WE Jr. Management of the neck in nasopharyngeal carcinoma (NPC). Otolaryngol Clin North Am. 1998;31(5):785-802.)

AJCC: American Joint Committee on Cancer (US)

UICC: Union Internationale Contre le Cancer (Europe)

view are older, and perhaps changes in treatment of NPC and regional lymph nodes has changed over time. Similarly, node size has been debated, with some contending that increased tumor burden worsens prognosis. In addition to the lack of attention to the retropharyngeal lymph nodes, the nodal staging systems also do not address several other disease features such as WHO histology type or viral serology, both of which have been shown to play a role in patient outcome.[52-55]

The cervical lymph nodes are almost universally included in the treatment fields during definitive radiation or chemoradiation. Post-treatment recurrence or persistence in the neck has been reported in up to 21% of patients. The treatment options in this group are re-irradiation and surgical salvage. The reports of persistence after re-irradiation are as high as 91% and the risk of radiation complications is higher after a second course. For these reasons, several authorities recommend neck dissection to manage recurrent or persistent nodal disease, including addressing the retropharyngeal nodes if involved.[56,57] If this is done, the neck dissection should proceed as any other salvage neck dissection for head and neck cancer would, and should include at least all levels initially involved with the disease. In most cases of surgical salvage for NPC, modified radical or radical neck dissection will be required to ensure adequate dissection.

CONCLUSION

Management of the cervical lymph nodes is an important topic that deserves consideration when treating paranasal sinus tumors. Similar to many other head and neck malignancies, metastasis to regional lymph nodes heralds a poorer prognosis and decreased survival. As treatment of the primary site is often multi-modality, so too is treatment of the neck. The first echelon of lymph node drainage from the nose and paranasal sinuses is to the perifacial and glandular nodes anteriorly and the retropharyngeal nodes posteriorly. These then continue to drain to the deeper jugular cervical lymph node groups. There are certain histologic subtypes, namely SCC and sinonasal undifferentiated carcinoma, which have shown a high propensity for lymph node metastasis, so elective treatment of the neck may be warranted, especially in advanced stage tumors. This treatment can be surgical or with radiotherapy, depending on the treatment modality of the primary site. Other subtypes, due to low probability of nodal metastasis, can most often be treated conservatively with treatment geared toward the primary site.

REFERENCES

1. Bachar G, Goldstein DP, Shah M, et al. Esthesioneuroblastoma: The Princess Margaret Hospital experience. Head Neck. 2008;30(12):1607-14.
2. Dulguerov P, Allal AS, Calcaterra TC. Esthesioneuroblastoma: a meta-analysis and review. Lancet Oncol. 2001;2(11):683-90.
3. Anatomic basis of tumor surgery. New York: Springer. 2009.
4. Robbins KT, Clayman G, Levine PA, et al. Neck dissection classification update: revisions proposed by the American Head and Neck Society and the American Academy of Otolaryngology-Head and Neck Surgery. Arch Otolaryngol Head Neck Surg. 2002;128(7):751-8.
5. Robbins KT, Medina JE, Wolfe GT, et al. Standardizing neck dissection terminology. Official report of the Academy's Committee for Head and Neck Surgery and Oncology. Arch Otolaryngol Head Neck Surg. 1991;117(6):601-5.
6. Cummings CW. Cummings otolaryngology head and neck surgery. 4th edition. Philadelphia: Elsevier Mosby; 2005.
7. Harrison LB, Sessions RB, Hong WK. Head and neck cancer: a multidisciplinary approach. 2nd edition. Philadelphia: Lippincott Williams & Wilkins. 2004; vol xvii. p. 1077.
8. Mancuso AA, Harnsberger HR, Muraki AS, et al. Computed tomography of cervical and retropharyngeal lymph nodes: normal anatomy, variants of normal, and applications in staging head and neck cancer. Part I: normal anatomy. Radiology. 1983;148(3):709-14.
9. Pan WR, Suami H, Corlett RJ, et al. Lymphatic drainage of the nasal fossae and nasopharynx: preliminary anatomical and radiological study with clinical implications. Head Neck. 2009;31(1):52-7.

10. Airoldi M, Garzaro M, Valente G, et al. Clinical and biological prognostic factors in 179 cases with sinonasal carcinoma treated in the Italian Piedmont region. Oncology. 2009;76(4):262-9.
11. Cantu G, Bimbi G, Miceli R, et al. Lymph node metastases in malignant tumors of the paranasal sinuses: prognostic value and treatment. Arch Otolaryngol Head Neck Surg. 2008;134(2):170-7.
12. Fasunla AJ, Lasisi AO. Sinonasal malignancies: a 10-year review in a tertiary health institution. J Natl Med Assoc. 2007;99(12):1407-10.
13. Blanch JL, Ruiz AM, Alos L, et al. Treatment of 125 sinonasal tumors: prognostic factors, outcome, and follow-up. Otolaryngol Head Neck Surg. 2004;131(6):973-6.
14. Le QT, Fu KK , Kaplan MJ, et al. Lymph node metastasis in maxillary sinus carcinoma. Int J Radiat Oncol Biol Phys. 2000;46(3):541-9.
15. Paulino AC, Fisher SG, Marks JE. Is prophylactic neck irradiation indicated in patients with squamous cell carcinoma of the maxillary sinus? Int J Radiat Oncol Biol Phys. 1997;39(2):283-9.
16. Jiang GL, Ang KK, Peters LJ, et al. Maxillary sinus carcinomas: natural history and results of postoperative radiotherapy. Radiother Oncol. 1991;21(3):193-200.
17. Robin PE, Powell DJ. Regional node involvement and distant metastases in carcinoma of the nasal cavity and paranasal sinuses. J Laryngol Otol. 1980;94(3):301-9.
18. Smith SR, Som P, Fahmy A, et al. A clinicopathological study of sinonasal neuroendocrine carcinoma and sinonasal undifferentiated carcinoma. Laryngoscope. 2000;110(10 Pt 1):1617-22.
19. Bradley PJ, Jones NS, Robertson I. Diagnosis and management of esthesioneuroblastoma. Curr Opin Otolaryngol Head Neck Surg. 2003;11(2): 112-8.
20. Zafereo ME, Fakhri S, Prayson R, et al. Esthesioneuroblastoma: 25-year experience at a single institution. Otolaryngol Head Neck Surg. 2008; 138(4):452-8.
21. Guzzo M, Grandi C, Licitra L, et al. Mucosal malignant melanoma of head and neck: forty-eight cases treated at Istituto Nazionale Tumori of Milan. Eur J Surg Oncol. 1993;19(4):316-9.
22. Patel SG, Prasad ML, Escrig M, et al. Primary mucosal malignant melanoma of the head and neck. Head Neck. 2002;24(3):247-57.
23. Stern SJ, Guillamondegui OM. Mucosal melanoma of the head and neck. Head Neck. 1991;13(1):22-7.
24. Temam S, Mamelle G, Marandas P, et al. Postoperative radiotherapy for primary mucosal melanoma of the head and neck. Cancer. 2005;103(2):313-9.
25. Yii NW, Eisen T, Nicolson M, et al. Mucosal malignant melanoma of the head and neck: the Marsden experience over half a century. Clin Oncol (R Coll Radiol). 2003;15(4):199-204.
26. Benlyazid A, Thariat J, Temam S, et al. Postoperative Radiotherapy in Head and Neck Mucosal Melanoma: A GETTEC Study. Arch Otolaryngol Head Neck Surg. 2010;136(12):1219-25.
27. AJCC cancer staging manual. New York: Springer; 2009.
28. Ballantyne AJ. Malignant melanoma of the skin of the head and neck. An analysis of 405 cases. Am J Surg. 1970;120(4):425-31.
29. Moreno MA, Roberts DB, Kupferman ME, et al. Mucosal melanoma of the nose and paranasal sinuses, a contemporary experience from the MD Anderson Cancer Center. Cancer. 2010;116(9):2215-23.
30. Wanebo HJ, Koness RJ, MacFarlane JK, et al. Head and neck sarcoma: report of the Head and Neck Sarcoma Registry. Society of Head and Neck Surgeons Committee on Research. Head Neck. 1992;14(1):1-7.
31. Farhood AI, Hajdu SI, Shiu MH, et al. Soft tissue sarcomas of the head and neck in adults. Am J Surg. 1990;160(4):365-9.
32. Freedman AM, Reiman HM, Woods JE. Soft-tissue sarcomas of the head and neck. Am J Surg. 1989;158(4):367-72.
33. Koka V, Vericel R, Lartigau E, et al. Sarcomas of nasal cavity and paranasal sinuses: chondrosarcoma, osteosarcoma and fibrosarcoma. J Laryngol Otol. 1994;108(11):947-53.
34. Benoit MM, Bhattacharyya N, Faquin W, et al. Cancer of the nasal cavity in the pediatric population. Pediatrics. 2008;121(1):e141-5.
35. Callender TA, Weber RS, Janjan N, et al. Rhabdomyosarcoma of the nose and paranasal sinuses in adults and children. Otolaryngol Head Neck Surg. 1995;112(2):252-7.

36. Wurm J, Constantinidis J, Grabenbauer GG, et al. Rhabdomyosarcomas of the nose and paranasal sinuses: treatment results in 15 cases. Otolaryngol Head Neck Surg. 2005;133(1):42-50.
37. Pitman KT, Johnson JT, Myers EN. Effectiveness of selective neck dissection for management of the clinically negative neck. Arch Otolaryngol Head Neck Surg. 1997;123(9):917-22.
38. Paulino AC, Marks JE, Bricker P, et al. Results of treatment of patients with maxillary sinus carcinoma. Cancer. 1998;83(3):457-65.
39. Day TA, Beas RA, Schlosser RJ, et al. Management of paranasal sinus malignancy. Curr Treat Options Oncol. 2005;6(1):3-18.
40. Myers LL, Oxford LE. Differential diagnosis and treatment options in paranasal sinus cancers. Surg Oncol Clin N Am. 2004;13(1):167-86.
41. Sisson GA Sr, Toriumi DM, Atiyah RA. Paranasal sinus malignancy: a comprehensive update. Laryngoscope. 1989;99(2):143-50.
42. Perez CA. Principles and practice of radiation oncology. 4th edition. Philadelphia: Lippincott Williams & Wilkins. 2004; vol xxiii. p. 25-27.
43. Gross ND, Ellingson TW, Wax MK, et al. Impact of retropharyngeal lymph node metastasis in head and neck squamous cell carcinoma. Arch Otolaryngol Head Neck Surg. 2004;130(2):169-73.
44. Hasegawa Y, Matsuura H. Retropharyngeal node dissection in cancer of the oropharynx and hypopharynx. Head Neck. 1994;16(2):173-80.
45. Morrissey DD, Talbot JM, Cohen JI, et al. Accuracy of computed tomography in determining the presence or absence of metastatic retropharyngeal adenopathy. Arch Otolaryngol Head Neck Surg. 2000;126(12):1478-81.
46. Bernier J, Domenge C, Ozsahin M, et al. Postoperative irradiation with or without concomitant chemotherapy for locally advanced head and neck cancer. N Engl J Med. 2004;350(19):1945-52.
47. Cooper JS, Pajak TF, Forastiere AA, et al. Postoperative concurrent radiotherapy and chemotherapy for high-risk squamous-cell carcinoma of the head and neck. N Engl J Med. 2004;350(19):1937-44.
48. Bernier J, Cooper JS, Pajak TF, et al. Defining risk levels in locally advanced head and neck cancers: a comparative analysis of concurrent postoperative radiation plus chemotherapy trials of the EORTC (#22931) and RTOG (# 9501). Head Neck. 2005;27(10):843-50.
49. Al-Sarraf M, LeBlanc M, Giri PG, et al. Chemoradiotherapy versus radiotherapy in patients with advanced nasopharyngeal cancer: phase III randomized Intergroup study 0099. J Clin Oncol. 1998;16(4):1310-7.
50. Lu H, Peng L, Yuan X, et al. Concurrent chemoradiotherapy in locally advanced nasopharyngeal carcinoma: a treatment paradigm also applicable to patients in Southeast Asia. Cancer Treat Rev. 2009;35(4):345-53.
51. Wee J, Tan EH, Tai BC, et al. Randomized trial of radiotherapy versus concurrent chemoradiotherapy followed by adjuvant chemotherapy in patients with American Joint Committee on Cancer/International Union against cancer stage III and IV nasopharyngeal cancer of the endemic variety. J Clin Oncol. 2005;23(27): 6730-8.
52. Brown JJ, Fee WE Jr. Management of the neck in nasopharyngeal carcinoma (NPC). Otolaryngol Clin North Am. 1998;31(5):785-802.
53. Lee AW, Foo W, Law CK, et al. N-staging of nasopharyngeal carcinoma: discrepancy between UICC/AJCC and Ho systems. Union Internationale Contre le Cancer. American Joint Committee for Cancer. Clin Oncol (R Coll Radiol). 1996;8(3): 155-9.
54. Nasopharyngeal cancer. New York: Springer; 2009.
55. Meyer JE, Wang CC. Carcinoma of the nasopharynx. Factors influencing results of therapy. Radiology. 1971;100(2):385-8.
56. Khafif A, Ferlito A, Takes RP, et al. Is it necessary to perform radical neck dissection as a salvage procedure for persistent or recurrent neck disease after chemoradiotherapy in patients with nasopharyngeal cancer? Eur Arch Otorhinolaryngol. 2010;267(7):997-9.
57. Wei WI, Lam KH, Ho CM, et al. Efficacy of radical neck dissection for the control of cervical metastasis after radiotherapy for nasopharyngeal carcinoma. Am J Surg. 1990;160(4):439-42.

14

Radiation Therapy for Sinonasal Cancers

Geoffrey A Geiger, MD; Alexander Lin, MD; Diana Stripp, MD; Harry Quon, MD, MS

INTRODUCTION

The mainstay of treatment for sinonasal cancers is surgical resection and postoperative radiation therapy, and is universally recommended in cases where the primary tumor cannot be completely resected. Radiation therapy can also be used definitively in advanced cases. Modern radiotherapy approaches have improved the conformality index, which is essential for minimizing doses to surrounding organs-at-risk (OAR) since treatment involves the use of high doses (66–70 Gy) in a region crowded with critical structures. Because of the steep dose gradients needed to protect critical adjacent normal structures, particle therapy represents a potential avenue to increase the therapeutic window in sinonasal malignancies. Despite these advances, local relapses continue to dominate the pattern of relapse.

HISTORICAL RADIATION THERAPY

The vast majority of treatment approaches for sinonasal cancers involve the use of surgery and radiation.[1-4] Unfortunately, due to the rarity of these cancers, the exact role of radiation therapy in the multimodality treatment of sinonasal cancers has never been assessed through prospective randomized trials. As such, the major barrier in advancing the management strategies including the role of radiotherapy continues to be the inevitable influence of patient selection factors confounding the interpretation of whether aspects of treatment may be improving the oncologic results. For example, evidence that improved local control rates may be seen with higher radiotherapy doses may be falsely due to an association between low radiotherapy doses administered to patients with poorer performance status (which may reflect more a more advanced cancer stage) or those treated palliatively. Similarly, series reporting on the role of radiotherapy alone typically have more advanced cancer that can adversely influence survival.

The ability to assess the influence of these potential confounding associations is traditionally addressed with a multivariate analysis but requires sufficient patient numbers for this to be possible. Only a limited number of retrospective reports have reported such an analysis.[4-11] One of the largest single institutional series reported an analysis of 308 patients treated with at least a craniofacial resection. With a mean follow-up duration of 63 months, tumor histology, orbital and brain invasion and not adjuvant therapy were the most dominant factors affecting survival.[10] However, details of the radiotherapy (e.g. dose) that was administered between 1978 to 2004 were not available but this data does suggest that at least historic radiotherapy approaches had a minimal impact on preventing relapses.

The use of radiation as a sole modality for the treatment of sinonasal cancers has been shown to be effective in retrospective reviews with locoregional control rates ranging from approximately 40–50%, which is lower than that achieved with surgery (locoregional) control of approximately 70%.[12,13] Doses higher than 66 Gy are felt to be necessary if radiation is to be used as a single modality for treatment.[14] As a result, past locoregional control rates have been limited due to the technical challenges with older radiation techniques to safely administer doses greater than 66 Gy without injuring surrounding normal OAR such as the eye. Modern technical radiotherapy advances, as described below have largely not been reflected in published institutional series to date and offer the promise of further improvements in locoregional control rates.

MODERN RADIATION THERAPY

Sinonasal cancers are challenging areas to irradiate given the location of these tumors between the optic nerves and their proximity to the optic chiasm and brainstem. The evolution from 2D to 3D conformal radiotherapy (3DCRT) and intensity-modulated radiotherapy (IMRT) has increasingly allowed for potentially curative doses of radiation to be given while minimizing the likelihood of significant long-term toxicities. Two-dimensional radiation typically employed a three-field technique using one anterior and two wedged lateral beams in an attempt to spare the brainstem and orbits but tolerances of the optic nerves were frequently exceeded. Quantification of doses to critical structures was rendered possible by 3DCRT and allowed for some optimization of field design utilizing multi-leaf collimation to reduce doses where possible, but the fundamental limitations of forward planning persisted. Some investigators advocated that a 4-beam technique utilizing a non-coplanar anterior-superior field produced a dose distribution that may be similar to coplanar intensity modulation.[15] Ultimately, modern IMRT, which is now regarded as the standard treatment technique, has facilitated the ability to generate concave dose distributions around target volumes and has the ability to spare the lacrimal apparatus, minimize visual impairment, and reduce the likelihood of the development of severe dry eye syndrome.[16,17]

Indications for Radiotherapy

A resectable treatment paradigm is most commonly used for sinonasal cancers. In part, this is due to the significant benefit of reducing the radiotherapy dose that is needed in the postoperative setting compared to that which would be favored for unresected cancer. While no prospective randomized studies have been conducted to establish the oncologic value of postoperative radiotherapy (PORT) to surgery alone, the retrospective evidence to date would suggest that this is associated with improved local control rates. This observation however must recognize that part of the improved cancer outcomes may come from the influence of the more favorable prognosis associated with resectable sinonasal cancers and not necessarily by this treatment approach.

Postoperative radiotherapy is typically favored after surgical resection for resectable sinonasal cancers due to the difficulties in achieving wide surgical margins given the anatomic density of the paranasal sinus and skull base. Moreover, while the development of modern transnasal endoscopic surgical approaches have greatly reduced the morbidity and cosmetic impact of traditional exposure techniques, the issue of potential tumor seeding from the piecemeal resection raises questions about whether or not PORT should be routinely indicated, has not been systematically evaluated. It is clear that there are circumstances in which PORT is not needed after endoscopic surgery. However, the specific indications have not been defined.

In one of the largest institutional series reported to date, Hanna et al. demonstrated that the risk of local relapse was 15% in 120 patients with a mixture of histologies endoscopically resected with 50% receiving PORT.[18] Details of how patients were selected for PORT were not described. We have favored PORT where the invasive base of the tumor limits confidence in the adequacy of the surgical resected margin. The risk of tumor seeding associated with current endoscopic resection cannot be completely excluded but the risk is likely to be sufficiently low such that PORT is not routinely indicated following endoscopic surgical approaches.

Preoperative radiotherapy has also been used as a treatment approach especially for advanced sinonasal cancers where the ability to achieve clear surgical margins is expected to be restricted. Examples include invasion through the periorbita or cavernous sinus. Proponents of this approach argue that preoperative radiotherapy may be more effective as the tissues are better oxygenated due to an undisturbed vascular supply. The risk of injury to critical OARs such as the eye is limited by prescribing a lower preoperative dose that does not exceed the risk of organ injury. Typically a dose of 50 Gy is administered. However, postoperative complications in wound healing, such as fistula formation, appear to be increased with this approach. How preoperative radiotherapy compares to a postoperative radiotherapy approach is not clear at this time, as institutional reports to date are influenced by the potential for selection bias, particularly where preoperative radiotherapy may be used for tumors of borderline resectability. In their retrospective review of 308 patients, Howard et al. found no difference in survival between preoperative and postoperative radiotherapy.[10]

An analysis of the locoregional control rates between preoperative and postoperative radiotherapy were not reported.

Definitive radiotherapy has also been used for unresectable disease.[19] In such cases, concurrent chemotherapy has typically been administered, but without any prospective randomized data to support its role. Similarly, concurrent preoperative and postoperative chemoradiotherapy have been used without any prospective randomized data to determine what incremental gains in treatment outcomes may be achieved despite the increased toxicities. Definitive chemoradiotherapy has also been used for resectable disease reserving surgery as a salvage approach for persistent disease identified with close follow-up.[20] This approach has been used especially for radioresponsive tumors such as sinonasal undifferentiated carcinomas.[21]

Radiation Treatment Planning

Organs-at-risk (OAR) are structures that are to be avoided where possible in treatment planning and which are given relative weights in inverse treatment planning (e.g. the optic chiasm should be protected more than the retinas). Although IMRT has not yet demonstrated a local control benefit over conventional techniques, multiple investigations have demonstrated a decrease in the radiation doses to OARs with intensity-modulation.[11,15,22] Anatomical structures that should be contoured as OARs include the optic nerves and chiasm, retinas, major lacrimal glands, brain, brainstem, and parotid glands. However, any important normal structure that may be at risk of injury given the orientation of the radiation beams should be considered an OAR and contoured to facilitate at least an evaluation of the dose delivered to the OAR assessing the safety of the radiation treatment. Recommended maximum doses adapted from Madani et al.[11] are provided in Table 14.1.

At this time, there are no accepted guidelines for the delineation of IMRT target volumes for the treatment of paranasal sinus malignancies. The proximity of critical OARs (e.g. optic nerves, lacrimal apparatus, chiasm, retinas, and brainstem) require precise delineation of all target treatment and avoidance volumes to allow the highest possible dose to be delivered to the tumor volumes while minimizing exposure of neighboring normal tissues. At the base of skull, the use of MRI to aid in the delineation of both tumor volumes and OARs

Table 14.1 Recommended maximum doses to organs-at-risk (OAR) (Adapted from Madani et al. (20))

Organ-at-Risk	*Dose-Volume Constraint*
Optic Nerve and Chiasm	Dmax <55–60
Brain	Dmax <60
Retina	Dmax <55–60, V55 <5%
Lacrimal Gland	D50 <30 Gy (median dose)
Spinal Cord	Dmax <50
Brainstem	Dmax <54 Gy
Parotid Gland	Mean Dose <26 (single)
Mandible	V70 <5%

Dmax = maximum dose received; V55 = relative volume receiving ≥55 Gy; D50 = dose level on dose–volume histograms above which 50% of contoured volume is exposed

can be extremely helpful.[23] MRIs are typically fused with the treatment planning CT such so that both can be visualized at the time of target and OAR contour delineation. The use of MRI-derived treatment volumes have been demonstrated to be smaller and have less inter-observer variation than CT-derived treatment volumes for locally advanced head and neck cancers.[24]

Practically, our group has observed that maintaining a consistent overlap of delineated target volumes with each progressive axial CT image slice employing gradual contour changes can help to ensure that the radiation doses are more accurately delivered within the target volumes and not outside in normal structures. The overlapping or stacking of target volumes on each slice ensures that good dosimetry is achieved in three-dimensions. To ensure achieving sharp radiotherapy dose gradients between target and normal structures, it is also important to remember that this may be more readily achieved if the isocenter for the radiation therapy is placed in the planes where the sharp dose gradient is desired. This can also be facilitated with the use of micro-multileaf collimation.

Both coplanar and non-coplanar beam arrangements for conformal irradiation have been described for the treatment of sinonasal cancers. Despite the limitations associated with only coplanar beam arrangements used with helical tomotherapy, a recent dosimetric analysis demonstrated that the increased number of beams that can be used with this technique may improve both the conformality index and hence offer lower radiotherapy doses to adjacent optic structures. The uniformity of the dose also appears to be improved with the target volumes.[25] Conceptually, similar dosimetric benefits may also be achieved with treatment on the linear accelerator with recent technical advances such as intensity modulated arc therapy (IMAT) and volumetric modulated arc therapy (VMAT) that can increase the number of beams that may be delivered. VMAT differs from existing techniques like helical tomotherapy or IMAT because it delivers dose to the whole volume, rather than slice by slice. To date, one dosimetric report suggests that multi-arc non-coplanar VMAT may in fact result in decreased dose between the orbits.[26]

PARTICLE THERAPY

Whether or not particle therapy such as protons can improve the radiotherapy dose gradient between the target volume and critical OARs due to its physical characteristics is unclear at this time and is a subject of active investigation.[27-30] The ability to successfully reduce the radiotherapy dose to critical OARs may be dependent on the physical distance from the OAR to the target volume. The use of current 3D proton beam arrangements may not provide sufficient dose conformality and sharp dose gradients to reduce the radiotherapy dose to adjacent OARs, such as the dose delivered to the ipsilateral optic structures for a tumor of the maxillary sinus.[30] In contrast, ongoing developments of the intensity modulated proton therapy (IMPT) technique may allow sufficient reduction of the dose delivered to adjacent OARs due to the improved conformality index of this technique.[31]

Dose inhomogeneity is inherent to IMRT treatment plans. For the skull base, it is critical to scrutinize the treatment plan not only for the magnitude of any dosimetric hotspots but also the location of the hotspots. Such inhomogeneities increase not only the total dose delivered to

OARs but the effective dose per fraction that is delivered. Both can influence the risk of late neurologic complications. Lastly, sinonasal cancers may involve tissue near or at the level of the skin, necessitating bolus or tissue equivalent material be placed in these regions to ensure adequate dose to these superficial regions.

Site-Specific Radiation Strategy and Orbital Radiation

For tumor involvement of the maxillary sinus, evaluation and possible irradiation of the masticator, parapharyngeal or pterygopalatine spaces should be considered. For example, if there is involvement of the pterygopalatine fossa where cranial nerve V2 courses through, it becomes important to evaluate the potential risk that subclinical microscopic disease may extend possibly in a perineural fashion extending more distally to foramen rotundum and possible to Meckel's cave in the middle cranial fossa. The adjacent nasal cavity and ethmoid sinus may also be considered for elective irradiation. Whether or not bilateral ethmoid sinuses should be electively irradiated for well confined early stage tumors in the maxillary sinus is unclear. Inferior maxillary involvement may require inclusion of a portion of the hard palate to allow for appropriate margin treatment. Involvement of the bone of the orbit does not necessitate irradiation of the entire orbital contents due to the fascial planes and muscles surrounding the globe which function as barriers for tumor infiltration.

For tumors involving the ethmoid sinus, a frequent treatment planning dilemma is when the orbital contents require irradiation especially when the lamina papyracea is involved. The lamina papyracea is the thin bony portion of the orbital plate of the ethmoid bone which forms part of the medial wall of the orbit. Underneath the bones of the orbit is a fascial sheet referred to as the periorbita to which it is loosely attached. Orbit preserving surgery has demonstrated that when the periorbita is not invaded, the risk of cancer recurrence within the orbit is low and survival is not compromised.[32] Even minimal invasion of the periorbita does not appear to increase this risk, with exenteration typically performed for extensive/full thickness periorbita invasion.[33] In the review by Howard et al. no statistically significant survival differences were observed with a policy of orbit preservation even with full thickness periorbita invasion.[11] While T2-weighted MRI appears to better facilitate evaluation of the periorbita,[34] some have argued that an additional fascial barrier exists between the periorbita and the periorbital fat allowing for orbit preservation even with periorbita invasion.[35]

Tumor extension to the orbital apex does not necessarily increase the risk of cancer extension into the orbit. However, when there is tumor invasion of the muscle and fat at the apex, an orbital exenteration is typically favored.[35] While the orbit may not require irradiation when the tumor does not invade beyond orbital apex, the ability to preserve vision in such cases may be limited due to the radiotherapy dose that is administered to the optic nerve and the retina. In a similar manner, tumors in the maxillary sinus and ethmoid sinus lying adjacent to the optic structures present challenges in preserving visual function even when the orbit does not require irradiation. In such circumstances, exploiting the principles of hyperfractionation may be beneficial when the radiotherapy dose cannot be adequately conformed around the optic structures.[36-38]

In a series of retrospective reviews of patients receiving definitive irradiation typically with non-conformal radiation techniques such as IMRT, investigators from the University of Florida have observed that the risk of radiation-induced optic neuropathy is not only significantly influenced by the total dose delivered to the retina[37] and optic nerve,[38] but that this risk may be reduced if a hyperfractionated schedule is used. Hence, in situations where the radiotherapy cannot be adequately conformed around optic structures such that the threshold dose for injury to the retina (>50 Gy)[37] and the optic nerve (>50 Gy)[38] is exceeded, the use of a hyperfractionated radiotherapy schedule may help to reduce the risk of injury.

In this regard, the IMRT technique can be exploited where a simultaneous in-field boost (SIB-IMRT or commonly referred to as dose painting) can be used to create a dose gradient such that the tumor mass receives a more conventional dose per fraction such as 1.8–2 Gy while the adjacent optic structures receives a lower dose per fraction. Bhandare et al. observed that the risk of optic neuropathy significantly increased for dose per fractions greater than 1.8 Gy.[37] As the hyperfractionated experience typically used at the University of Florida ranged from 1.1–1.2 Gy, the relationship between the risk of optic neuropathy and specific dose per fraction delivered to the optic nerve could not be evaluated. For the retina, hyperfractionation was shown to significantly reduce the risk of radiation induced retinopathy observed with daily fractionated total doses greater than 50 Gy (15–46%).[37] Again, the majority of the hyperfractionation schedules used, employed a dose per fraction of 1.1–1.2 Gy.

An accelerated fractionation schedule designed to offset the influence of tumor repopulation to radiotherapy as a stress response has been suggested to improve local control rates for unresectable paranasal sinus cancers.[39] Consistent with this have been reports identifying that prolonged radiotherapy treatment time may adversely influence survival.[7] For these reasons, the dose painting advantages of the IMRT technique may further aid in improving local control rates. To date, no reports have evaluated this fractionation schedule for paranasal sinus cancers specifically though it is commonly employed for cancers in other anatomic sites of the head and neck including the nasopharynx.[40]

Radiotherapy for the Neck

The improved radiotherapy conformality seen with IMRT can also be exploited to more readily administer radiotherapy to the draining cervical nodes while still ensuring that the dose delivered to the parotid glands are sufficiently low (parotid sparing) to reduce the risk of permanent xerostomia. The issue of elective nodal irradiation remains a controversial issue and has been influenced largely by the risk of nodal metastases at presentation. These observations suggest that the risk of occult nodal metastases is low (2–10%)[41-45] to not warrant elective management be it surgery or radiation. For these reasons elective nodal irradiation has not historically been advocated. Elective nodal irradiation has however been advocated for patients presenting with nodal metastases who consistently have been noted to have an adverse prognosis.[46,47]

In contrast, when the risk of nodal relapse is evaluated, several high-risk situations have been reported prompting considerations of elective nodal irradiation even in the N0 neck. These include high-risk histologies such as poorly differentiated carcinoma even in anatomic sites not typically considered at high-risk,[47] advanced T3/4 ethmoid[48] and maxillary sinus cancers,[49] unresectable paranasal sinus carcinomas[19] and possibly for SNUCs.[50] For esthesioneuroblastomas, nodal relapses ranging from 20–30% have been reported leading some to recommend elective irradiation especially for Kadish B and C disease. If disease has spread to involve the adjacent nasopharynx, the retropharyngeal nodes should be included in the treatment volume. Jeremic et al. reported in a study of 49 maxillary sinus patients with T3–4N0 carcinomas, ipsilateral elective nodal irradiation (ENI) was associated with a 10-year regional recurrence-free survival rate of 94% and 5-year and 10-year survival rates of 66% and 60% respectively.[51] Despite local relapses still dominating the relapse pattern, these investigators suggest that ENI may offer a strategy to improve survival rates for advanced T-stage maxillary carcinomas.

Optimal Radiation Dosing

The optimal total dose both for definitive and postoperative irradiation is unknown at this time. Complicating the dose that is actually delivered is the potential for the air cavities that arise from modern endoscopic surgeries contributing to underdosing of the mucosa. Hence, inhomogeneity correction in the treatment planning algorithm should be applied. The doses that have been used have largely been extrapolated from the treatment of epithelial malignancies in the head and neck. With the IMRT technique using a "shrinking field technique" whereby smaller fields are sequentially treated to allow for a boost dose to the smallest volume, 70 Gy in 35 fractions has been reported and used for both definitive and postoperative patients. Alternatively, a simultaneous in-field boost (SIB) technique can be used such that a single plan is used throughout the entire treatment whereby various volumes receive different doses per fraction (e.g. one volume receives 2.12 Gy/fraction to a total dose of 70 Gy over 33 fractions, a second volume receives 1.8 Gy/fraction to a dose of 59.4 Gy and the lowest risk volume receives a dose of 1.64 Gy/fraction to a dose of 54 Gy).[52]

TREATMENT OUTCOMES

Nasal Cavity and Paranasal Sinus

Both surgery and radiation have historically been used for these tumors with curative intent although results of single modality techniques have been disappointing. Table 14.2 outlines the results of surgery alone for treatment of maxillary sinus primaries. Unfortunately, no randomized trials have been performed assessing surgery versus radiation or the optimal sequencing of these treatment options. Early studies comparing radiation in the preoperative and postoperative setting for maxillary sinus tumors revealed advantages of preoperative radiation in terms of survival rates[53,54] (Table 14.3), although there were notable disadvantages in terms of poorer wound healing and increased risk of infections, particularly in an era with limited antimicrobials. Despite early data suggesting an advantage to preoperative radiation therapy, more recently, radiation has been increasingly offered in the postoperative setting to allow for more accurate staging and pathological assessment and a higher likelihood of encompassing all potential residual disease within reasonable radiation fields.[55,56]

Table 14.2 Selected results of surgery alone in maxillary sinus malignancies

Author	*Published*	*Period*	*No. Patients*	*5-yr Survival*
Gallagher[71]	1970	1955–1964	8	50
Tabb	1971	1958–1968	19	62
St. Pierre[72]	1983	1964–1975	10	20

* Adapted from Chen et al. 2010[73]

Table 14.4 outlines the results of nonrandomized trials assessing combined modality treatment. Based on the available data, most investigators recommend surgery followed by postoperative radiation although preoperative radiation may be considered for the treatment of tumors that are not resectable at the time of diagnosis. Radiation alone has the capacity for high cure rates when utilized alone, but at curative doses may risk optic nerve injury.

Esthesioneuroblastoma

The favored treatment of this disease is typically surgical resection followed by postoperative external beam radiation therapy.[57,58] Treatment of earlier stage tumors is associated with excellent outcomes when surgery is followed by postoperative radiation: up to 96% 5-year survival for Kadish A tumors and above 80% for Kadish B tumors.[59] The locoregional and distant control numbers are significantly lower for Kadish C tumors with a 5-year overall survival of approximately 50%.

A prospective study utilizing chemotherapy, surgery and combined photon/proton radiation

Table 14.3 Selected results of preoperative versus postoperative radiation therapy for maxillary sinus primary malignancies

Author	*Published*	*Period*	*No. Patients*	*Technique*	*Preop OS (%)*	*Postop OS (%)*
Jesse[54]	1965	1952–1961	41	2D	45 (3 yr)	37 (3 yr)
Tabb	1971	1958–1968	54	2D	32 (5 yr)	12 (5 yr)
Hu[53]	1982	1958–1974	50	2D	64 (5 yr)	26 (5 yr)

* Adapted from Chen et al. 2010[73]

Table 14.4 Outcome of locally advanced patients treated with combined modality treatment

Author	Published	Period	Site	No. patients	Technique	5 yr OS (%)
Lavertu[74]	1989	1977-1986	PNS	54	2D	38
Zaharia[56]	1989	1963-1980	MS	149	2D	36
Spiro[75]	1995	1966-1982	NC/PNS	106	2D	38
Jiang[76]	1998	1969-1993	ES	34	2D	55
Paulino[1]	1998	1969-1995	MS	48	2D	47
Le[7]	1999	1959-1996	MS	97	2D	34
Myers[43]	2002	1980-1997	PNS	141	2D+BT+P*	52
Duthoy[77]	2005	1998-2003	NC/PNS	39	IMRT	59 (4 yr)
Bristol[55]	2007	1969-2002	MS	146	2D, 3DCRT or IMRT	55
Hoppe[78]	2007	1987-2005	PNS	85	3DCRT or IMRT	67
Hoppe[79]	2008	1990-2006	PNS	37	2D, 3DCRT or IMRT	51
Truong[30]	2009	1991-2005	SS	20	Proton	53 (2 yr)
Madani[11]	2009	1998-2006	NC/PNS	84	IMRT	59

Abbreviations: PNS = Paranasal Sinus (includes more than one subsite); NC: Nasal Cavity; MS: Maxillary Sinus; ES: Ethmoid Sinus; SS: Sphenoid Sinus.

* 2D+BT+P: 2D Radiation Therapy plus Brachytherapy (some) plus Particle Therapy (helium and neon ion).

at Massachusetts General Hospital of four patients with Kadish Stage B disease and 15 patients with Kadish Stage C disease reported a 5-year local control rate of 88% and a 5-year overall survival rate of 74%.[60] This aggressive multimodality therapy was well tolerated with no patient sustaining more than grade 3 hematologic toxicity. Thirteen patients showed a partial or complete response to chemotherapy. Interestingly, radical surgery was reserved for non-responders and in many patients, neoadjuvant chemotherapy and high-dose proton-photon radiotherapy represented a successful treatment approach for patients

Sinonasal Undifferentiated Carcinomas

Sinonasal undifferentiated carcinomas (SNUCs) are a type of primitive neuroendoscrine tumor which demonstrate aggressive behavior and a high rate of distant metastases.[61] These tumors are thought to arise from Schneiderian epithelium and early reports on treatment results reported very poor outcomes.[62,63] More recent reports suggest the incorporation of combined modality treatment utilizing chemotherapy for SNUC tumors may improve survival (5-year overall survival rate of 64%).[61] The records of 21 patients with SNUC at UCSF treated between 1990 and 2004 were analyzed and reported on multimodality therapy including surgery followed by postoperative radiotherapy with or without adjuvant chemotherapy for 17 patients, neoadjuvant chemoradiotherapy followed by surgery for two patients, and definitive chemoradiotherapy for two patients. Median follow-up among surviving patients was 58 months with 2- and 5-year local control rates of 60% and 56% respectively without any difference in local control according to initial treatment approach. But among the 19 patients who underwent surgery, the 5-year local control rate was 74% for those with gross total tumor resection, compared with 24% for those with subtotal tumor resection (p =0.001) suggesting that gross total resection should be the goal of all treatments whenever possible.[64,65]

TOXICITIES OF TREATMENT

Orbital and Optic Nerve Injury

Radiation-induced injury to the retinas, optic nerves and/or chiasm represent some of the most dreaded complications of treatment for sinonasal cancers. One report from the MD Anderson Cancer Center on 219 patients, some of which were treated in the pre-IMRT era, demonstrated corneal injury in 24 of the 49 patients treated with a three-field technique without orbital shielding and symptomatic retinopathy in 7 of 77 patients treated to a relatively large retinal surface.[66] Eight patients developed ipsilateral blindness due to optic neuropathy and 11 patients had bilateral visual impairment secondary to chiasm injury. The total radiation dose was identified as the predominant determinant. Zero patients receiving a dose of less than 50 Gy developed optic neuropathy or chiasm injury. In contrast, the 10-year actuarial incidences of optic nerve-chiasm injury were 5% and 30% for patients receiving 50–60 Gy and 61–78 Gy, respectively.[66]

A more recent publication reporting on an IMRT technique to reduce the likelihood of complications in these critical structures looked at 36 patients and reported conjunctivitis in 29 patients, only 11 of which were grade 2+.[22] Other reported complications in the acute setting included keratitis in one patient. All of the acute toxicities observed in that retrospective series resolved with conservative medical management.

A longitudinal examination of the UCSF experience with sinonasal cancers revealed that the incidence of chronic grade 3+ toxicity differed significantly between the conventionally irradiated patients as compared to those treated with IMRT. Only 13% of patients treated with IMRT developed high grade late toxicity compared to 54% and 22% of those treated with conventional and 3DCRT, respectively.[67] It should be noted that caution should be applied to contouring OARs and to setting dose constraints for the IMRT algorithm, as inverse planning is only as good as the contours and constraints set by the physician and executed by the physicist or dosimetrist.

Severe Dry Eye Syndrome

Injury to the lacrimal apparatus and/or minor glands can lead to an increased risk of a permanent dry eye that can result in vision loss and possible need for enucleation.

The conformal nature of IMRT treatment planning appears to be reducing the risk of dry eye syndrome. With 2D non-conformal treatment planning, Parsons et al. reported that all 17 patients who received doses greater than equal to 57 Gy to the lacrimal apparatus developed severe dry-eye syndrome compared to 3 (19%) of 16 patients who received doses less than equal to 45.[68] In their retrospective review, they defined the severe dry-eye syndrome as resulting in vision loss. Most patients who developed complications were symptomatic within one month after completing the radiotherapy. They concluded that the incidence of severe dry syndrome, from their experience and a review of the literature injury, increases from 0% after doses less than 30 Gy to 100% after doses greater than 57 Gy.[68]

In contrast, Claus et al. reported the risk of dry eye syndrome in a prospective cohort of 32 patients with sinonasal cancers treated with IMRT.[16] The mean dose to the major lacrimal glands was 23 Gy (median 25 Gy, range 6 and 40 Gy). Using the NCI common toxicity criteria, no patients developed grade 3 (impaired vision) lacrimal gland injury at one month or greater in follow-up (mean 15 months, range 3–33 months).

FUTURE DIRECTIONS

While the IMRT technique is the accepted standard when irradiating sinonasal cancers, the increasing use and commercial development of particle therapy such as proton radiotherapy offers the promise of further improvements in the therapeutic ratio. The use of proton or carbon ion beams takes advantage of the Bragg peak. When a charged particle moves quickly through matter, it ionizes atoms of the material and deposits a dose along its path. A peak occurs because the interactional cross section increases as the charged particle's energy decreases resulting in a peak deposition of energy before the particles come to rest. When a range of ion energies are used ("spread out Bragg peak" or SOBP), a broad flattened beam can generate a clinically useful beam which has essentially no exit

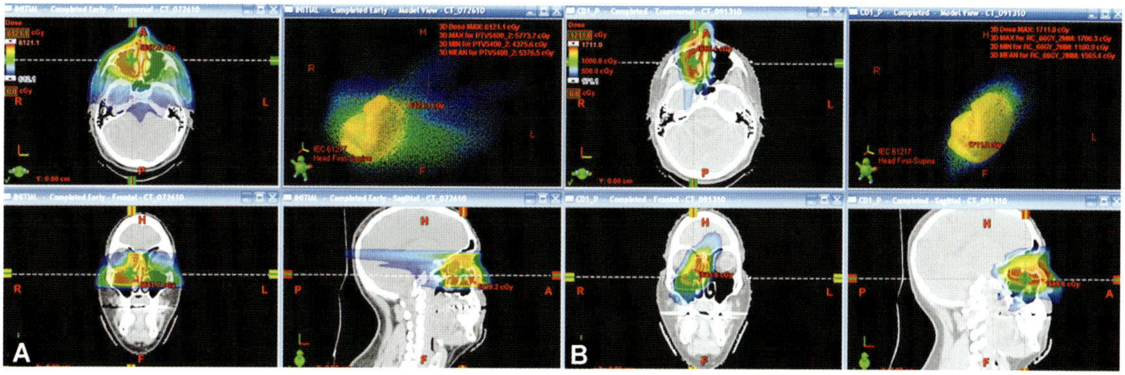

Figs 14.1A and B: Difference in conformality of photon IMRT and passive scattering protons. (A) Initial photon intensity-modulated plan with representative axial, coronal and sagittal images with accompanying dose cloud; (B) Conedown volume in same planes using double scattering passive protons. Note: Treated volumes differ between A and B, proton plan with smaller treatment volume in (B) than initial plan (A).

dose, which distinguish these beams from X-rays. Carbon ions possess an additional radiobiological advantage over protons.

Use of these beams has been largely restricted to theoretical dosimetric comparisons of ions versus X-rays and publications of results of proton beam therapy for sinonasal cancers are very limited. Nonetheless, the use of proton and carbon ion beams has the potential to further increase conformality with sparing of OARs, particularly in head and neck sites, as compared to conventional, 3D and IMRT techniques.[69] Figures 14.1A and B demonstrate the difference in conformality of photon IMRT and passive scattering protons between an initial and conedown (second phase) plan for a sinonasal cancer.

Limited centers have experience utilizing intensity-modulated proton therapy (IMPT), which have an even greater conformality index than passive-scattering proton beams. Lomax et al. found that compared to IMRT, only IMPT provided a method by which critical structures could be spared at all dose levels, while simultaneously providing acceptable dose homogeneity within the target volume.[28] A combination of IMRT and carbon ions has also been utilized to deliver high doses to the base of skull for patients with adenoid cystic carcinomas. In one series, 21 patients were treated with photon IMRT plus carbon ion resulting in a 3-year locoregional control and disease-specific survival of 62% and 40%, respectively.[70]

CONCLUSIONS

The optimal management for sinonasal cancers remains to be defined and continues to be limited by the many histologies and treatment heterogeneity that has been reported to date. Technical radiotherapy advances now offer the ability to improve the radiotherapy dose delivery and conformality achieving the steep dose gradients needed to achieve adequate target volume dosing while sparing nearby critical structures. The advent of intensity-modulated and particle therapies have clearly led to an enhanced ability to reduce the risk of late toxicity and appear to be associated with improved treatment outcomes. Local control rates continue to be a major relapse pattern and future directions require more consistent treatment approaches and cooperative efforts between practitioners and institutions.

REFERENCES

1. Paulino AC, Marks JE, Bricker P, et al. Results of treatment of patients with maxillary sinus carcinoma. Cancer. 1998;83(3):457-65.
2. Tiwari R, Hardillo JA, Mehta D, et al. Squamous cell carcinoma of maxillary sinus. Head Neck. 2000;22(2):164-9.

3. Tran L, Sidrys J, Horton D, et al. Malignant salivary gland tumors of the paranasal sinuses and nasal cavity. The UCLA experience. Am J Clin Oncol. 1989;12(5):387-92.
4. Waldron JN, O'Sullivan B, Warde P, et al. Ethmoid sinus cancer: twenty-nine cases managed with primary radiation therapy. Int J Radiat Oncol Biol Phys. 1998;41(2):361-9.
5. Alvarez I, Suarez C, Rodrigo JP, et al. Prognostic factors in paranasal sinus cancer. Am J Otolaryngol. 1995;16(2):109-14.
6. Giri SP, Reddy EK, Gemer LS, et al. Management of advanced squamous cell carcinomas of the maxillary sinus. Cancer. 1992;69(3):657-61.
7. Le QT, Fu KK, Kaplan M, et al. Treatment of maxillary sinus carcinoma: a comparison of the 1997 and 1977 American Joint Committee on cancer staging systems. Cancer. 1999;86(9):1700-11.
8. Grau C, Jakobsen MH, Harbo G, et al. Sinonasal cancer in Denmark 1982-1991–a nationwide survey. Acta Oncol. 2001;40(1):19-23.
9. Jakobsen MH, Larsen SK, Kirkegaard J, et al. Cancer of the nasal cavity and paranasal sinuses. Prognosis and outcome of treatment. Acta Oncol. 1997;36(1):27-31.
10. Howard DJ, Lund VJ, Wei WI. Craniofacial resection for tumors of the nasal cavity and paranasal sinuses: a 25-year experience. Head Neck. 2006;28(10):867-73.
11. Madani I, Bonte K, Vakaet L, et al. Intensity-modulated radiotherapy for sinonasal tumors: Ghent University Hospital update. Int J Radiat Oncol Biol Phys. 2009;73(2):424-32.
12. Dulguerov P, Allal AS, Calcaterra TC. Esthesioneuroblastoma: a meta-analysis and review. Lancet Oncol. 2001;2(11):683-90.
13. Katz TS, Mendenhall WM, Morris CG, et al. Malignant tumors of the nasal cavity and paranasal sinuses. Head Neck. 2002;24(9):821-9.
14. Lee N, Chen AM. Cancer of the nasal cavity and paranasal sinus: radiation therapy and chemotherapy management. In: Harrison LB, Sessions RB, Hong WK (Eds). Head and neck cancer: a multidisciplinary approach. 3rd edition. Philadelphia: Lipppincott Williams & Wilkins; 2009. p. 475-90, 500-1.
15. Pacholke HD, Amdur RJ, Louis DA, et al. The role of intensity modulated radiation therapy for favorable stage tumor of the nasal cavity or ethmoid sinus. Am J Clin Oncol. 2005;28(5):474-8.
16. Claus F, Boterberg T, Ost P, et al. Short term toxicity profile for 32 sinonasal cancer patients treated with IMRT. Can we avoid dry eye syndrome? Radiother Oncol. 2002;64(2):205-8.
17. Claus F, De Gersem W, De Wagter C, et al. An implementation strategy for IMRT of ethmoid sinus cancer with bilateral sparing of the optic pathways. Int J Radiat Oncol Biol Phys. 2001;51(2):318-31.
18. Hanna E, DeMonte F, Ibrahim S, et al. Endoscopic resection of sinonasal cancers with and without craniotomy: oncologic results. Arch Otolaryngol Head Neck Surg. 2009;135(12):1219-24.
19. Hoppe BS, Nelson CJ, Gomez DR, et al. Unresectable carcinoma of the paranasal sinuses: outcomes and toxicities. International journal of radiation oncology, biology, physics. 2008;72(3):763-9.
20. Logue JP, Slevin NJ. Carcinoma of the nasal cavity and paranasal sinuses: an analysis of radical radiotherapy. Clin Oncol (R Coll Radiol). 1991;3(2):84-9.
21. Rischin D, Porceddu S, Peters L, et al. Promising results with chemoradiation in patients with sinonasal undifferentiated carcinoma. Head Neck. 2004;26(5):435-41.
22. Daly ME, Chen AM, Bucci MK, et al. Intensity-modulated radiation therapy for malignancies of the nasal cavity and paranasal sinuses. Int J Radiat Oncol Biol Phys. 2007;67(1):151-7.
23. Raghavan P, Phillips CD. Magnetic resonance imaging of sinonasal malignancies. Top Magn Reson Imaging. 2007;18(4):259-67.
24. Rasch C, Keus R, Pameijer FA, et al. The potential impact of CT-MRI matching on tumor volume delineation in advanced head and neck cancer. Int J Radiat Oncol Biol Phys. 1997;39(4):841-8.
25. Sheng K, Molloy JA, Larner JM, et al. A dosimetric comparison of non-coplanar IMRT versus Helical Tomotherapy for nasal cavity and paranasal sinus cancer. Radiother Oncol. 2007;82(2):174-8.
26. Guckenberger M, Richter A, Krieger T, et al. Is a single arc sufficient in volumetric-modulated arc therapy (VMAT) for complex-shaped target volumes? Radiother Oncol. 2009;93(2):259-65.

27. Chera BS, Malyapa R, Louis D, et al. Proton therapy for maxillary sinus carcinoma. Am J Clin Oncol. 2009;32(3):296-303.
28. Lomax AJ, Goitein M, Adams J. Intensity modulation in radiotherapy: photons versus protons in the paranasal sinus. Radiother Oncol. 2003;66(1): 11-8.
29. Mock U, Georg D, Bogner J, et al. Treatment planning comparison of conventional, 3D conformal, and intensity-modulated photon (IMRT) and proton therapy for paranasal sinus carcinoma. Int J Radiat Oncol Biol Phys. 2004;58(1):147-54.
30. Truong MT, Kamat UR, Liebsch NJ, et al. Proton radiation therapy for primary sphenoid sinus malignancies: treatment outcome and prognostic factors. Head Neck. 2009;31(10):1297-308.
31. Pommier P, Liebsch NJ, Deschler DG, et al. Proton beam radiation therapy for skull base adenoid cystic carcinoma. Arch Otolaryngol Head Neck Surg. 2006;132(11):1242-9.
32. Carrau RL, Segas J, Nuss DW, et al. Squamous cell carcinoma of the sinonasal tract invading the orbit. Laryngoscope. 1999;109(2 Pt 1):230-5.
33. Perry C, Levine PA, Williamson BR, et al. Preservation of the eye in paranasal sinus cancer surgery. Arch Otolaryngol Head Neck Surg. 1988;114(6): 632-4.
34. Kim HJ, Lee TH, Lee HS, et al. Periorbita: computed tomography and magnetic resonance imaging findings. Am J Rhinol. 2006;20(4):371-4.
35. Tiwari R, van der Wal J, van der Waal I, et al. Studies of the anatomy and pathology of the orbit in carcinoma of the maxillary sinus and their impact on preservation of the eye in maxillectomy. Head Neck. 1998;20(3):193-6.
36. Gras Cabrerizo JR, Sarandeses Garcia A, Montserrat IGJR, et al. [Revision of carcinomas in paranasal sinuses]. Acta otorrinolaringologica espanola. 2007;58(6):266-75.
37. Monroe AT, Bhandare N, Morris CG, et al. Preventing radiation retinopathy with hyperfractionation. Int J Radiat Oncol Biol Phys. 2005;61(3): 856-64.
38. Bhandare N, Monroe AT, Morris CG, et al. Does altered fractionation influence the risk of radiation-induced optic neuropathy? Int J Radiat Oncol Biol Phys. 2005;62(4):1070-7.
39. Harrison LB, Pfister DG, Kraus D, et al. Management of unresectable malignant tumors at the skull base using concomitant chemotherapy and radiotherapy with accelerated fractionation. Skull Base Surg. 1994;4(3):127-31.
40. Wolden SL, Chen WC, Pfister DG, et al. Intensity-modulated radiation therapy (IMRT) for nasopharynx cancer: update of the Memorial Sloan-Kettering experience. Int J Radiat Oncol Biol Phys. 2006;64(1):57-62.
41. Cantu G, Bimbi G, Miceli R, et al. Lymph node metastases in malignant tumors of the paranasal sinuses: prognostic value and treatment. Arch Otolaryngol Head Neck Surg. 2008;134(2):170-7.
42. Dulguerov P, Jacobsen MS, Allal AS, et al. Nasal and paranasal sinus carcinoma: are we making progress? A series of 220 patients and a systematic review. Cancer. 2001;92(12):3012-29.
43. Myers LL, Nussenbaum B, Bradford CR, et al. Paranasal sinus malignancies: an 18-year single institution experience. Laryngoscope. 2002;112(11):1 964-9.
44. Monroe AT, Hinerman RW, Amdur RJ, et al. Radiation therapy for esthesioneuroblastoma: rationale for elective neck irradiation. Head Neck. 2003; 25(7):529-34.
45. Gras-Cabrerizo JR, Montserrat-Gili JR, Leon-Vintro X, et al. Treatment results for ethmoid sinus carcinoma. J Laryngol Otol. 2009;123(10):1120-4.
46 Choussy O, Ferron C, Vedrine PO, et al. Adenocarcinoma of Ethmoid: a GETTEC retrospective multicenter study of 418 cases. Laryngoscope. 2008;118(3):437-43.
47. Dirix P, Nuyts S, Geussens Y, et al. Malignancies of the nasal cavity and paranasal sinuses: long-term outcome with conventional or three-dimensional conformal radiotherapy. Int J Radiat Oncol Biol Phys. 2007;69(4):1042-50.
48. Lin CY, Chen HH, Fang SY, et al. Ethmoid sinus cancer: results of treatment with surgery and combined therapy. Acta Otolaryngol. 2004;124(10): 1220-5.
49. Le QT, Fu KK, Kaplan MJ, et al. Lymph node metastasis in maxillary sinus carcinoma. Int J Radiat Oncol Biol Phys. 2000;46(3):541-9.
50. Lin EM, Sparano A, Spalding A, et al. Sinonasal undifferentiated carcinoma: a 13-year experience

at a single institution. Skull Base. 2010;20(2):61-7.
51. Jeremic B, Shibamoto Y, Milicic B, et al. Elective ipsilateral neck irradiation of patients with locally advanced maxillary sinus carcinoma. Cancer. 2000;88(10):2246-51.
52. Chien PC, Missett B, Yom SS. Nasal cavity and paranasal sinus. In: Hansen EK, Roach M. (Eds). Handbook of evidence-based radiation oncology. 2nd edition. New York: Springer; 2010. pp. 109-16.
53. Hu YH, Tu GY, Qi YQ, et al. Comparison of pre- and postoperative radiation in the combined treatment of carcinoma of maxillary sinus. Int J Radiat Oncol Biol Phys. 1982;8(6):1045-9.
54. Jesse RH. Preoperative versus postoperative radiation in the treatment of squamous carcinoma of the paranasal sinuses. Am J Surg. 1965;110(4):552-6.
55. Bristol IJ, Ahamad A, Garden AS, et al. Postoperative radiotherapy for maxillary sinus cancer: long-term outcomes and toxicities of treatment. Int J Radiat Oncol Biol Phys. 2007;68(3):719-30.
56. Zaharia M, Salem LE, Travezan R, et al. Postoperative radiotherapy in the management of cancer of the maxillary sinus. Int J Radiat Oncol Biol Phys. 1989;17(5):967-71.
57. Levine PA, Frierson HF Jr, Stewart FM, et al. Sinonasal undifferentiated carcinoma: a distinctive and highly aggressive neoplasm. Laryngoscope. 1987;97(8 Pt 1):905-8.
58. Schwaab G, Micheau C, Le Guillou C, et al. Olfactory esthesioneuroma: a report of 40 cases. Laryngoscope. 1988;98(8 Pt 1):872-6.
59. Elkon D, Hightower SI, Lim ML, et al. Esthesioneuroblastoma. Cancer. 1979;44(3):1087-94.
60. Fitzek MM, Thornton AF, Varvares M, et al. Neuroendocrine tumors of the sinonasal tract. Results of a prospective study incorporating chemotherapy, surgery, and combined proton-photon radiotherapy. Cancer. 2002;94(10):2623-34.
61. Rosenthal DI, Barker JL Jr, El-Naggar AK, et al. Sinonasal malignancies with neuroendocrine differentiation: patterns of failure according to histologic phenotype. Cancer. 2004;101(11):2567-73.
62. Deutsch BD, Levine PA, Stewart FM, et al. Sinonasal undifferentiated carcinoma: a ray of hope. Otolaryngol Head Neck Surg. 1993;108(6):697-700.
63. Frierson HF Jr, Mills SE, Fechner RE, et al. Sinonasal undifferentiated carcinoma. An aggressive neoplasm derived from schneiderian epithelium and distinct from olfactory neuroblastoma. Am J Surg Pathol. 1986;10(11):771-9.
64. Chen AM, Daly ME, El-Sayed I, et al. Patterns of failure after combined-modality approaches incorporating radiotherapy for sinonasal undifferentiated carcinoma of the head and neck. Int J Radiat Oncol Biol Phys. 2008;70(2):338-43.
65. Tanzler ED, Morris CG, Orlando CA, et al. Management of sinonasal undifferentiated carcinoma. Head Neck. 2008;30(5):595-9.
66. Jiang GL, Tucker SL, Guttenberger R, et al. Radiation-induced injury to the visual pathway. Radiother Oncol. 1994;30(1):17-25.
67. Chen AM, Daly ME, Bucci MK, et al. Carcinomas of the paranasal sinuses and nasal cavity treated with radiotherapy at a single institution over five decades: are we making improvement? Int J Radiat Oncol Biol Phys. 2007;69(1):141-7.
68. Parsons JT, Bova FJ, Fitzgerald CR, et al. Severe dry-eye syndrome following external beam irradiation. Int J Radiat Oncol Biol Phys. 1994;30(4):775-80.
69. Miralbell R, Crowell C, Suit HD. Potential improvement of three dimension treatment planning and proton therapy in the outcome of maxillary sinus cancer. Int J Radiat Oncol Biol Phys. 1992;22(2):305-10.
70. Schulz-Ertner D, Nikoghosyan A, Thilmann C, et al. Results of carbon ion radiotherapy in 152 patients. Int J Radiat Oncol Biol Phys. 2004;58(2):631-40.
71. Gallagher TM, Boles R. Symposium: Treatment of malignancies of paranasal sinuses. I Carcinoma of the maxillary antrum. Laryngoscope. 1970;80(6):924-32.
72. St-Pierre S, Baker SR. Squamous cell carcinoma of the maxillary sinus: analysis of 66 cases. Head Neck Surg. 1983;5(6):508-13.
73. Chen AM, Ryu J, Donald PJ, et al. Cancer of the nasal cavity and paranasal sinuses. In: Hoppe RT, Phillips TL, Roach M. (Eds). Leibel and Phillips textbook of radiation oncology. Philadelphia: Elsevier Sanders; 2010. p. 700-23.
74. Lavertu P, Roberts JK, Kraus DH, et al. Squamous cell carcinoma of the paranasal sinuses: the Cleveland

Clinic experience 1977-1986. Laryngoscope. 1989;99(11):1130-6.

75. Spiro JD, Soo KC, Spiro RH. Nonsquamous cell malignant neoplasms of the nasal cavities and paranasal sinuses. Head Neck. 1995;17(2):114-8.
76. Jiang GL, Morrison WH, Garden AS, et al. Ethmoid sinus carcinomas: natural history and treatment results. Radiother Oncol. 1998;49(1):21-7.
77. Duthoy W, Boterberg T, Claus F, et al. Postoperative intensity-modulated radiotherapy in sinonasal carcinoma: clinical results in 39 patients. Cancer. 2005;104(1):71-82.
78. Hoppe BS, Stegman LD, Zelefsky MJ, et al. Treatment of nasal cavity and paranasal sinus cancer with modern radiotherapy techniques in the postoperative setting-the MSKCC experience. Int J Radiat Oncol Biol Phys. 2007;67(3): 691-702.
79. Hoppe BS, Wolden SL, Zelefsky MJ, et al. Postoperative intensity-modulated radiation therapy for cancers of the paranasal sinuses, nasal cavity, and lacrimal glands: technique, early outcomes, and toxicity. Head Neck. 2008;30(7): 925-32.

15

Chemotherapy for Sinonasal Cancers

Kena Desai, MD; Madeleine A Kane, MD, PhD

INTRODUCTION

Sinonasal tumors represent less than 1% of all malignancies; however, they are comprised of a wide diversity of histological types and it is not uncommon to find more than one histological type in an anatomically isolated area.[1] It is for this reason that sinonasal tumors are often treated as a single entity.[2] Craniofacial resection followed by postoperative radiation have been the mainstay of treatment for early stage disease. However, because the presenting symptoms are often indolent and nonspecific, the majority of sinonasal tumors are diagnosed in advanced stages. Previously, chemotherapy was reserved for metastatic disease and palliation. Currently it is frequently utilized in the multimodality approach to minimize the size of borderline resectable tumors to treat unresectable tumors and to prevent locoregional recurrence.[3] Unfortunately, due to the rarity of sinonasal tumors, much of what is known about the benefits of chemotherapy comes from relatively small case series and prospective studies. Additionally, these studies have not added chemotherapy to standard surgery plus radiation but to advanced types of surgery and more sophisticated radiation regimens. Therefore, the conclusive benefits of chemotherapy have been difficult to discern.

From review of the literature, the 5-year survival rates of sinonasal malignancies have been estimated to be between 30–50%.[1,2,4,5] In a larger case series of 125 patients with sinonasal tumors primarily treated with surgery +/- radiation, the 5-year survival rate was only 37%.[4] In this series 50% of the patients had T1 disease, 29% had T2 disease and 20% had T3 disease. This population of patients had less advanced disease than most case series, in which chemotherapy has been used as a part of the multimodal approach.

USES OF SYSTEMIC THERAPY

Systemic therapy may be used in a variety of ways for cancers of the sinonasal locations and each approach has a different purpose. Neoadjuvant therapy is administered prior to definitive treatment in an effort to reduce the size of the primary tumor and local extension and/or regional lymph nodes so that the definitive therapy may be potentially less extensive and more likely to have a curative outcome. Induction chemotherapy has been used in this fashion. Chemotherapy has also been used with radiation treatment prior to planned surgical resection. Systemic therapy may also be considered in the adjuvant setting, where definitive therapy has eradicated all detectable tumor, but prognostic factors predict high likelihood of recurrence. The purpose of adjuvant therapy is to reduce the likelihood of recurrence and improve long-term complete response rates and thus overall survival. If surgical treatment is used as a primary modality and no preoperative radiation has been administered, radiation together with systemic therapy may be recommended as adjuvant therapy. Systemic therapy alone may be recommended as adjuvant therapy if radiation and/or surgery have already been administered. Systemic therapy is the only treatment for widely metastatic cancer, although radiation and/or surgery may play a limited role in reduction of tumor burden and palliation. In these cancers, chemotherapy is not considered as a curative treatment by itself. Systemic therapy has also been studied as a chemoprevention approach for some tumors of the sinonasal region but no studies have demonstrated a benefit in recurrence rates or overall survival on average.[6,7]

Commonly Used Agents

Cisplatin

Cisplatin, dichloro-, diamino-platinum, binds to DNA and intercalates itself, causing strand breaks, aberrant DNA synthesis, induction of apoptosis and cell death. Cisplatin is administered IV and is most often used in combination with other systemic drugs. Doses are calculated as mg/m^2 (of body surface area, a calculation based on height and weight of the patient). Doses of cisplatin alone every 3–4 weeks, with or without radiation, range from 75–100 mg/m^2. Major potential toxicities are nausea/vomiting, acute renal failure, ototoxicity, moderate myelosuppression and mild to severe acute or subacute hyponatremia, hypokalemia and hypomagnesemia. Peripheral neuropathy is another potential toxicity. Nausea and vomiting are successfully prevented or significantly reduced with the use of modern antiemetic agents. Renal toxicity may be prevented by aggressive hydration with normal saline prior to, during and after administration of the cisplatin. Inclusion of mannitol in the cisplatin infusion as an osmotic diuretic or the use of small doses of intravenous furosemide, have largely eliminated severe acute renal failure. Ototoxicity manifests as high frequency hearing loss and/or persistent tinnitus, and rarely toxicity to the vestibular system causing persistent dizziness. Amifostine is Food and Drug Administration (FDA) approved for administration prior to cisplatin in order to prevent or reduce severity of these toxicities, especially renal failure, ototoxicity and peripheral neuropathy. Since amifostine itself is highly emetogenic, it is not routinely used in all patients receiving cisplatin.

Carboplatin

Carboplatin delivers platinum chelated with an organic molecule to the DNA of cells. In comparative studies, outcomes with cisplatin vs. carboplatin seem similar with respect to overall survival. Carboplatin toxicities differ somewhat from those of cisplatin. Myelosuppression and peripheral neuropathy are more prevalent, whereas nausea/vomiting, renal failure and electrolyte abnormalities are seldom seen. Although most treatment regimens prefer the use of cisplatin, carboplatin may be substituted for cisplatin if the side effects of cisplatin are poorly tolerated.

Fluorouracil

Fluorouracil (5-FU) is a nucleoside analog which inhibits DNA synthesis by inhibiting the conversion of uridine to thymidine by thymidylate synthetase. 5-FU has been most often used as a 96–120 hour continuous IV infusion together with cisplatin in head and neck cancers including sinonasal cancers. Capecitabine is an oral drug that is converted to 5-FU intracellularly. Capecitabine has been minimally studied in head and neck cancers, but potentially could replace the continuous intravenous administration of 5-FU, which requires a semipermanent IV access, such as a peripherally inserted central catheter (PICC) line or a mediport. Potential toxicities of 5-FU include diarrhea, mucositis, severe fatigue, skin photosensitivity and less likely nausea/vomiting and myelosuppression.

Etoposide

This drug is an inhibitor of topoisomerase II, which results in DNA strand breaks and ultimately apoptosis. It is generally used in combinations with other chemotherapeutic agents. Common side effects include bone marrow suppression, mucositis, alopecia and infusion-related blood pressure variations. It is strongly bound to albumin and its use in patients with low albumin results in greater proportion of unbound drug and greater associated toxicity.

Taxanes (Paclitaxel and Docetaxel)

These are usually included in combination regimens with platinum compounds and 5-FU. Their mechanism of action is prevention of microtubule disassembly into tubulin monomers, thus disturbing mitosis. Potential toxicities are myelosuppression, fatigue, asthenia and peripheral neuropathy. Nausea and vomiting are generally mild. Hypersensitivity reactions may also occur, and premedication routinely with corticosteroids, antihistamines and histamine receptor-2 blockers greatly reduces the likelihood of this side effect. Efficacy of the taxanes is similar. Docetaxel may have slightly less likelihood of causing peripheral neuropathy.

Methotrexate

Methotrexate, a dihydrofolate reductase inhibitor, impedes DNA synthesis by depleting intracellular reduced folates, which are needed for thymidylate synthetase conversion of uridine to thymidine. Potential toxicities of methotrexate include fatigue, myelosuppression, nausea, mucositis and diarrhea. Toxicities are dose dependent.

Doxorubicin and Daunorubicin

These are anthracyclines. They intercalate between base pairs, inhibit topoisomerase II and generate free radicals. Their toxicity profile includes bone marrow suppression, gastrointestinal distress and severe alopecia. This class is also associated with myocardial toxicity, resulting in cardiomyopathy and heart failure. Their effects on the myocardium are dose dependent with the cumulative dose limit being 450 mg/m^2 in most regimens. Previous cardiovascular disease and irradiation of the heart may result in cardiotoxicity at even lower doses.

Application of Systemic Therapy in Different Types of Sinonasal Cancer

Sinonasal tumors can be divided into two broad histological categories, which are epithelial and nonepithelial. The epithelial tumors are comprised of squamous cell carcinomas (SCC), adenocarcinomas, adenoid cystic carcinomas and undifferentiated carcinomas.[8] Nonepithelial tumors includes the important subset of tumors of neuroendocrine origin, which are esthesioneuroblastoma, neuroendocrine carcinoma and small cell carcinoma.[1,9,10] Cisplatin-based therapies have been used in the treatment of both epithelial tumors and tumors of neuroendocrine origins (Table 15.1).

Table 15.1 Summary of selected chemotherapy studies of sinonasal cancers

Tumor Type	*Chemotherapy*	*Survival rates*	*Reference*
Epithelial	Neoadjuvant, intra-arterial Cisplatin + radiation	5 year – 81%	5
Epithelial	Intra-arterial 5-FU + surgery and radiation	5 year – 76%	9
Epithelial	Systemic cisplatin, 5-FU and leucovirin followed by sugery and radiation	3 year – 63%	15
Epithelial	Surgical debulking followed by a topical 5% 5-FU emulsion	5 year – 87%	10
Neuroendocrine	Cisplatin, etoposide + high dose proton-photon radio therapy and sugery	5 year – 74%	4

In the earlier studies, investigating the benefits of adding chemotherapy to surgery plus radiation, the results were unimpressive. There was only a small but statistically significant improvement in survival with the addition of chemotherapy, however, the systemic side effects outweighed the benefits.[11] In a novel study, neoadjuvant, intra-arterial cisplatin with concurrent radiation followed by conservative craniofacial resection was investigated in 11 patients with T3 and T4 epithelial sinonasal tumors.[8] In this protocol, branches of the external carotid artery supplying the tumor were infused with cisplatin at a dose of 150 mg/m^2. Sodium thiosulfate was administered simultaneously with the cisplatin to neutralize the systemic effects, most notably nephrotoxicity and ototoxicity. This form of selective, locoregional chemotherapy was estimated to allow for a ten-fold increase in the delivery of cisplatin to the tumor bed. The patients underwent four weekly cycles of cisplatin infusions with concurrent radiation for five weeks, followed by conservative craniofacial resection. The authors reported a 5-year overall survival of 81% and a progression free survival of 67% in this study population. When compared with the author's reported survival rates of 27–45% for resection +/– radiation, this was a dramatic improvement in the treatment.

In a similar study, 78 Japanese patients with carcinoma of the maxillary sinus (the majority being SCC) were treated with surgery, intra-arterial 5-FU and radiation.[5] In this trial, the patients received an intra-arterial infusion of 250 mg of 5-FU at the time of the surgery, followed by an additional 5 days of infusions with concomitant radiation.[5] These authors reported a 5-year overall survival rate of 76% and local control rates of 74%.[5] Again, these were significantly better results than with surgery plus radiation alone.

Systemic use of cisplatin in combination with 5-FU and leucovirin has also shown benefits. In a study of 49 patients with predominantly adenocarcinoma of the paranasal sinus, induction with cisplatin, 5-FU and leucovorin was used prior to surgery and radiation. Of the 49 patients, 32 (65%) completed a minimum of three cycles of the induction chemotherapy and 21 (43%) had a response. Four patients had a complete radiological response, as defined by complete disappearance of the tumor and 17 patients had a partial response as defined by at least 50% reduction of the measurable lesion's two greatest perpendicular diameter. Three of the four patients who had a complete response received five cycles of induction chemotherapy. Of the 17 patients that did not complete the minimum three cycles of induction chemotherapy, two patients died due to thrombotic complications and eight patients were withdrawn from the study due to adverse cardiac events. These incidences occurred during the first cycle and all of the cardiac events occurred during the infusion of 5-FU. Regardless of response to induction chemotherapy, 42 patients (86%) underwent anterior craniofacial resection. Of these, eight patients (16%) were found to have complete pathological remission on biopsy. Unfortunately, the authors did not report, which percent of these patients were responders to chemotherapy. The authors reported an overall three-year survival rate of 69% and event-free survival of 57%. Of the patients who had completed pathological response, the three-year event-free survival and overall survival rate was 100%.[12]

Fluorouracil (5-FU) has also been used topically in the treatment of adenocarcinoma of the ethmoidal sinuses. Sixty-two patients underwent surgical debulking, followed by generous application of a 5% fluorouracil emulsion to the resection bed.[11] The patients then underwent eight dressing changes with meticulous debridement of necrotic tissue and reapplication of the 5-FU emulsion. Disease free survival at 5-years was reported as 87%.

Although nonepithelial tumors of the sinonasal cavity comprise only a small percentage, neuroendocrine tumors have been the subject of several small case series. Nineteen patients with neuroendocrine tumors, neuroblastoma or neuroendocrine carcinoma were treated with two courses of neoadjuvant cisplatin at a dose of 33 mg/m^2 and etoposide at a dose of 100 mg/m^2.[9]

This regimen was followed by high-dose proton-photon radiotherapy and surgical resection. Responders to the initial neoadjuvant therapy proceeded to receive four additional cycles of cisplatin and etoposide after surgery, whereas non-responders did not. Of the responders, three had complete remission of disease and ten had partial remission, defined as a greater than 50% reduction in tumor dimensions. Of the six patients that had no response to chemotherapy 50% progressed to metastatic disease, while only one of the responders progressed to metastatic disease. The overall 5-year survival rate was 74% and 5-year local control rate was 88%. Complete or partial response to chemotherapy directly correlated with increased overall survival ($p = 0.02$), as well as metastasis-free survival ($p = 0.04$) but not with local control of disease.

TARGETED AGENTS IN SINONASAL CANCER

Chemotherapy in all malignancies is associated with systemic toxicity and acquired drug resistance, therefore, the need for targeted agents is evident.[13] The use of targeted agents in sinonasal tumors has only recently started to be investigated. What is known has been extrapolated from data from the treatment of head and neck SCC in advanced disease states. Like head and neck carcinomas, SCC comprises 75–90% of the histological type of sinonasal malignances; therefore, the aberrant biochemical pathways are likely to be the same.

The majority of SCC over-express the epidermal growth factor receptor (EGFR).[13,14] Over-expression of EGFR is a strong prognostic indicator of locoregional recurrence, as well as shortened disease-free survival. Currently, there are two classes of targeted agents that module EGFR activity, first, monoclonal antibodies and second, tyrosine kinase inhibitors.

Cetuximab is the best studied of the monoclonal antibodies. It binds to EGFR with greater affinity then its physiological ligands, epidermal growth factor (EGF) and tumor necrosis factor-alpha (TNF-α). The EGFR-cetuximab complex is then endocytosed and degraded by the cell without activation of downstream signal transduction pathways.[13] Cetuximab has also been shown to potentiate the activity of both chemotherapy and radiation therapy.[13-15]

Several case series have investigated the benefits of adding cetuximab to a cisplatin based chemotherapy +/– radiation. In a pilot study conducted by Pfister et al. the combination cisplatin and cetuximab with simultaneous high-dose radiation therapy was used to treat patients with stage III and VI squamous cell head and neck cancer without metastasis.[14] The authors reported 3-year survival rates of 76% and progression-free survival rate of 56%. Unfortunately, this series only contained 22 patients and was prematurely terminated due to significant adverse events. It retrospect the authors concluded that adverse events were unlikely to be related to the treatment. Two randomized, placebo controlled trials have also been conducted. In the earlier trial, 117 patients with recurrent/metastatic SCC of the head and neck were randomized to treatment with cisplatin at a dose of 100 mg/m^2 every 4 weeks alone or with cetuximab at an initial dose of 200 mg/m^2 and all following doses of 125 mg/m^2.[16] Although, an increase in progression free survival was observed in the cisplatin plus cetuximab arm, it was not statistically significant. Also, a correlation was observed between cetuximab skin toxicity, which manifests as an acne-like rash and increased survival. This has been noted in other studies with cetuximab.

In the more recent randomized, placebo-controlled, clinical trial of 442 patients, the combination of cisplatin, 5-FU and cetuximab was found to be superior to just cisplatin and 5-FU alone in the treatment of recurrent or metastatic head and neck SCC.[15] In this study, patients received cisplatin 100 mg/m^2 on day one and 5-FU 1000 mg/m^2 on day four. The cycles were repeated every 3 weeks for a maximum of six cycles. In the cetuximab arm, cetuximab 400 mg/m^2 was initiated on the first cycle and repeated at a dose of 250 mg/m^2 weekly for every additional cycle. The results showed an increase in disease-free survival of 2.3 months ($p<0.001$) and overall survival of 2.7 months ($p=0.04$) in the cetuximab group. This success of this study compared to the previous was likely multifaceted. This study was better powered, it used high doses of both cisplatin and cetuximab, and 5-FU was added to the treatment regimen. Of interest, this study did not find a statistical significance between the cetuximab-induced skin toxicity and overall survival.

SUMMARY

Sinonasal tumors are rare, histologically diverse groups of malignancies, which are associated with considerable morbidity and mortality. The morbidity of these tumors arises largely from their intricate and compact anatomical location, as well as their proximity to other vital structures. They are challenging to treat surgically and with irradiation without causing appreciable collateral damage. Locoregional recurrence is the predominant cause of mortality. The treatment complexities of sinonasal tumors have prompted the evolution of multimodality treatment regimens. Many of these regimens are now routinely including chemotherapy. The goals are to reduce the size of the tumor to facilitate complete resection, mimimize regional and systemic collateral damage and treat the surrounding tissue in order to prevent locoregional recurrence. The initial failures of chemotherapy were due to inadequate dosing and the rapid development of resistance. Today, the use of novel techniques to administer chemotherapy, synergistic combinations of chemotherapy, and the addition of targeted agents to further potentiate the chemotherapeutic effects, are creating an evolving role for chemotherapy in the multimodality treatment of sinonasal tumors. It is likely in the near future that an approach that includes chemotherapy will be considered the standard of care.

REFERENCES

1. Rischin D, Coleman A. Sinonasal Malignancies of Neuroendocrine Origin. Hematol Oncol Clin N Am. 2008;1297-316.
2. Resto VA, Deschler DG. Sinonasal Malignancies. Otolarynol Clin N Am. 2004;37:473-87.
3. Blanch JL, Ruiz AM, Alos L, et al. Treatment of 125 sinonasal tumors: prognostic factors, outcomes and follow-up. Otolaryngol Head Neck Surg. 2004;973-6.
4. Fitzek MM, Thornton AF, Varvares M, et al. Neuroendocrine tumors of the sinonasal tract: results of a prospective study incorporating chemotherapy, surgery and combined proton-photon radiotherapy. Cancer. 2001;94(10):2623-34.
5. Micheal LM, Sorenson JM, Samant S, et al. The Treatment of Advanced Sinonasal Malignancies with Preoperative Intra-arterial Cisplatin and Concurrent Radiation. J NeuroOncol. 2005;72:67-75
6. Wade PM, Smith RE, Johns ME. Response of Esthesioneuroblastoma to Chemotherapy: Report of Five Cases and Review of the Literature. Cancer. 1984;53:1036-41.
7. Khademi B, Moradi A, Hoseini S, et al. Malignant Neoplasms of the Sinonasal Tract: Report of 71 patients and literature review and analysis. Oral Maxillofac Surg. 2009;13:191-9.
8. Sayed S, Nelson N. Adjuvant and Adjunctive Chemotherapy in the Management of Squamous Cell Carcinoma of the Head and Neck Region: Meta-Analysis of Prospective and Randomized Trials. J Clin Oncol. 1996;14(3):838-47.
9. Nishino H, Miyata M, Morita M, et al. Combined therapy with conservative surgery, radiotherapy, and regional chemotherapy for maxillay sinus carcinoma. Cancer. 2000;89(9):1925-32.
10. Knegt PP, Ah-See KW, Velden L, et al. Adenocarcinoma of the Ethmoidal Sinus Complex. Arch Otolaryngol Head Neck Surg. 2001;127:141-6.
11. Specenier PM, Vermorken JB. Targeted therapies in head and neck cancer. Tag Oncol. 2007;2:73-88.
12. Pfister DG, Su YB, Kraus DH, et al. Concurrent cetuximab, cisplatin and concomitant boost

radiotherapy for locoregionally advanced, squamous cell head and neck cancer: A pilot phase II study of a new combined-modality paradigm. J Clin Oncol. 2006;24:1072-8.

13. Burtness B, Goldwasser MA, Flood W, et al. Phase III randomized trial of cisplatin plus placebo compared with cisplatin plus cetuximab in metastatic/ cooperative oncology group study. J Clin Oncol. 2005;23:8646-54.

14. Vermorken JB, Mesia R, Rivera F, et al. Platinum-based chemotherapy in head and neck cancer. N Eng J Med. 2008;359(11):1116-27.

15. Licitra L, Locati LD, Cavina R, et al. Primary chemotherapy followed by anterior craniofacial resection and radiotherapy for paranasal cancer. Annals Oncol. 2003;14:367-72.

16. Marur S, Forastiere A. Head and neck cancer: changing epidemiology, diagnosis and treatment. Mayo Clin Proc. 2008;83(4):489-501.

16

Recurrence and Surveillance for Sinonasal Cancers

Nithin D Adappa, MD; Jeremy T Reed, MD, MPH; James N Palmer, MD

INTRODUCTION

Malignant paranasal sinus tumors are a heterogeneous group that account for approximately 3% of all head and neck cancers.[1] Paranasal sinus cancers most commonly include the following pathologic subtypes: Squamous cell carcinoma (SCC) which represent approximately 50–80% of malignancies, adenocarcinoma, adenoid cystic carcinoma, olfactory neuroblastoma, sinonasal undifferentiated carcinoma, minor salivary tumors, mucosal melanoma, sarcoma and other rare tumors.[2-4] Sinonasal tumors most commonly originate from the maxillary sinus (70–80%), followed by the ethmoid sinuses (10–20%) and rarely sphenoid and frontal sinuses.[2-4]

While much of this textbook centers on the importance of diagnosis and proper surgical management, the focus of this chapter is on post-treatment management and tumor surveillance for long-term survival. Due to the relative paucity of sinonasal tumors and multiple sites of origin and various histological types, there are no multi-institutional prospective, randomized trials looking at treatment modalities for primary tumors. Similarly, no uniform post-treatment protocol has been developed for surveillance of this patient population. For all head and neck cancers, there is mixed data in the literature looking at the efficacy of routine surveillance. It has been demonstrated that routine surveillance is associated with a survival benefit. De Visscher demonstrated in a large cohort study mean survival after detection of events (154 recurrences, 58 second primaries and 56 distant metastases) was significantly improved with routine follow-up as compared to self-referral (58 versus 32 months) in 428 patients.[5] Conversely, other studies that have found no survival benefit from detecting asymptomatic recurrence.[6-8] Ritoe et al. looked at 402 patients who underwent curative-intent therapy for laryngeal cancer and were followed with routine surveillance. They found no difference in either overall survival or tumor-related mortality rates for patients with and without symptoms. They did demonstrate a small difference in whether salvage therapy was done with curative intent but this did not translate into a survival benefit.[9] Unfortunately, even in the general head and neck literature, there are no controlled, prospective studies demonstrating a survival benefit for any follow-up protocol.

Despite the lack of conclusive data on routine surveillance, nearly all cancer surgeons believe that regular post-treatment follow-up is an essential part of long-term cancer management. The goal of surveillance is to pick up locoregional recurrences that are detected early and are more likely to be successfully salvaged, thus resulting in overall improved outcomes.[10,11] Additionally, close surveillance has benefits beyond improved survival including dealing with treatment-related complications such as nasal obstruction, crusting, xerostomia and orbital related issues.

POST-TREATMENT SURVEILLANCE

In most cases of sinonasal tumors, treatment is surgical with or without adjuvant chemoradiation. Whether the surgical resection is performed open or endoscopically, it is critical that all sinuses are opened up for maximal post-treatment surveillance. The goal is a large, wide-open nasal cavity, where clear visualization for any evidence of recurrence is possible and any areas of concern may be easily biopsied (Figs 16.1A and B). In addition to the endoscopic examination, routine history and physical examination is critical for post-treatment surveillance.

History and Physical Examination

The key points covered during a focused history highlight any changes in sinonasal symptoms. These include epistaxis, nasal congestion, rhinorrhea, increasing postnasal drip, epiphora, and new onset pain. Additionally, patients should be screened for overall health changes, including weight loss and fatigue, which may raise suspicion for recurrent disease.

A complete physical examination should be performed on every visit. Otologic examination looking specifically for evidence of eustachian tube dysfunction or obstruction such as serous otitis media or acute otitis media should be noted. Eye examination will evaluate for any evidence of restricted extraocular movements or proptosis. As many sinonasal tumors involve the region surrounding the pterygopalatine fossa and cavernous sinus, tests of cranial nerve (CN) II, III, IV and VI as well as branches of the trigeminal nerve should be tested. Additionally, the neck should be carefully palpated for lymphadenopathy.

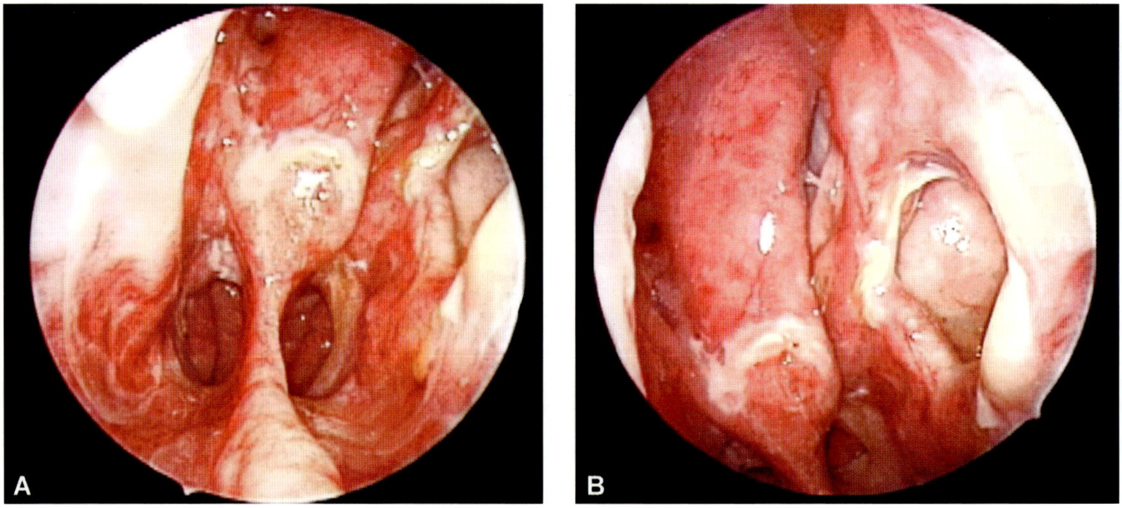

Figs 16.1A and B: (A) Patient's status post-resection and reconstruction with a nasoseptal flap with subsequent radiation therapy for an esthesioneuroblastoma. He has a large patent cavity for clear endoscopic surveillance; (B) Visualization with 30° endoscope demonstrating healthy appearing mucosa along the skull base with widely patent sphenoid and maxillary ostium with no evidence of recurrence.

Examination of the nasal cavity should include an anterior rhinoscopy followed by nasal endoscopy. The advent of angled endoscopes has improved our in-office surveillance. Use solely of a 0-degree endoscope limits visualization past the nasal cavity. Both direct visualization into maxillary sinuses as well as the skull base and frontal sinuses are not possible with the 0-degree field of view. 30-degree scopes add an improved view of the maxillary sinuses and skull base. They generally afford adequate visualization into the frontal sinuses as well. When special attention is required for the frontal sinus, the 70-degree scope will provide a clear field of view (Figs 16.2A to F). If any crusting or purulence is present, it should be aggressively suctioned away for clear visualization of the underlying mucosa. In many cases of tumor recurrence, the surrounding mucosa becomes inflamed. This will manifest as thickened mucosa and purulent secretions. Hence, any focal areas of infection should be closely examined to rule out a local recurrence.

Equally as important as angled endoscopes is the availability of straight and angled instruments in the office setting. The importance in detecting recurrent sinonasal cancer in its early stages should give the surgeon little hesitation to biopsy any concerning areas. The paranasal sinuses, when previously operated and if provided with adequate instrumentation, allows for biopsy of the majority of areas in the office setting. This further highlights the importance of opening up all sinuses widely for long-term surveillance. If patients present with fullness or the appearance of submucosal changes

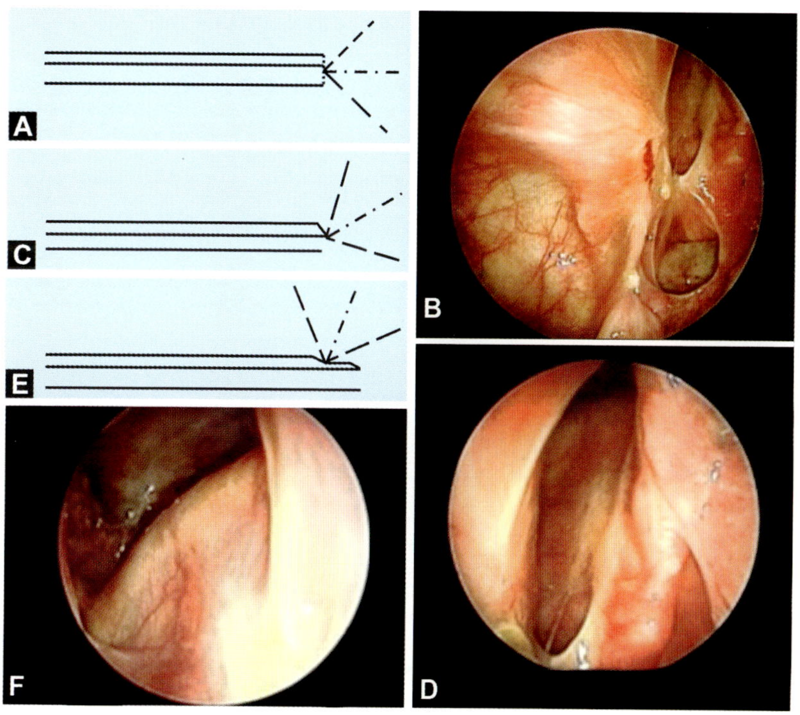

Figs 16.2A to F: (A) Schematic of 0° scope demonstrating its field-of-view; (B) Field-of-view of 0° scope. Visualization of maxillary sinus as well as posterior ethmoid cells; (C) Schematic of 30° scope demonstrating field-of-view; (D) Field-of-view of 30° scope. Visualization of skull base as well as posterior aspect of frontal recess; (E) Schematic of 70° scope demonstrating field of view; (F) Field-of-view of 70° scope. Visualization of patent frontal recess.

or has a suspicious area adjacent to a major blood vessel or critical area, i.e. clivus, pterygopalatine fossa, the patient may require an intraoperative biopsy and imaging is recommended prior to intervention.

Figure 16.3 highlights the importance of surveillance nasal endoscopy. This is a patient with a history of mucosal melanoma who underwent complete resection but refused post-treatment chemoradiation. Approximately one year post-surgical treatment, she presented for routine follow-up. On nasal endoscopy she had multiple sites of recurrence. This was confirmed with in-office biopsies. This was easily seen due to the widely opened sinus cavities allowing clear visualization. These small, local recurrences may have been difficult to assess on imaging studies. She subsequently underwent chemoradiation therapy (Fig. 16.3).

Frequency of Post-Treatment Examination

In the literature, there is limited evidence on optimal timing between follow-up appointments. Currently, multiple expert groups are attempting to address post-treatment surveillance protocols as part of practice guidelines for head and neck cancers.[6,12] The National Comprehensive Cancer Network (NCCN) has developed the current guidelines for follow-up protocols.[13] The NCCN guidelines include follow-up for the vast majority of head and neck cancers, which includes those of the paranasal sinus. These guidelines stress close surveillance over the course of the first 2 years, as this is the period where 80–90% of recurrence occur.[9] Sinonasal tumor patients should be seen every 1–3 months in the first year after treatment, and then stretched out to eventually every 6–12 months after 5 years. (Table 16.1) Although clear evidence of benefit from follow-up after 3 years is lacking, continued follow-up beyond 5 years is generally suggested since the risk of recurrence remains elevated beyond 5 years. This is especially true for cancers of the hypopharynx, larynx, nasopharynx, and salivary glands.[12,14,15]

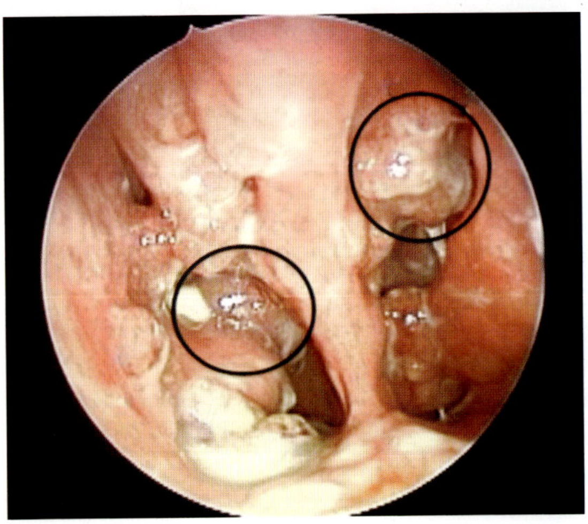

Fig. 16.3: Nasal endoscopy with a 30° endoscope demonstrates two sites of tumor recurrence (black circles). These were treated with chemoradiotherapy.

Post-Treatment Imaging

Long-term surveillance is not complete without routine imaging in addition to complete history and physical examination. Generally, computed tomography (CT) and magnetic resonance imaging (MRI) are used to evaluate treatment response and evaluate for residual disease.

The difficulty encountered in patients who have completed chemoradiotherapy is the differentiation between residual tumor and treatment-induced edema and postoperative changes. Imaging should not be performed for at least 4 weeks after treatment to minimize false positive interpretation.

Computed tomography and MRI are useful post-treatment screening modalities to detect

Table 16.1 Frequency of physical examination of all head and neck cancer sites including paranasal sinuses according to NCCN

Post-treatment year	*Physical examination frequency*
1	Every 1–3 months
2	Every 2–4 months
3–5	Every 4–6 months
>5	Every 6–12 months

recurrence after treatment. Although nasal endoscopy provides direct visualization into tumor recurrence sites, imaging provides information on areas that are not accessible clinically. MRI is generally the more commonly used imaging modality as it allows for greater delineation of soft tissues planes in the previously treated field. In addition, MRI provides early evidence of dural involvement or perineural invasion. (Please see Chapter 3 for further details) The proper time period for scans is unclear in the head and neck literature. What is clear is that the initial 2–3 years after treatment is critical as this is the greatest time point for recurrent disease to appear.[7,9] During this time, it is important to continue periodic imaging due to the difficulty in scan interpretation. Comparison among imaging studies obtained over time is more informative in excluding recurrent tumor than a single study due to the difficulty in radiographic evaluation in the early post-treatment period. Figures 16.4A and B illustrate a case where imaging identified tumor recurrence in the face of a normal endoscopic examination. This is a patient with a paranasal sinus neuroendocrine tumor. She underwent an endoscopic resection and post-surgical radiation therapy. She followed up routinely and underwent complete nasal endoscopy on each follow-up. Her endoscopy demonstrated well-healed, normal appearing mucosa. Despite this normal appearance, a routine surveillance MRI demonstrated a large submucosal recurrence. She was subsequently treated with palliative chemotherapy.

Positron emission tomography (PET) or CT scan is another modality of post-treatment surveillance that is gaining wide spread use. PET scans are particularly useful in differentiating post-treatment changes from recurrent tumor. Physiologically, tumor cells are metabolically more active than surrounding normal tissue thus retaining more of the18F-flourodeoxyglucose (FDG) and demonstrating increased uptake. The difficulty with CT and MRI post-treatment are that they have limited ability to identify small areas of recurrence in the setting of post-treatment change when anatomic or fascial planes have been disrupted. The exact timing of initial post-treatment PET scans is of continued debate. Scan completed within 1–2 months of treatment have a high false positive rate due to continued inflammatory changes.[16] Generally, PET scans performed 3–4 months after treatment

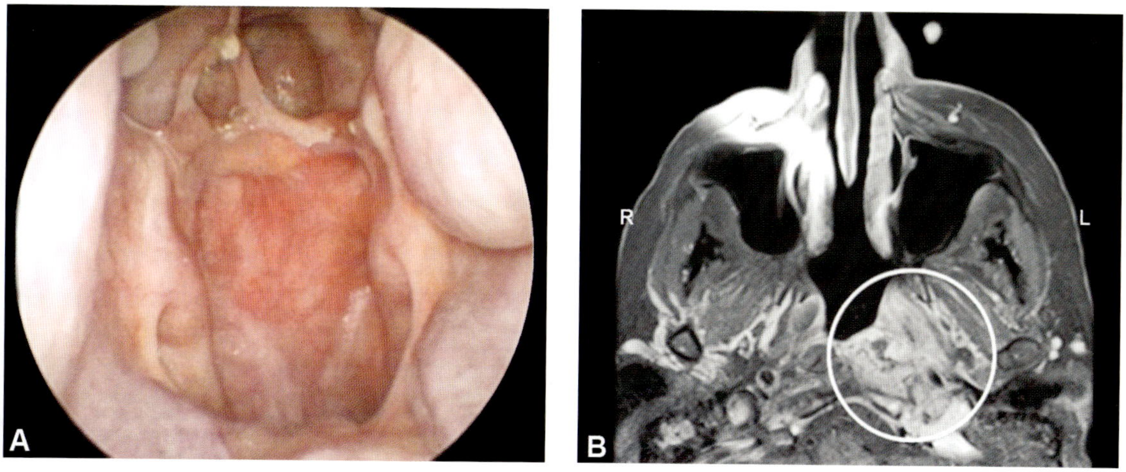

Figs 16.4A and B: (A) Patient with a paranasal sinus neuroendocrine tumor after endoscopic resection and radiation therapy. She has a well-mucosalized nasal cavity with no evidence of recurrence on examination; (B) An axial T1-weighted postgadolinium-MRI demonstrating a large submucosal recurrence (white circle) extending from the left nasopharynx into the skull base, retropharyngeal, parapharyngeal, prevertebral and carotid spaces. It had encased the left carotid artery.

minimize false positive results.[16,17] Based on FDG avidity in metabolically active tumor cells, a number of studies are also currently looking at the utility of PET scans in benign tumors such as inverted papilloma (IP) attempting to quantify increased FDG avid regions that may correlate to squamous cell originating from an IP.[18] Future research will be continued in this direction attempting to stratify PET scan uptake in correlation with risk of malignancy. Although there is no clear literature on the timing and frequency of post-treatment radiographic imaging, it is clear that 80–90% of recurrence occurs in the first 2–4 years and thus the majority of scans should be performed during this time period.

Post-Treatment Protocol

Currently the dilemma clinicians face in post-treatment surveillance for sinonasal cancer is secondary to the lack of clear-cut data or guidelines regarding optimal timing for various surveillance modalities. Additionally, the majority of the literature is focused on general head and neck cancers and not specifically on sinonasal malignancies.

The key factor in regards to paranasal sinus malignancies as opposed to other oropharyngeal carcinomas is our vastly superior postoperative visualization. Oropharyngeal recurrence is often difficult to assess due to the challenge in evaluating tissue following surgery and radiation. Patients generally have a large amount of edema and secretions that pose a problem with evaluation. Additionally, suspicious areas in the upper aerodigestive tract, unless in the oral cavity, generally cannot be biopsied in the office and require evaluation in the operating room. After creating a wide surgical field for sinonasal tumor surgery, postoperative surveillance is aided by accurate visualization with endoscopes. Furthermore, even with adjuvant chemoradiation, the sinonasal mucosa generally heals well with minimal post-treatment edema. Crusting of the cavity can be an issue, but these areas can be suctioned to evaluate underlying mucosa quite readily. Finally, with the use of angles scopes and instruments, just about every area in the paranasal sinus can be safely biopsied in the office, allowing for evaluation of even questionable regions that may otherwise be observed closely in other aerodigestive tract locations.

At our institution, we emphasize direct visualization of the sinonasal cavity with frequent nasal endoscopy. Following surgery, we will follow the patient with nasal endoscopy every 1–2 weeks until the nasal cavity has completely mucosalized. At this point, we will perform nasal endoscopy once every 2 months for the first year, once every 3 months for the second year and every 6 months after that. We use post-treatment imaging less frequently than surveillance on other head and neck cancers as we feel our visualization in this location is far superior. We perform a PET/CT scan approximately 3-4 months following full treatment and then annually thereafter. In addition, we will perform an annual MRI and if any clinical suspicion arises in the interim, we will perform an MRI and/or CT scan at that time.

Recurrent Disease

Patient developing recurrent disease generally have a poor outcome.[19] Treatment options are limited based on previous treatment modalities employed for primary therapy.

When recurrence is demonstrated, the decision should be made as to whether to employ aggressive therapy with curative intent or to plan for palliative treatment and supportive care. This decision is based on (1) location and extent of recurrence; (2) previous treatment modality; (3) overall health of the patient and desire for various treatment protocols.

In addition, the initial disease-free interval plays an important role in determining the treatment modality. Patients with disease recurrence within one year of initial treatment have a significantly worse survival than patients who recur later.[20]

Any patient with locoregional recurrent disease should be worked up for distant metastases with a

PET/CT. If they demonstrate distant disease, they will likely to be candidates for palliative chemotherapy. If the disease is confined locoregionally, they may be candidates for curative treatment with either surgical salvage or chemoradiation depending on the previous modality of treatment. In patients who can tolerate aggressive therapy but have tumors not amendable to surgical resection, reirradiation protocols with chemotherapy may be an option. The toxicity in this therapy, especially considering the surrounding structures including the eye, optic nerve, brain and spinal cord must be taken into consideration.

CONCLUSION

Paranasal sinus tumors pose a difficult dilemma in both initial treatment as well as optimal post-treatment surveillance. The challenge remains in providing regimented surveillance with a lack of literature studies and guidelines. Much of the data regarding follow-up and even salvage treatment is extrapolated from the general head and neck literature despite the obvious anatomic and pathologic differences in the disease process. Despite these facts, certain tenants of post-treatment care remain. These include long-term patient follow-up with thorough history and physical examination, careful nasal endoscopy, and post-treatment surveillance imaging. The overall benefit of imaging is magnified with multiple post-treatment scans leading to improved interpretation through careful comparison of images. And finally, recurrence must be dealt in a systematic fashion including a complete new work-up with biopsy results, CT and MRI as well as a metastatic evaluation.

REFERENCES

1. Day TA, Beas RA, Schlosser RJ, et al. Management of paranasal sinus malignancy. Curr Treat Options Oncol. 2005;6(1):3-18.
2. Blanch JL, Ruiz AM, Alos L, et al. Treatment of 125 sinonasal tumors: prognostic factors, outcome, and follow-up. Otolaryngol Head Neck Surg. 2004;131(6):973-6.
3. Myers LL, Nussenbaum B, Bradford CR, et al. Paranasal sinus malignancies: an 18-year single institution experience. Laryngoscope. 2002;112(11):1964-9.
4. Dulguerov P, Jacobsen MS, Allal AS, et al. Nasal and paranasal sinus carcinoma: are we making progress? A series of 220 patients and a systematic review. Cancer. 2001;92(12):3012-29.
5. de Visscher AV, J.J. Manni. Routine long-term follow-up in patients treated with curative intent for squamous cell carcinoma of the larynx, pharynx, and oral cavity. Does it make sense? Arch Otolaryngol Head Neck Surg. 1994;120(9):934-9.
6. Schwartz DL, Barker J Jr, Chansky K, et al. Postradiotherapy surveillance practice for head and neck squamous cell carcinoma--too much for too little? Head Neck. 2003;25(12):990-9.
7. Boysen M, Lövdal O, Tausjö J, et al. The value of follow-up in patients treated for squamous cell carcinoma of the head and neck. Eur J Cancer. 1992;28(2-3):426-30.
8. Francis DO, Yueh B, Weymuller EA Jr, et al. Impact of surveillance on survival after laryngeal cancer in the medicare population. Laryngoscope. 2009;119(12):2337-44.
9. Ritoe SC, Krabbe PF, Kaanders JH, et al. Value of routine follow-up for patients cured of laryngeal carcinoma. Cancer. 2004;101(6):1382-9.
10. Snow GB. Follow-up in patients treated for head and neck cancer: how frequent, how thorough and for how long? Eur J Cancer. 1992;28(2-3):315-6.
11. Manikantan K, Khode S, Dwivedi RC, et al. Making sense of post-treatment surveillance in head and neck cancer: when and what of follow-up. Cancer Treat Rev. 2009;35(8):744-53.
12 Joshi A, Calman F, O'Connell M, et al. Current trends in the follow-up of head and neck cancer patients in the UK. Clin Oncol (R Coll Radiol). 2010;22(2):114-8.
13. Network, N.C.C. 2010 [cited 2010 12/1/10].
14. Spector JG, Sessions DG, Haughey BH, et al. Delayed regional metastases, distant metastases, and second primary malignancies in squamous cell carcinomas of the larynx and hypopharynx. Laryngoscope. 2001;111(6):1079-87.
15. Chen AM, Garcia J, Granchi PJ, et al. Late recurrence from salivary gland cancer: when does "cure" mean cure? Cancer. 2008;112(2):340-4.
16. Ryan WR, Fee WE Jr, Le QT, et al. Positron-emission tomography for surveillance of head and neck cancer. Laryngoscope. 2005;115(4):645-50.

17. Greven KM, Williams DW 3rd, McGuirt WF Sr, et al. Serial positron emission tomography scans following radiation therapy of patients with head and neck cancer. Head Neck. 2001;23(11):942-6.
18. Jeon TY, Kim HJ, Choi JY, et al. 18F-FDG PET/CT findings of sinonasal inverted papilloma with or without coexistent malignancy: comparison with MR imaging findings in eight patients. Neuroradiology. 2009;51(4):265-71.
19. Goodwin WJ Jr. Salvage surgery for patients with recurrent squamous cell carcinoma of the upper aerodigestive tract: when do the ends justify the means? Laryngoscope. 2000;110(3 Pt 2 Suppl 93):1-18.
20. Spencer SA, Harris J, Wheeler RH, et al. Final report of RTOG 9610, a multi-institutional trial of reirradiation and chemotherapy for unresectable recurrent squamous cell carcinoma of the head and neck. Head Neck. 2008;30(3):281-8.

17

Benign Neoplasms of the Sinonasal Tract

Devyani Lal, MD

INTRODUCTION

Benign tumors of the sinonasal tract are rare. These tumors arise from the osteo-cartilaginous skeleton, lining skin and respiratory mucosa, and the rich population of glandular, vascular and neural structures within the sinuses. Some tumors primarily arise from adjacent structures such as the skull base, and involve the sinonasal cavity by extension.

Table 17.1 Benign Tumors of the sinonasal cavity (WHO classification)

Origin of Tumor	*Tumor*
Fibro-osseous	Osteoma, fibrous dysplasia, ossifying fibroma, chondroma
Epithelial	Sinonasal papillomas (Inverted, exophytic, oncocytic), salivary adenomas (pleomorphic, oncocytoma, myoepithelioma)
Vascular	Hemangioma, juvenile nasopharyngeal angiofibroma, pyogenic granuloma, hemangiopericytoma
Neural	Schwanomma, neurofibroma, meningioma
Soft tissue	Fibroma, myxoma, leiomyoma
Hamartoma	Respiratory epithelial adenoid hamartoma (REAH)
Neuro-ectodermal	Ameloblastoma, craniopharyngioma

As such, the range of tumors that can occur in the sinonasal cavity is diverse (Table 17.1). Tumors can arise from epithelial, neural, fibro-osseous, hamartomatous, vascular and odontogenic tissue.[1] The most common tumor diagnosed in this location is osteoma, followed by inverted papilloma.[2,3]

Most benign tumors present relatively late. The location of these tumors is in close proximity to the orbit, cranial cavity and the external facial skeleton. Therefore, traditional methods of resection resulted in significant functional and cosmetic morbidity from collateral injury to these surrounding structures. The evolution of minimally invasive access routes via endoscopic approaches has not only addressed some of these issues, but has also provided equivalent rates of success when compared to traditional approaches.[3]

CLINICAL FEATURES

Tumors present with symptoms similar to inflammatory pathology of the sinonasal cavity.[3] Nasal obstruction, congestion and drainage are common symptoms, although these may occur late in presentation, and some tumors may remain asymptomatic for long periods of time. Symptoms are often unilateral and the presence of unilateral symptoms should always alert the physician to the possibility of a neoplastic mass. Unilateral epistaxis can often represent a vascular tumor such as a JNA or hemangioma or as a sign of a large tumor with surface necrosis. Tumors located in the anterior or superior nasal cavity, ethmoid sinuses and frontal recess may also cause loss of smell due to obstruction and/or concomitant mucosal inflammation. Tumors that involve the lateral maxillary wall, such as an inverted papilloma, can obstruct the nasolacrimal duct and lead to epiphora. Facial pain is rare, although obstruction of sinuses by a bulky tumor can lead to recurrent or chronic sinusitis. Facial deformity and orbital proptosis occur very late when early symptoms are ignored and the tumor causes bony expansion. This is most commonly seen with fibro-osseous lesions that can expand the medial orbital wall, anterior table of the frontal sinus or anterior maxillary wall.

WORK-UP

A complete head and neck examination followed by nasal endoscopy should be performed. On endoscopy, the mass may be surrounded by polypoid tissue. Tumor may push the septum to the contralateral side. The oral cavity should be inspected to look for palatal expansion, erosion or loosening of teeth. Frank invasion is usually not a feature of benign tumors. Tumors that grow posteriorly into the nasopharynx may be visible in the oropharynx or as a bulge in the soft palate. Telecanthus and proptosis may be seen due to expansion of the ethmoid labyrinth due to the tumor. Nerve involvement with benign tumors is rare, although fibro-osseous tumors such as fibrous dysplasia can compress nerves at cranial foramina. Neural impingement can result in visual field deficits (optic nerve), diplopia (oculomotor, trochlear and abducens nerves) or sensory deficits in the face (trigeminal nerve).[4]

Radiographic imaging with computerized tomography (CT) and/or magnetic resonance (MR) is necessary.[5] These are complementary and used to characterize the tumor, determine the sites of extension and possible site of origin.[3] One of the main principles for surgical resection of benign tumors is to identify the site of attachment. Failure to do so, whether it is a fibro-osseous lesion or inverted papilloma, can lead to residual and/or recurrent disease. CT scans can be helpful in not only identifying extent of disease, but focal areas of bony osteitis that can lead to the site of attachment for an inverted papilloma. This information is useful for surgical planning, as there are occasions where an external adjunctive approach is needed to fully address the site of attachment. Fine-cut axial CT scans may also be used for intraoperative image-guidance. Like for most sinus pathology, CT scan is used for the initial evaluation. The bony detail is excellent for the diagnosis of fibro-osseous lesions, and is superior to MR in demonstrating bony erosion. Soft tissue tumors, such as inverted papilloma and JNA, are better appreciated with the use of MR. MR can help distinguish solid mass from obstructed secretions, and can help to identify cranial nerve involvement and to distinguish CSF from cysts.[6] Radiology for sinonasal tumors is discussed in detail in Chapter 3.

A broad differential diagnosis may be narrowed based on clinical examination and imaging, but final diagnosis is based on histopathological examination. Tumors may be difficult to distinguish from benign polyp on endoscopy (Figs 17.1A to C). An office biopsy is, therefore, performed to obtain tissue and confirm diagnosis, unless it is contraindicated or the tumor is inaccessible. For some tumors such as osteoma or fibrous dysplasia, radiographic imaging may suffice for diagnosis, and a biopsy may not be indicated. For vascular tumors such as angiofibroma or hemangioma, office biopsy is contraindicated due to risk of causing major hemorrhage. If the tumor erodes through the skull base, one should consider the possibility of causing cerebrospinal (CSF) leak due to the biopsy.

A discussion of specific benign tumors will follow, focusing on the more commonly encountered pathology.

FIBRO-OSSEOUS TUMORS

The commonest fibro-osseous tumors are osteoma, ossifying fibroma and fibrous dysplasia. Other

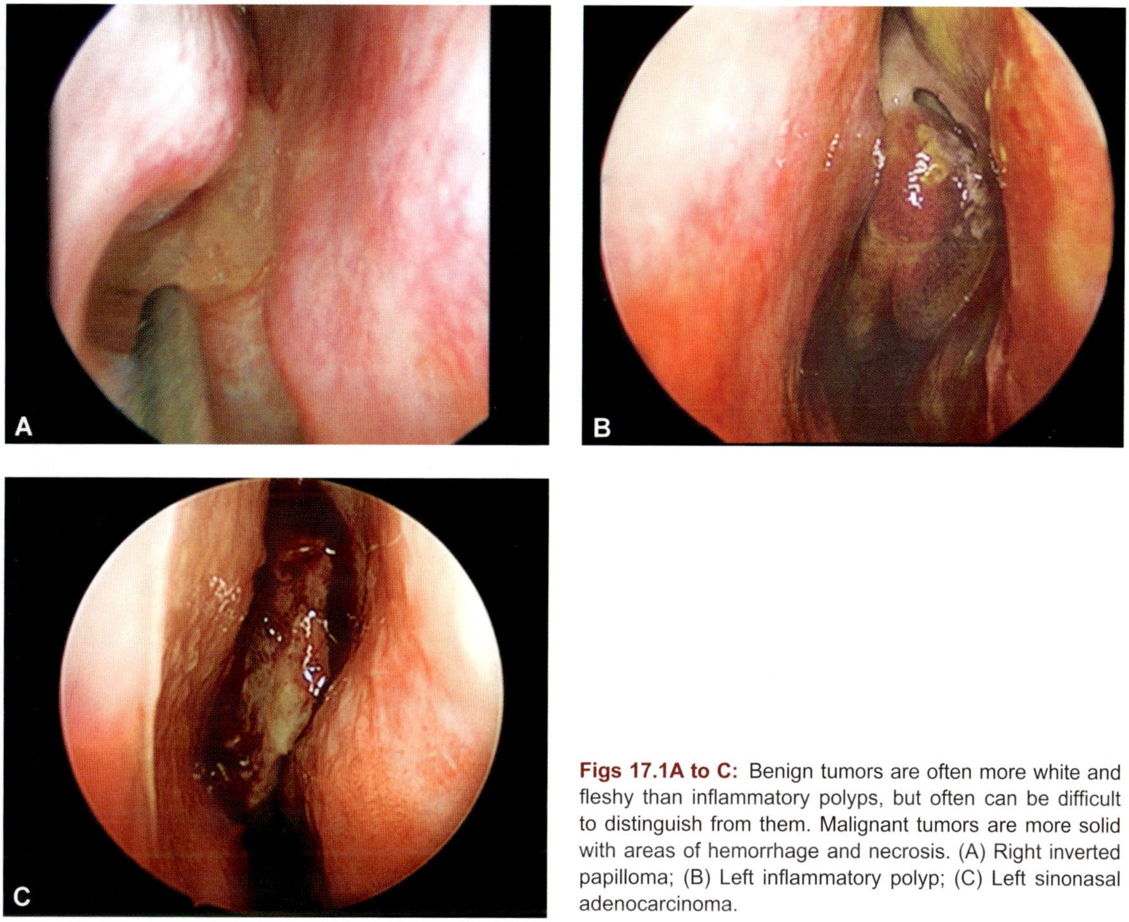

Figs 17.1A to C: Benign tumors are often more white and fleshy than inflammatory polyps, but often can be difficult to distinguish from them. Malignant tumors are more solid with areas of hemorrhage and necrosis. (A) Right inverted papilloma; (B) Left inflammatory polyp; (C) Left sinonasal adenocarcinoma.

lesions include chondroma, fibromyxoma and osteoblastoma.

Osteoma

Osteoma is reported to be the most common benign sinonasal tumor. It has been reported to be seen in up to 3% of routine CT sinus imaging.[2] Sinonasal osteoma was first reported by Viega in 1506.[3] Osteomas are slow-growing tumors. They are most frequently located in the frontal sinus (57%), followed by the maxillary (20%), ethmoid and sphenoid sinuses[3] (Fig. 17.2). The etiology of osteomas is controversial. The developmental theory proposes that embryonic stem cells become activated, causing new bone growth. An inflammatory process is believed to stimulate bone growth in the traumatic and infectious theories.[3] Histologically, osteoma can be distinguished into three types: Ivory/compact (composed of dense cortical bone); mature (composed of cancellous bone) and mixed (Fig. 17.3). Osteomas can be associated with Gardner's syndrome, an autosomal dominant disorder with a triad of multiple osteomas, soft tissue tumors (epidermal inclusion cysts, fibroma) and colonic polyposis. If suspected, a prompt gastroenterological consultation is warranted, as the colonic polyps in Gardner's syndrome are prone to malignant degeneration in 40%.[7,8]

Osteomas usually present in the fifth or sixth decades, and are more common in men.[2] The most common presenting symptom is frontal headache or facial pain, present in 60% of patients with frontal

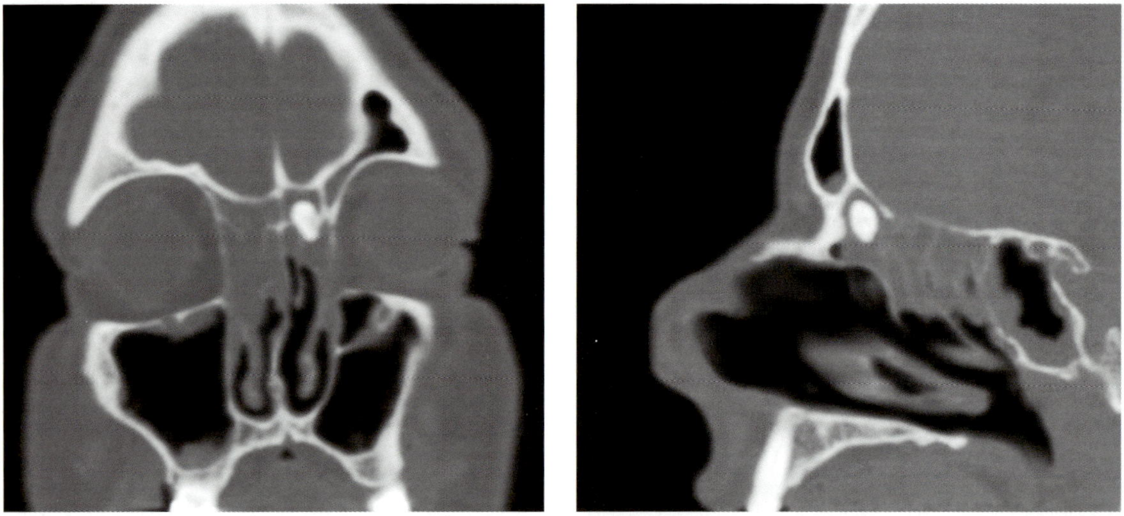

Fig. 17.2: Left frontal osteoma. Osteomas are often discovered incidentally on CT scans. They are most commonly located around the frontal recess.

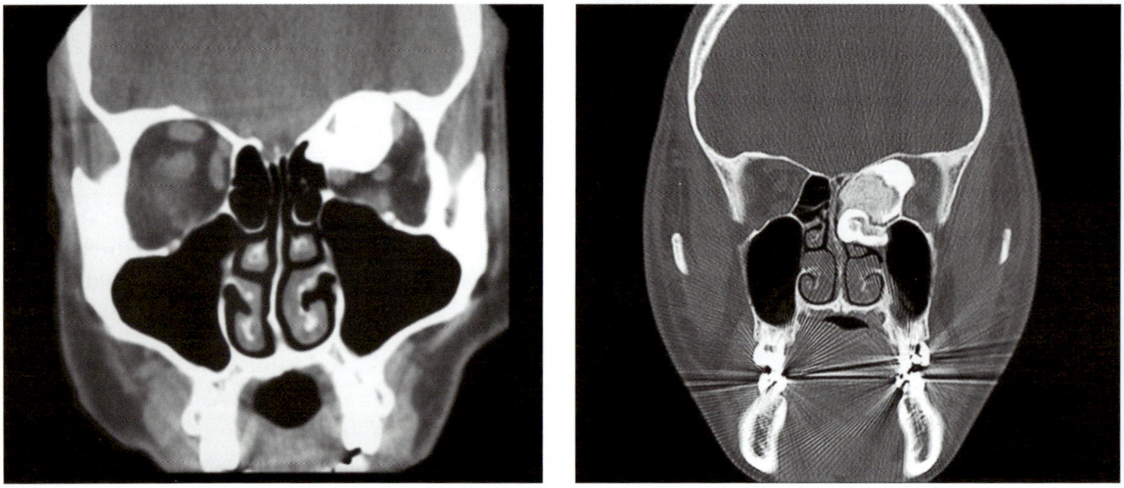

Fig. 17.3: Osteomas are of three types: Ivory/compact (composed of dense cortical bone); mature (composed of cancellous bone) and mixed.

sinus osteoma.[7] This is likely secondary to frontal recess obstruction from the expanding tumor causing sinusitis. Osteomas can expand causing orbital symptoms such as diplopia, epiphora, exophthalmos and even blindness. Cosmetic deformities may also appear on the forehead and face. Intracranial complications can occur due to impingement on the dura; this can lead to formation of intracranial mucocele, CSF leak, meningitis, and brain abscess. However, most patients remain asymptomatic, with the diagnosis being incidental on radiographic studies done for unrelated reasons.[8] On CT scans osteomas appear to homogeneous, very dense and well-circumscribed lesions. If visible on nasal endoscopy, osteomas appear mucosa-covered and hard on palpation. The growth rate of osteomas ranges from 0.44–6.0 mm/year.[9] Malignant transformation of osteomas has never been described.

The management of an osteoma depends on the symptoms, location and rate of growth. Small, asymptomatic lesions can be watched. If there is rapid growth, or the patient is symptomatic, surgery is advocated. Surgical approaches to the tumor can be endonasal, external or combined, based on the size and location of the tumor.[7,9] Those located within the ethmoid and sphenoid sinus can be approached with an endoscopic approach alone. A posterior septectomy can be useful to access large fibro-osseous lesions in the sphenoid, as in many cases an endoscopic drill needs to be used for long periods of time to debulk the tumor. In many instances, debulking the central portion of the fibro-osseous lesion will leave a thin shell of bone around the periphery. This thin bone can then be collapsed upon itself, thus allowing a large lesion to be removed intra-nasally without having to make an external incision to deliver the specimen. Surgical access to the posterior ethmoids and sphenoid can also be improved by performing a posterior septectomy. A posterior septectomy will allow both nostrils to be used for instrumentation and will facilitate the drilling, as one surgeon can suction and drill while the other can hold the endoscope.

Fibro-osseous lesions of the frontal sinus can be removed through a standard endoscopic frontal recess approach if they are pedicled on the posterior frontal recess and have a site of attachment medial to a sagittal plane through the medial orbital wall. Larger lesions growing in the lateral frontal sinus, attached superiorly onto the intersinus septum or involving a large portion of the frontal sinus, are likely best approached through an extended frontal recess approach, i.e. modified Lothrop or Draf III. Removing the intersinus septum, superior nasal septum and floor of the frontal recess allows better access to the tumor. Much like lesions of the sphenoid sinus, an endoscopic drill can be used to core out the middle of the tumor until a bony shell remains. If the lesion is pedicled on the anterior table of the frontal sinus or fills the entire sinus, an external adjunct such as an osteoplastic flap or trephination, may be needed to ensure a complete removal of the lesion.

Fibrous Dysplasia

Fibrous dysplasia was first described by Lichtenstein in 1938. It is usually present in the first two decades of life with equal sex distribution.[3] Two classic forms are described: polyostotic (15–30%), involving more than one bone, and monostotic (70–85%), involving only one bone.[10] McCune-Albright syndrome is a very rare disorder of young girls associated with the presence of polyostotic fibrous dysplasia, precocious puberty, and cutaneous pigmentation.[11] The maxilla and mandible are the most commonly involved sites in the skull.[10] Asymptomatic fibrous dysplasia is often an incidental finding on radiologic studies obtained for unrelated reasons, with the sphenoid and central skull base being frequently involved in such cases. The progression of disease is variable. Growth usually slows after puberty. A low rate of malignant transformation has been reported, occurring in 0.5% of polyostotic forms and in 4% of lesions in patients with McCune-Albright syndrome.[3,10]

The etiology of fibrous dysplasia is not understood, although estrogen may play a role in tumor pathogenesis.[12] Mutations in the GNAS1 gene, located on chromosome 20q13.2, coding for a G-protein subunit has been noted in both fibrous dysplasia and McCune-Albright syndrome.[13] Histologically, the medullary bone appears to be gradually replaced by abnormal fibrous tissue and bone metaplasia.[14] CT scan with a homogeneous "ground-glass" appearance on the bone window is almost diagnostic[4] (Fig. 17.4). The most common clinical presentation is facial asymmetry, followed by facial pain, ocular and neurological changes.[4]

Patients with monostotic fibrous dysplasia are usually asymptomatic, and can be kept under observation. Medical therapy is indicated only to provide symptomatic relief. Bisphosphonates can decrease rate of fractures and bony pain.[15] Appropriate supplementary hormonal therapy is employed in McCune-Albright syndrome. Surgical therapy is chosen based on the patient's symptoms and age, and the location and extent of the tumor.[4]

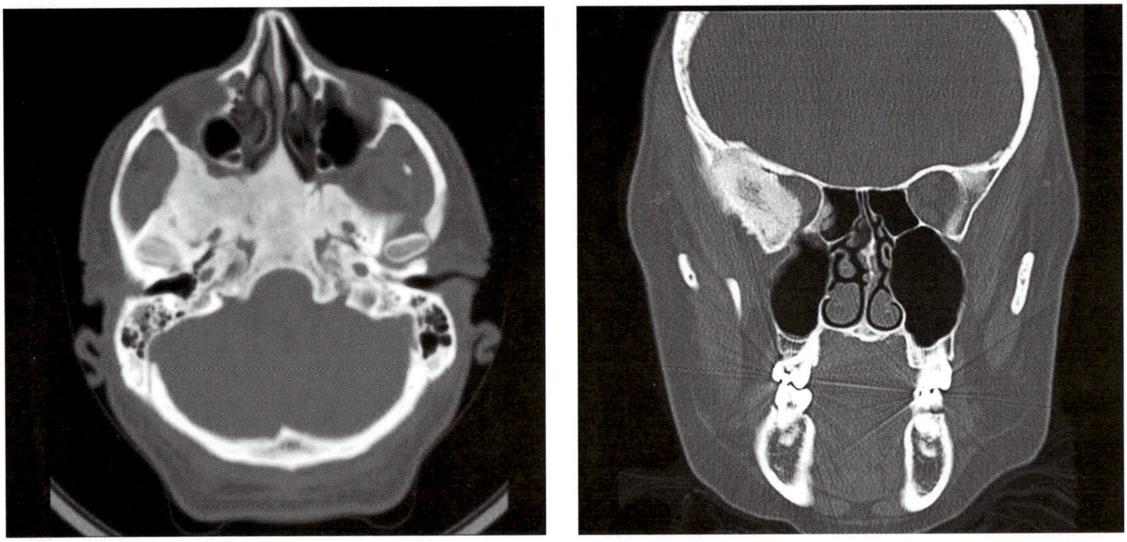

Fig. 17.4: Fibrous dysplasia has a relatively homogeneous, "groundglass" appearance on the bone window. Ossifying fibroma show a characteristic sharply demarcated, expansile mass covered by a thick shell of bone; the tumor mass appears to be multiloculated and is of varying density.

Some authors have reported endonasal endoscopic treatment of fibrous dysplasia, especially for the relief of ocular symptoms (optic nerve decompression) or chronic rhinosinusitis.[4,16]

Ossifying Fibroma

Ossifying fibroma was first described by Montgomery in 1927.[3] It is a benign tumor composed of bone, fibrous tissue, calcification and cementum.[14] It is more commonly found in the mandible (75%) or maxilla (10–20%) and lesions in the nasoethmoidal region are rare.[3] The etiology of ossifying fibroma is unclear, but trauma has been proposed to play a major role. Histologically, the tumor shows distinct regions consisting of fibrous tissue with varying amounts of mineralized or calcified psammomatoid bodies.[17]

Patients usually present between the second and fourth decades of life, with females being involved more often.[3] Symptoms depend on the extent of the tumor, with patients complaining of facial pain, swelling, nasal obstruction, rhinosinusitis and ocular symptoms. An aggressive variant termed "juvenile ossifying fibroma", has an earlier age of onset, and is seen more often in male children.[17] CT images of ossifying fibroma show a sharply demarcated, expansile mass covered by a thick shell of bone. The tumor mass appears to be multiloculated and is of varying density.[18]

Treatment depends on tumor location. Tumors invading the midface and sinonasal tract behave more aggressively when compared to more asymptomatic mandibular lesions behavior. They may need surgical resection. Most authors recommend complete resection when possible, as recurrence is high. Larger series on pure endonasal resection are not reported, though there are case reports and small series, including for optic nerve decompression.[16,19] In large tumors, most authors recommend a combined approach including craniofacial resection.[20]

EPITHELIAL TUMORS

Inverted Papilloma

Introduction

Papillomas (inverted, oncocytic, fungiform) are the most common sinonasal tumors for which surgery is conducted. Inverted papilloma is found in 0.5–4%

of surgically resected nasal tumor specimens.[21,22] Ward was the first to describe a nasal papilloma in 1854. Reingertz in 1935 was the first to describe the inverted appearance of the epithelium.[3] Hyams' work in 1971, based on the review of 315 cases was seminal in describing and solidifying the terminology and pathology of sinonasal papillomas. He subdivided sinonasal papillomas into inverted, fungiform, and cylindrical cell types.[23] Of these, it is inverted papilloma that generates the most interest. As opposed to exophytic (Fig. 17.5) and cylindrical papillomas, these have a locally aggressive behavior. They can be associated with malignancy, and tend to recur after surgery. Numerous other terms used to refer to inverted papilloma include inverting papilloma, Schneiderian papilloma, and transitional cell papilloma.

The incidence of inverted papilloma in the general population has not been formally studied. By extrapolating data from the number of local patients seen in a tertiary care institution, the incidence was estimated to be 4.3 cases per million per year.[24] Inverted papilloma can occur in the very young to the very old, ranging from 15–96 years old. The highest incidence is seen in patients in the 5th and 6th decades of life. It is more common in males (2–5:1) and has no racial predilection. Patients may be symptomatic for months to decades before diagnosis is established.

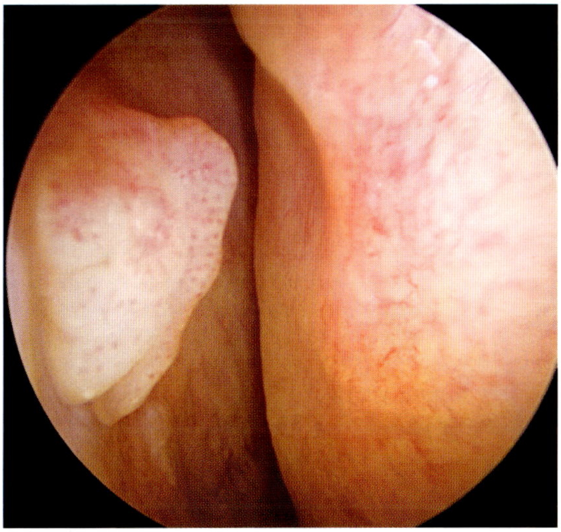

Fig. 17.5: Everted papilloma has a frond-like appearance and commonly located at the anterior end of the septum.

Clinical Features

Inverted papilloma can present with the usual symptoms of nasal obstruction, epistaxis, and drainage. As the tumor grows, it causes obstruction of the sinuses and the nasolacrimal duct, resulting in sinusitis and epiphora. Inverted papilloma should be suspected in anyone with a unilateral nasal polyp. Inverted papillomas tend to be more fleshy, white and vascular when compared to the boggy, translucent appearance of nasal polyps (Figs 17.1A to C).

Imaging

Computed tomography is the primary preoperative imaging modality. Often hyperostosis or sclerosis is noted in an area adjacent to the tumor. Some authors have proposed that this corresponds to the site of tumor attachment.[25] Erosion and invasion through bone should raise the concern of malignancy, although long-standing inverted papilloma can also cause bony erosion. Calcification within the inverted papilloma is also occasionally noted (Fig. 17.6). MR is useful for delineating tumor from retained secretions and inflammatory changes (Fig. 17.7). MR studies noting "cerebriform" or "columnar" pattern, on T2 and contrast-enhanced T1 sequences have been proposed to reflect the histological architecture of the underlying lesion. The loss of the cerebriform pattern thus has been thought to be a sign of a concomitant carcinoma.[26,27] However, there are no reliable features that differentiate inverted papilloma from inverted papilloma with malignancy or squamous cell carcinoma (SCC) on MR alone.

It is not always possible to determine the site of origin of inverted papillomas. Most arise from the lateral nasal wall and extend into the adjacent sinuses and nasopharynx. The ethmoid sinuses are the next more frequent site of origin (48%), followed

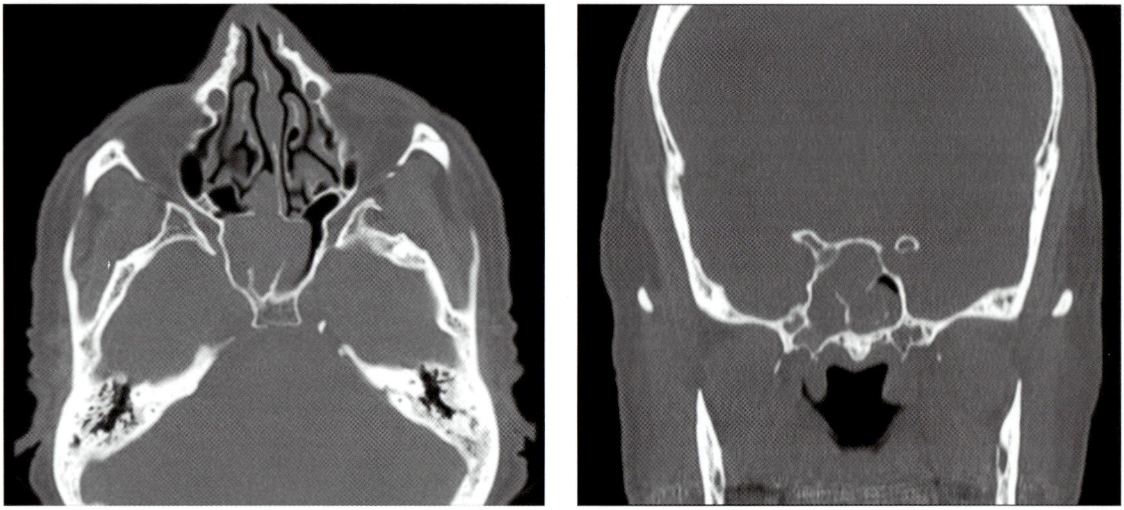

Fig. 17.6: Right sinonasal inverted papilloma. The plain CT (axial, coronal sagittal cuts) show intact skull base and lamina papyracea. Note the presence of an Onodi cell with and erosion of the bony margin. Subtle calcification is seen in the coronal scan.

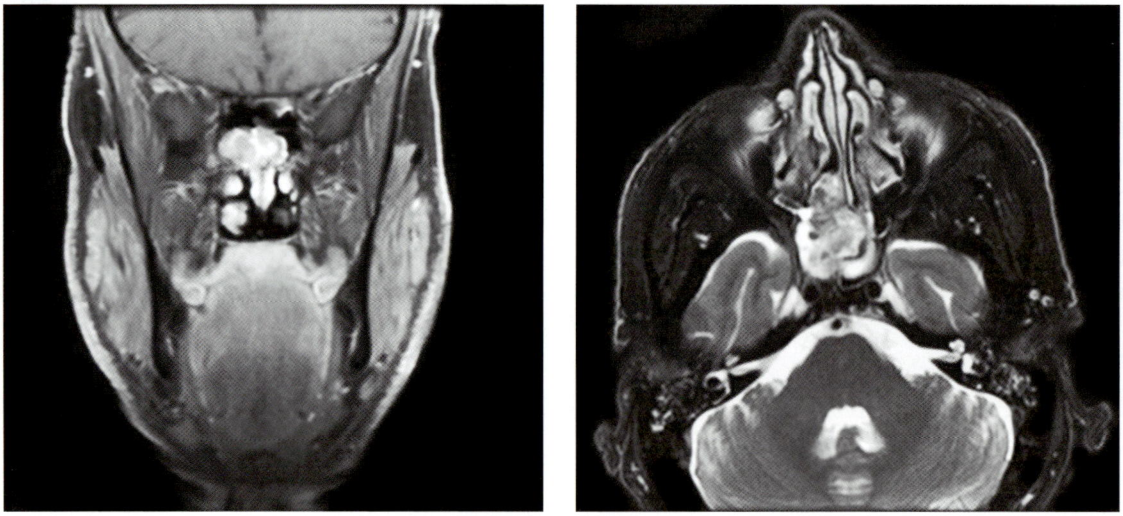

Fig. 17.7: MR of same right sinonasal sphenoid inverted papilloma. The T1 sequence shows contrast enhancing tumor in the sphenoid and the spheno-ethmoid recess. The T2 weighted sequence shows the presence of fluid in the lateral aspects of the sphenoid.

by the maxillary (28%), sphenoid (7.5%) and frontal (2.5%) sinuses. The inferior turbinate (2.5%) and septum (2.5%) are rarely sites of origin.[28] Bony erosion through the cribriform plate or lamina papyracea is rare, and when present, should alert the clinician to the possibility of a malignant tumor. Inverted papilloma is usually unilateral; bilateral involvement is very rare (1–9%).[28,29] The frequency of inverted papilloma is detected in bilateral nasal polyposis is very rare (0–0.92%).[30,31]

Pathogenesis

Outdoor and industrial occupations have been found to be risk factors for inverted papilloma in a case-control study; tobacco, smoking, allergy, sinusitis and polyps were not found to be significantly associated.[32] The reported incidence of SCC associated with inverted papilloma varies widely between 0–53%.[33] In reviewing the literature, Mirza et al. found that the rates of synchronous and metachronous carcinomas associated with inverted papilloma to be 7.1–3.6% respectively. The rate of malignant transformation in recurrent inverted papillomas was higher, at 11%.[24] Studies have proposed that SCC in inverted papilloma is triggered by human papilloma virus (HPV) infection. HPV infection is presumed to reduce cellular apoptosis.[34] Though a viral etiology for inverted papilloma itself has been sought because of the association of HPV with other papillomas, the premise has remained controversial.[35] Some experts think HPV may cause multi-centric disease, dysplasia and malignancy.[36] Since HPV DNA has been found in both the inverted papilloma and the neighboring normal mucosa, some advocate removing the neighboring normal-appearing mucosa to reduce the rate of inverted papilloma recurrence.[37] This may be important, as when previously excised tumor recurs, the risk of subsequent recurrence has been reported to be as higher.[24,37,38] However, the current state of evidence is not enough to offer conclusive support for a viral etiology for inverted papilloma.[35]

Histology

The term "inverted papilloma" is used to describe the histological appearance of the tumor. The epithelial lining of the tumor inverts into the underlying stroma. The stroma is separated from the epithelium by an intact and well-defined basement membrane. The epithelium of the inverted papilloma is distinct from the normal surrounding respiratory epithelium (pseudostratified ciliated columnar). Inverted papilloma epithelial cells may be squamous, transitional, or respiratory. The epithelium in inverted papilloma is proliferative and thickened, and lacks mucus-secreting cells and eosinophils. The nuclear to cytoplasm ratio is normal. Atypia, dysplasia, carcinoma *in situ*, as well as frank SCC may be present within the tumor. As such, as much of the tumor specimen as possible should be sent for histopathological examination during surgery.[23,38,39]

Atypia and dysplasia are seen in 1–2% of specimens. One study found 163 (7.1%) cases of synchronous carcinoma out of 2297 specimens.[24] The majority was SCCs, but transitional cell carcinoma, adenocarcinoma, mucoepidermoid carcinoma and verrucous carcinoma were also found in association with inverted papilloma.

Staging

The most common and new classification systems have been proposed by Krouse, Han, Oikawa and Cannady.[40-43] Staging is based on the extent of the tumor. However, even very bulky and extensive tumors can have a relatively narrow pedicle and site of attachment, and other authors advocate that inverted papilloma staging should depend on the site of tumor attachment, not on their volume.[44] The system proposed by Kamel takes into account the site of attachment and not volume.[45] Table 17.2 summarizes the classification systems.

Treatment

The choice of surgical technique needs to weigh completeness of resection versus the desire to reduce surgical morbidity. Historically, the gold standard was an external approach comprising a medial maxillectomy (via a lateral rhinotomy or midfacial degloving).[46,47] Vrabec reported a recurrence rate of only 2% using a lateral rhinotomy on mean follow-up of 8.9 years.[46,47] However, the use of endoscopic techniques for resection has been gaining favor (Figs 17.8A to D). This is in part to reduce morbidity associated with external approaches, but most importantly due to results comparable to external approaches. Improvements in imaging, image guidance, access routes and availability of angled scopes and specialized instruments have allowed endoscopic techniques to achieve complete tumor resection even in unfavorable locations, such as the frontal sinus and anterior wall or floor of the maxillary sinus.[3]

Table 17.2 Staging systems for inverted papilloma

(Krouse[42])	
Type 1	Tumor totally confined to nasal cavity; must not extend into sinuses or any extranasal structure. No concurrent malignancy
Type 2	Tumor involving ostiomeatal complex, ethmoid sinus, and/or medial part of maxillary sinus, with/without nasal cavity. No concurrent malignancy
Type 3	Tumor involving lateral, inferior, superior, anterior, or posterior walls of maxillary sinus; sphenoid sinus, and/or frontal sinus, with/without involvement of medial maxillary sinus, ethmoid sinus, or nasal cavity. No concurrent malignancy
Type 4	All tumors with extranasal/extrasinus extension (orbit, intracranial or pterygomaxillary space). All tumors with concurrent malignancy
(Han[41])	
Group 1	Tumor limited to nasal cavity, lateral nasal wall, medial maxillary sinus, ethmoid sinus, and sphenoid sinus
Group 2	Group 1 plus tumor extends lateral to the medial maxillary wall
Group 3	Tumor extends to involve frontal sinus
Group 4	Tumor extends outside sinonasal cavity (orbital or intracranial extension)
Oikawa[43]	
T1	Tumor limited to nasal cavity
T2	Tumor limited to ethmoid sinus and/or medial and superior maxillary sinus
T3	Tumor involves lateral, inferior, anterior, or posterior walls of maxillary sinus, sphenoid sinus, or frontal sinus T3-A: without extension to frontal sinus or supraorbital recess T3-B: involving frontal sinus or supraorbital recess
T4	Tumor extends outside sinonasal cavity (orbit/ intracranial) or associated with malignancy
Cannady[40]	
Group A	Inverted papilloma confined to the nasal cavity, ethmoid sinuses, or medial maxillary wall
Group B	Inverted papilloma with involvement of any maxillary wall (other than the medial wall), or frontal sinus, or sphenoid sinus
Group C	Inverted papilloma with extension beyond the paranasal sinuses
Kamel[45] (Classification focuses on origin and not size/extent)	
Type 1	Tumor originating from the nasal septum or lateral nasal wall
Type 2	Tumor originating from the maxillary sinus

Recurrence of inverted papilloma is secondary to either incomplete tumor removal, or perhaps a field change in mucosa. Polypectomy or local excision are unsuitable and have a recurrence rate—as high as 78%.[48] Complete resection of the involved mucosa and mucoperiosteum is therefore advocated. Some surgeons also drill the osteitic bone where the tumor is attached.[25]

External surgical approaches include headlight-assisted intranasal polypectomy, Caldwell Luc procedure, medial maxillectomy, lateral rhinotomy and external procedures of the frontal sinus.

Endoscopic transnasal approaches can be used to perform tumor removal (Figs 17.8A to D). The advantage of the endoscopic technique is cosmesis secondary to absence of an external facial incision, shorter inpatient stay, reduction in postoperative pain and swelling, and decreased morbidity from avoiding injury to the infraorbital nerve. Newer angled scopes with wide angles, modern camera and high-definition monitors afford improved visualization and magnification. This allows for improved discrimination of tumor from normal tissue. Angled lenses allow visualization around corners (anterior wall and

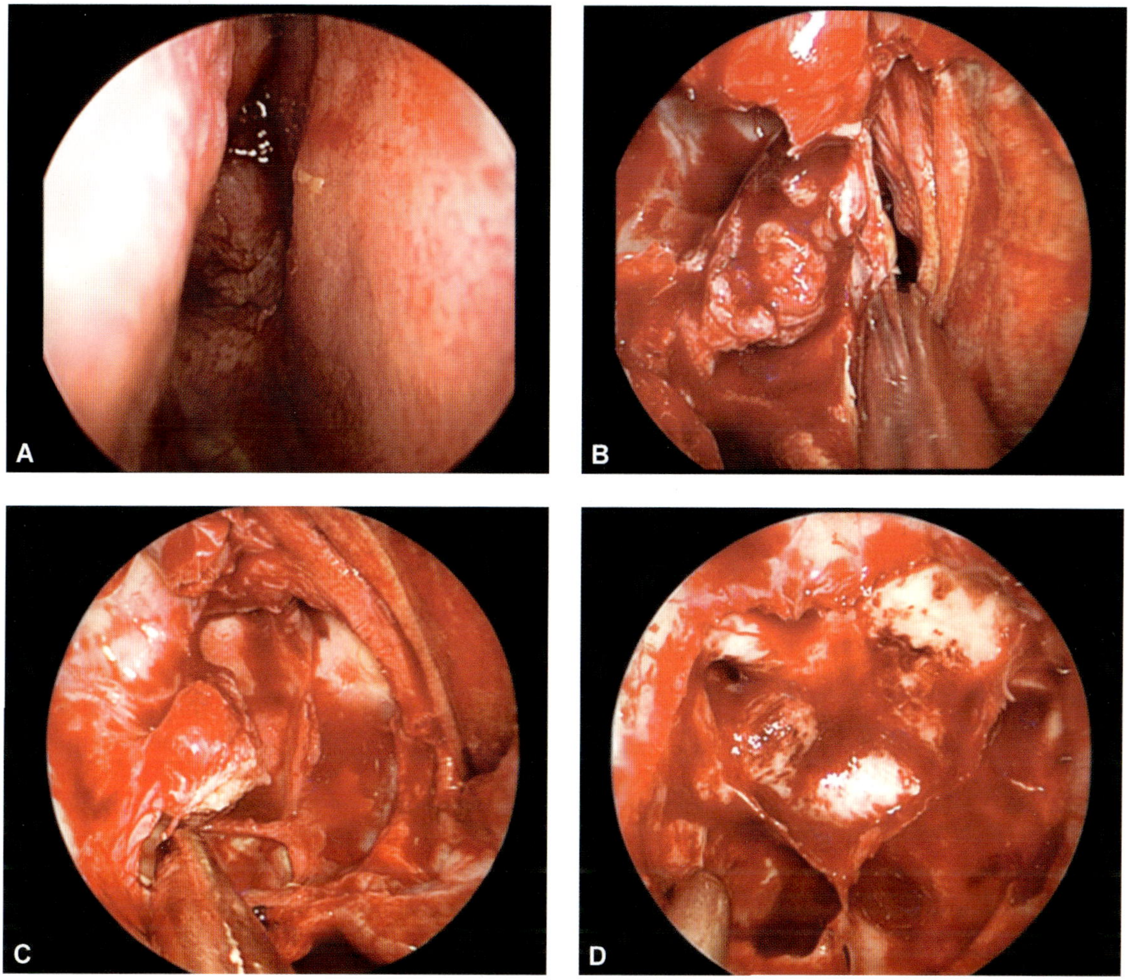

Figs 17.8A to D: Intraoperative endoscopic resection of the same inverted papilloma. (A) Tumor in right sphenoethmoid recess; (B) Tumor in right sphenoid; (C) Tumor is traced to be attached to bony septation on the right side; (D) The sphenoid and Onodi cell are widely opened, tumor resected and mucosa was removed. Note the denuded bone in the area of the planum and the clival and optico-carotid recess.

floor of the maxillary sinus and within frontal sinus). Newly described surgical approaches and techniques such as endoscopic medial maxillectomy, transpterygoid sphenoidotomy and Draf type III procedures allow removal of tumor from difficult areas in the maxillary, sphenoid and frontal sinuses.[44,49-53]

Results

The reported recurrence rate of inverted papilloma varies widely. Bielamowicz et al found a statistically significant difference between recurrences in patients treated with medial maxillectomy (20%) versus those treated with a conservative resection (47%).[48] Results of endoscopic tumor resection have been compared to open medial maxillectomy.[28,54] Mirza et al. found that recurrence rates in 63 case series was 12.8% for endoscopic procedures (n = 484), 17.0% for lateral rhinotomy with medial maxillectomy (n =1025) and 34.2% for limited resections such as nasal polypectomy (n = 600).[24] Recurrence depends on several factors including tumor location, extent, histology, multicentricity, method of removal and length of follow-up. The principal cause of recurrence is the incomplete resection at site of origin.[28,54] Recurrence rates are higher in revision cases and this may be due to the nature of the disease as well as difficulty in surgical access.[55]

Recent reviews of the literature show success is comparable by both external and endoscopic techniques.[3,56] The endoscopic technique may perhaps be even slightly better.[3] Most cases recur within the first 9 months. Recurrence rates for the endoscopic group (14.5%) compare favorably with the external group (16.7%) with follow-up of 3 years and 5 years, respectively. When comparing results, it should be noted that the postoperative follow-up period was shorter in the endoscopic group.[3] Recurrence was higher in cases of scarred frontal recess, distortion from previous surgery, very advanced disease and associated malignancy.[28] Therefore, relative contraindications for the endoscopic technique are where disease involves the frontal sinus and there is scarring or new bone formation in the frontal recess and if there is associated malignancy.

Angiofibroma (Juvenile Nasopharyngeal Angiofibroma)

Juvenile angiofibroma is a benign vascular tumor accounting for 0.5% of all head and neck tumors. This is a rare tumor, with the incidence in the general population estimated to be approximately 1:150,000. In the United States, the incidence is reported to be between 1:5,000–1:60,000, being amongst the most frequent tumor of the adolescents. In the Middle East and in India, the incidence seems to be much higher than in Europe.[3] The median age at diagnosis is 18.5 years (range 8–35 years) and all patients are males.[57] Only 30 female patients have been reported in the literature to have juvenile angiofibroma. However, whether all these cases were, in fact, juvenile angiofibroma or other vascular tumors has been questioned. A review of 299 juvenile angiofibroma cases from six studies showed no female patients.[3]

The hormonal influence of gonadosteroid hormones on juvenile angiofibroma is still controversial although studies have found androgen and/or estrogen receptors in tumor tissue and hormonal disorders in patients with juvenile angiofibroma. However, serum levels of these hormones are not abnormal in juvenile angiofibroma patients.[58] Recent genetic studies have found partial or complete loss of the Y chromosome, with gains in the X chromosome. The gain in X chromosome is associated with gain of the androgen receptor gene, supporting an androgen-related pathophysiologic process.[59] Other chromosome deletions and gene aberrations have also been reported.[60-65] In another school of thought, some believe juvenile angiofibroma to be a vascular malformation from non-resorption of a primitive artery of the first brachial arch.[66]

Juvenile angiofibroma likely originates from near the pterygopalatine fossa, starting from the basisphenoid and the sphenopalatine foramen.[67] They then have a gradual expansile growth into the nasal cavity and nasopharynx. They can be locally aggressive and destroy bone, thus growing into the paranasal sinuses, orbit, and through the skull base into the intracranial compartment. Dumb-belling of the tumor around the sphenopalatine foramen and basisphenoid may be noted, with growth into the pterygopalatine fossa and subsequently the infratemporal fossa, the cavernous sinus or intracranial.[68] Histologically, they are vascular tumors with large ectatic vessels, which branch into progressively smaller capillary-sized vessels. The cells of angiofibroma are bland, evenly spaced and stellate. The tumor has a variable component of fibrous stroma[69] (Fig. 17.9).

Clinical Presentation

The disease is seen primarily in adolescent males. Patients complain of increasing unilateral nasal obstruction (80–90%), drainage and recurrent epistaxis (45–60%). Paranasal sinus and eustachian tube obstruction may present as headache and otitis media with effusion. Swelling of the face and cheek may be noted with tumor extension through the sinuses, and also with a large extension into

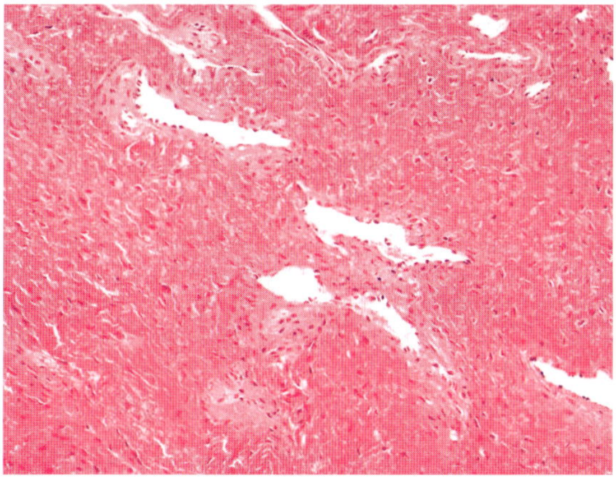

Fig. 17.9: Angiofibroma: Histopathology shows them to be vascular tumors with large ectatic vessels, which branch into progressively smaller capillary-sized vessels. The cells are bland, evenly spaced and stellate. The tumor has a variable component of fibrous stroma.

the infratemporal fossa (10–18%). Extension into the orbit and intracranial cavity can cause visual and neural symptoms.[3] Endoscopic examination and imaging are used to confirm diagnosis. Biopsy is not recommended if juvenile angiofibroma is suspected for risk of causing major hemorrhage.

Diagnosis and Imaging

Angiofibromas are very vascular tumors with a fibrous component. They have a characteristic pattern of growth that can be recognized on imaging. Both CT and MR (with contrast) are useful and complementary (Figs 17.10A to D). CT defines bony anatomy and is also useful for intraoperative image guidance. The characteristic patterns on imaging are the presence of several signal voids within the lesion on both T1 and T2 weighted images that reflect its rich vascularity. Finger-like projections of tumor extending into cranial foramina and the sinonasal cavity are also noted. Intradiploeic spread can be detected on post-contrast T1-weighted MR images. Submucosal growth and invasion of the cancellous bone of the basisphenoid are distinct features that are noted on CT or MR.[67,70,71] MR angiogram can also be used to further define vascular supply. MR angiography has now supplanted angiography for diagnostic angiography, but traditional angiography is still used for embolization prior to surgery. Intracranial extension is also better defined on MR. MR is preferred for follow-up for these reasons, and so excessive radiation to these young patients can be limited.[67]

Preoperative assessment may include angiography to study the tumor vascular supply. Angiography is usually performed with embolization to decrease intraoperative blood loss, and should be performed within 24–48 hours of the planned resection depending on the material used. The vascular supply comes mainly from branches of the internal maxillary artery, the ascending pharyngeal artery and the vidian artery. Occasionally, supply from other branches of the external carotid, the internal carotid artery, the vertebral arteries and branches of the contralateral carotid system can be noted. When using resorbable materials, the interval between embolization and surgery should not exceed 48 hours as the supplying artery can quickly be recanalized.[3] Branches from the internal carotid artery are rare in extracranial tumors, but can be seen with involvement of the cavernous sinus. Control of major vascularization from the internal carotid artery can be difficult on angio-embolization because of risk of major neurologic complications.[72] Alternatively, direct intra-tumoral embolization under general anesthesia and radiographic control has been proposed.[47,73] In the rare event of complete encasement of the internal carotid artery, balloon occlusion test, stenting and sacrifice of the ICA may become necessary. Embolization provides a 60–70% reduction of the intraoperative bleeding and decreases the need for blood transfusions. Many surgeons prefer not to carry out preoperative embolization, citing risks of the procedure, similar risk of tumor recurrence, and potential difficulty in defining the tumor planes. Alternatives to embolization include direct intraoperative identification and ligation of vessels, and hypotensive anesthesia. Embolization, preoperative autologous donation and the cell saver system help deal with blood loss during surgery.[3]

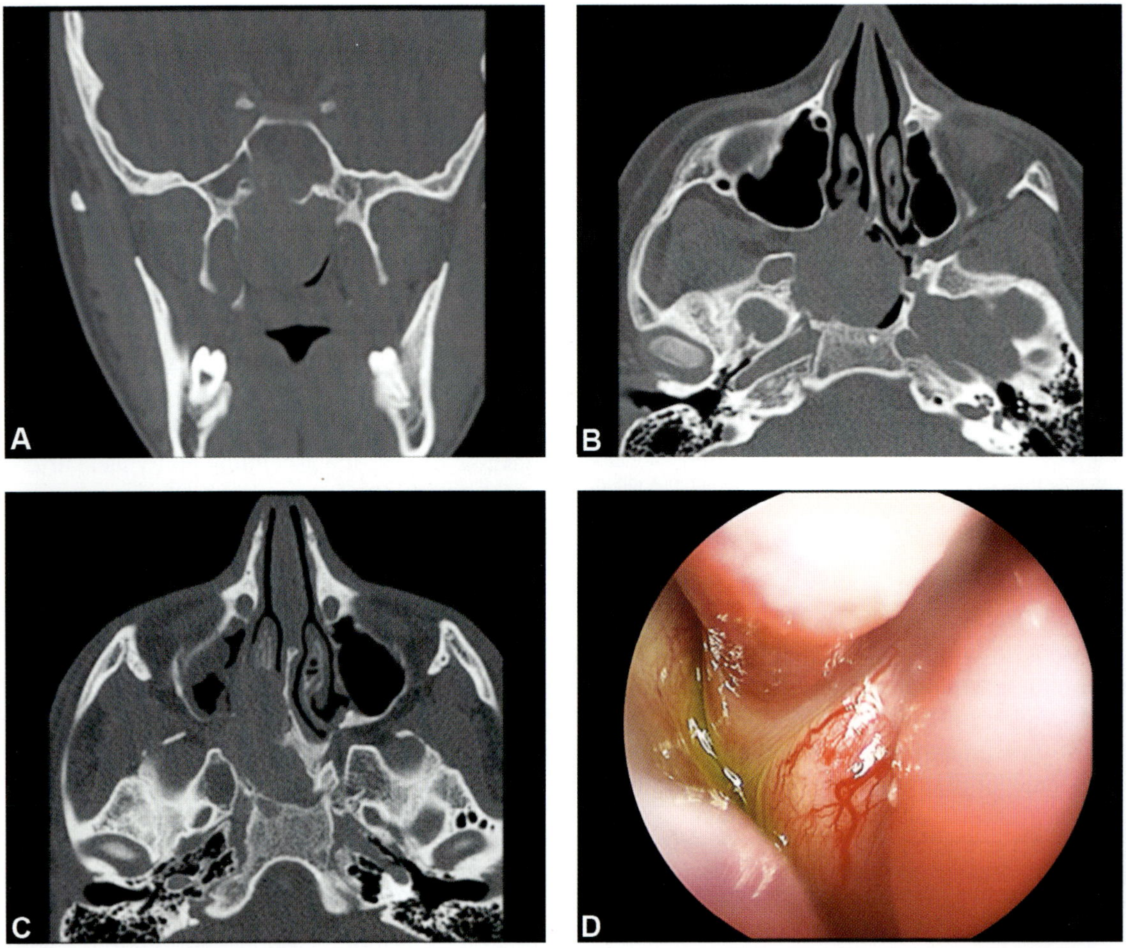

Figs 17.10A to D: Right sinonasal angiofibroma. The plain CT (axial, coronal and sagittal cuts) and endoscopic appearance. (A to C): Note erosion of the right basisphenoid and vidian canal, as well as the subtle expansion of the right pterygopalatine fossa. (A) Large part of the tumor dumb-bells into the nasopharynx; (D) The tumor appears to be more fleshy and vascular compared to an inflammatory polyp.

Staging

Various authors have proposed staging systems based on the tumor extension.[3] The Sessions classification from 1981[74] was modified in1996 by Radkowski.[75] Fisch proposed another system in 1983.[76] The 1984 classification of Chandler[68] bases staging on that used for nasopharyngeal carcinomas. Bremer,[77] in 1986 and Antonelliin 1987[78] presented other staging systems. These staging systems did not account for the route of intracranial extension and the vascularity of the tumor. New staging systems seem to better predict morbidity from blood loss or tumor recurrence. Recently, Onerci,[79] Carrillo,[80] and Snyderman[81] have made proposals for new classifications reflecting these. A complete discussion of these is beyond the scope of this chapter. Table 17.3 highlights some classic, commonly used and new staging systems for angiofibroma.

Treatment

The conventional surgical approach is resection by open approaches. However, the endoscopic approach is being increasingly utilized now for selected juvenile angiofibroma tumors (Figs 17.11A to D).

Table 17.3 Selected staging systems for angiofibroma

Author/ Stage	*Session (1981)*	*Fisch (1983)*	*Radkowski (1996)*	*Snyderman (2010)*
I	IA: limited to posterior nasal cavity and choana IB: IA plus involvement of at least one paranasal sinus	Limited to nasal cavity and nasopharynx; without any bony destruction	IA: limited to posterior nasal cavity and choana IB: IB: IA plus involvement of at least one paranasal sinus	No significant extension beyond site of origin; tumor remains medial to the mid-point of pterygopalatine space
II	II A: Minimal lateral extension to the pterygopalatine fossa IIB: Extension into entire pterygopalatine fossa with or without orbital bone erosion	Invading the pterygopalatine fossa and the maxillary, ethmoid and sphenoid sinus with bone destruction	II A: Minimal lateral extension to the pterygopalatine fossa IIB: Extension into entire pterygopalatine fossa with or without orbital bone erosion II C: Extension posterior to pterygoid plates	Extension to the paranasal sinuses and lateral to the midpoint of the pterygo palatine space
III	III A: Skull base erosion (e.g. middle fossa, pterygoid plates) with minimal intracranial invasion III B: Extensive intracranial extension with or without cavernous sinus invasion	Invasion of infratemporal fossa, orbit and parasellar region remaining lateral to the cavernous sinus	III A: Erosion of the skull base with minimal intracranial extension III B: Extensive intracranial extension with or without cavernous sinus invasion	Locally advanced with skull base erosion or extension to additional extracranial spaces, including orbit and infratemporal fossa; no residual vascularity following embolization
IV		Massive invasion of cavernous sinus, the optic chiasmal region or pituitary fossa		IV: Skull base erosion or extension to additional extracranial spaces, including orbit and infratemporal fossa; Residual vascularity following embolization
V				V: Intracranial extension, residual vascularity M: medial extension L: lateral extension

As with other tumors such as inverted papilloma, this is due to increased experience with endoscopic skills, superior understanding of the anatomy and disease process, advances in radiological imaging and intraoperative imaging, more accurate image navigational systems, newer endoscopic instruments and improvements in techniques such as embolization. The availability of radiofrequency devices such as ultrasonic aspirators and coblation, as well as better-designed cautery and clip systems have resulted in a shift from the classic en-bloc removal to "piecemeal" resection by endoscopic techniques.

The first reports on endoscopic resections were published during the 1990s for smaller tumors. These demonstrated not only the feasibility of the technique, but efficacy similar to open techniques in recurrence rate.[3] With increasing experience, the indications for resecting larger tumors endoscopically are expanding.[82,83] Direct endoscopic approaches to the pterygopalatine fossa and the infratemporal space have been proposed, showing the potential range of purely endoscopic tumor access.[84,85] For larger tumor extensions into the infratemporal fossa a combined, endoscopic assisted antral window approach can be used.[86]

When performing an endoscopic approach, it is best to first perform a large maxillary antrostomy and remove the posterior fontanelle posteriorly to the palatine bone. Removing the middle turbinate will also increase the working space within the nasal cavity. With or without preoperative embolization, the vascular pedicle within the pterygopalatine fossa should be identified and ligated prior to debulking or removing the tumor. Exposing the back wall of the maxillary sinus allows for dissection to continue into the pterygopalatine fossa. Identification of the vascular pedicle can often be done after developing a mucosal flap over the palatine bone and identifying the crista ethmoidalis bone. Removing this bone will expose the vascular pedicle. Once the pedicle is identified, the bone of the posterior maxillary wall should be removed from a medial to lateral direction until the surgeon

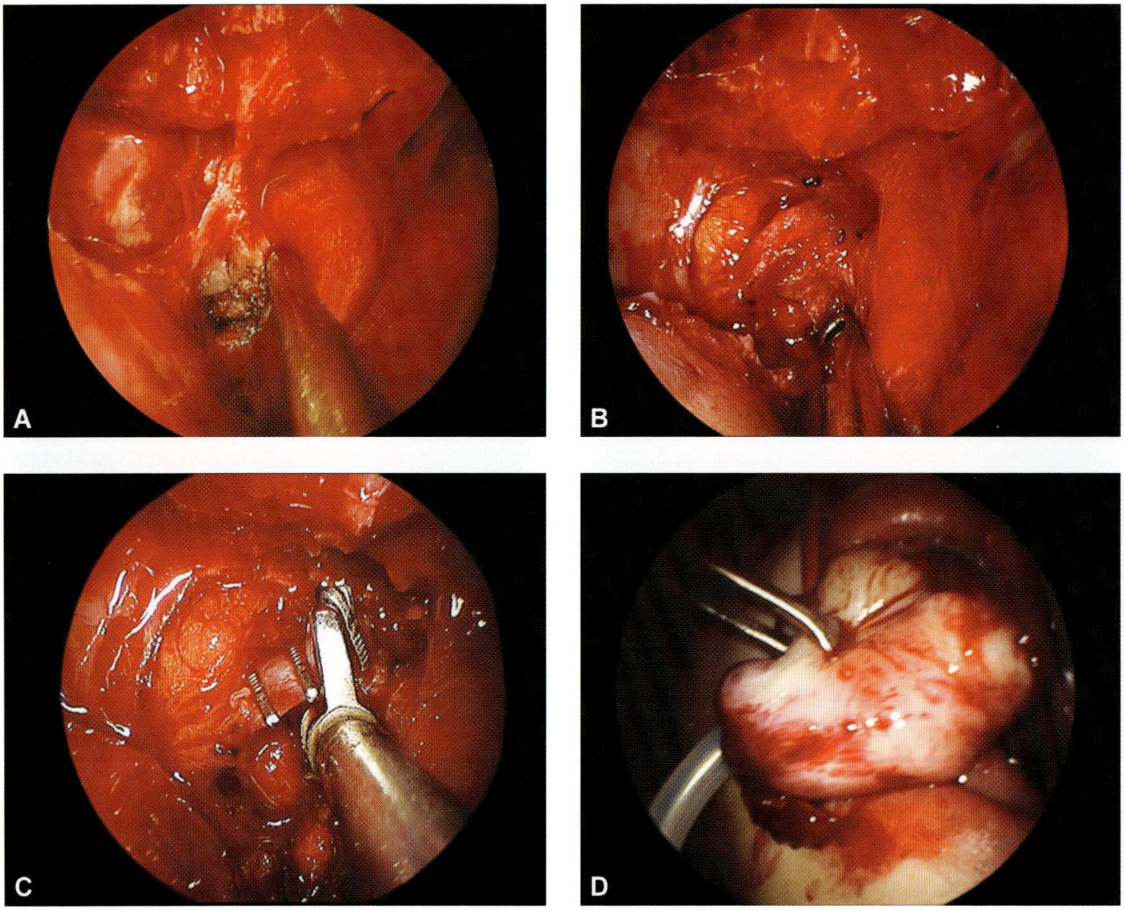

Figs 17.11A to D: Post-embolization, an endoscopic resection of the above right sinonasal angiofibroma was performed. (A) A wide maxillary antrostomy is performed. Pterygopalatine fossa dissection is initiated by opening the sphenopalatine foramen; (B) The pterygopalatine fossa is opened (note fat) and the lateral aspect of the tumor is defined and pushed medially; (C) The internal maxillary artery is identified and ligated; (D) Due to the large nasopharyngeal component, the tumor is delivered trans-orally after freeing all its attachments.

is lateral to the extent of tumor. The internal maxillary artery should then be clipped and ligated and the contents of the tumor can be swept medially into the nose.

Endoscopic resection by removing the tumor in a piece-meal fashion helps define and remove extensions meticulously and is not associated with any increase in recurrence.[87] Key to preventing recurrences is subperiosteal dissection of the tumor attachment at the basisphenoid with drilling of the denuded bone to remove any residual disease.[70,71,87] Lloyd found that in their series, 60% of juvenile angiofibromas expanded posteriorly along the pterygoid canal with invasion of the cancellous bone of the pterygoid base and greater wing of the sphenoid. They determined that 93% of recurrences occurred in patients with imaging evidence of invasion of the sphenoid diploe through the pterygoid canal.[71]

Non-surgical treatment options include external-beam therapy and stereotactic radiation. These are recommended as adjuvant therapy for unresectable tumors, residual and recurrent tumor and for extensive intracranial extension. Radiotherapy can control tumor in 85% with 30–35 Gy.[88] Recurrent tumors need either further surgery or radiation. Adverse effects of radiation for angiofibroma in young adolescents include cataracts years after radiotherapy, transient central nervous system syndrome growth impairment, and malignant transformation of juvenile angiofibroma.[3] Chemotherapy has been proposed for aggressive recurrences, but the experience is limited.[89] Despite promising early studies, a hormonal therapy has not yet been found effective. The number of cases studied in both were too few and hormonal therapy has yet to be formally evaluated.[3]

Results

A recent literature review found the rate of recurrent tumors to be low for smaller lesions, and increasing with higher staged tumors.[3] The results may be skewed when comparing open and endoscopic approaches since larger tumors tend to be resected using open or combined techniques. In the pre-endoscopic series, initial tumor control rate was around 97%, but with a symptomatic recurrence rate of about 50%. Preoperative embolization is considered to be a risk factor showing a higher recurrence rate and earlier recurrences.[90] However, the recurrence rate seems to be more related to the involvement of specific sites, such as the basisphenoid, anterior skull base, the infratemporal fossa and the cavernous sinus, the pterygoids, vidian canal and pterygopalatine fossa indicating that more extensive tumors tend to develop a higher rate of recurrence.[3,70,71] Synderman reported recurrence to be higher in those with residual vascularity after embolization.[81]

Endoscopic surgery can be undertaken for recurrent juvenile angiofibromas from any previous approaches. Dry eye can occur due to injury to the sphenopalatine ganglion or its branches. The duration of the endoscopic technique is a relative disadvantage, although this likely decreases with increasing experience. Complications of the external approach which are usually less common in endoscopic techniques are numbness and trismus. The need of blood transfusions depends on the extent of surgery.[3] This may be related to tumor volume and the success of embolization and residual vascularity following embolization.[81] Hospital stays appear to be shorter after endoscopic juvenile angiofibroma removal compared to external surgery, but again this may reflect a bias in selecting smaller tumors.[3]

Extensive tumors remain a surgical challenge. However, there is increased experienced-based evidence that endoscopic resection of large or an extended tumor is feasible in expert hands.[3]

Other Vascular Tumors

Lobular capillary hemangioma (pyogenic granuloma) is relatively common in the nasal cavity (Fig. 17.12). It mainly affects females in the third decade (range 11–65 years). They are usually located in the anterior aspects of the nasal septum and the turbinates.[3,69] Etiologic factors that have

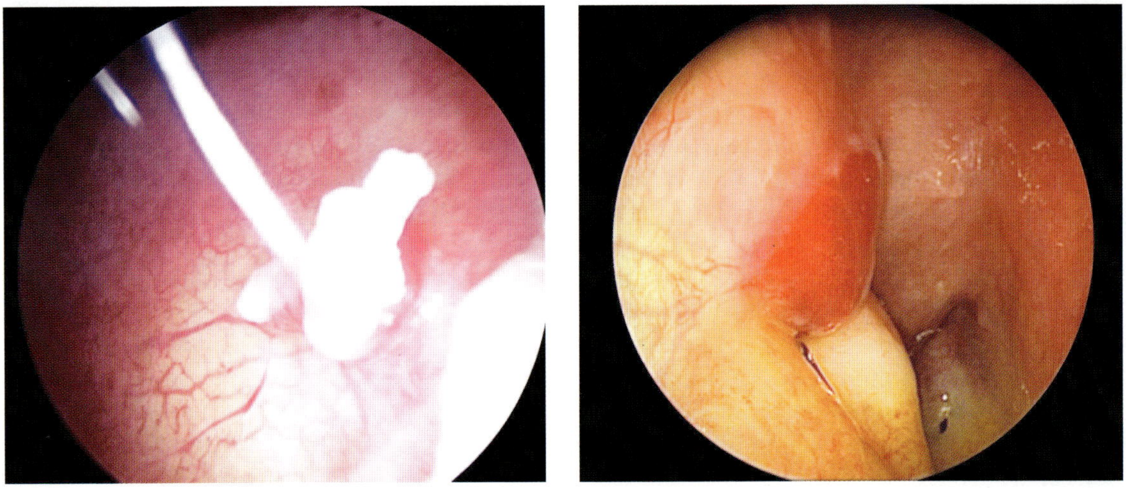

Fig. 17.12: Pyogenic granuloma (lobular capillary hemangioma) typically arises in the anterior septum as a polypoid vascular submucosal mass with intact surface mucosa. On the right, hemangioma has a very vascular appearance, as in this small recurrence on the right anterior skull base.

been postulated include nasal trauma and hormonal alterations. The tumor typically is a polypoid vascular submucosal mass with intact surface mucosa and effacement of submucosal structures. It is a cellular tumor with prominent vasculature, including large irregular ectatic vessels, and it may have stromal hemorrhage. These lesions are cured by surgical excision and rarely recur.[69]

Glomangiopericytoma are borderline, low-malignant-potential tumors of the nose and paranasal sinuses.[69] It is a soft tissue tumor with characteristic vascular proliferation. These tumors light up brightly on T1 sequences on MR, and may show flow voids similar to hemangioma. T2 weighted sequences delineate tumor from secretions (Fig. 17.13). This lesion was thought to fall in the spectrum between glomus tumors and capillary hemangioma and thus initially termed hemangiopericytoma. Sinonasal-type hemangiopericytoma, now termed glomangiopericytoma, represents a lesion separate from traditional soft tissue hemangiopericytoma since they have a more indolent pattern of growth. Glomangiopericytomas are rare, accounting for less than 1% of sinonasal tumors. They usually arise in the nasal cavity, and may extend into the paranasal sinuses. Peak incidence is in the seventh decade of life with a slight female preponderance. Glomangiopericytoma is an indolent tumor, associated with 5-year survival greater than 90% after surgical resection. Local recurrence has been reported in 7–40% of cases, usually secondary to incomplete resection. Aggressive behavior is rare. Large tumors that invade bone have profound nuclear pleomorphism, necrosis, and high mitotic rate, and are more likely to behave aggressively.[69]

NEURAL RELATED TUMORS

Meningiomas

They are usually benign and slow growing tumors, accounting for 15% of primary intracranial tumors. The peak age at presentation is 40–60 years with a female preponderance. Their incidence is increased by radiation, with increasing age, and by the presence of neurofibromatosis type 2 (NF_2). They originate from arachnoid cap cells and may be located anywhere where arachnoid cells are found.[3,91] Meningiomas are encountered infrequently in the nose and paranasal sinuses. They arise from ectopic arachnoid tissue. They are expansile in nature, and can, at times, be difficult to distinguish from extensions of intracranial

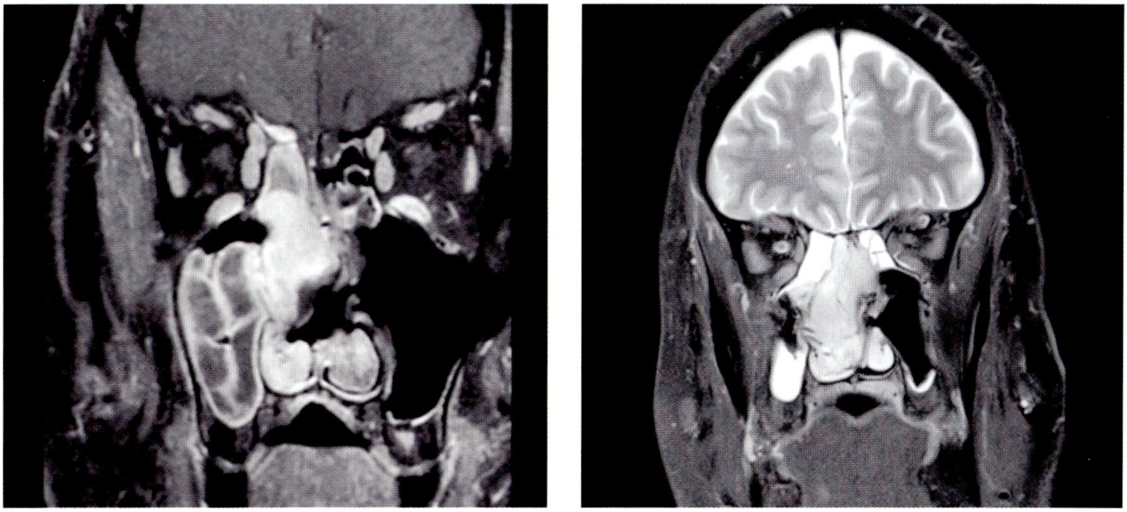

Fig. 17.13: Both hemangioma and glomangiopericytoma light up brightly onT1 sequences on MR, and may show flow voids similar to hemangioma. T2 weighted sequences differentiate tumor from secretions. Secretions appear dark on T1 and bright on T2 weighted sequences.

meningioma. The skull base usually remains intact in sinonasal cases, with bony expansion toward the skull base. Anterior skull base meningiomas account for 40% of all intracranial meningiomas. These include locations in the tuberculum sellae, sphenoidal ridge, and olfactory groove. Olfactory groove meningiomas arise in the midline along the cribriform plate; approximately 15% grow into the ethmoid sinuses. Presenting features are neurologic depending on the tumor location.

Meningiomas are encapsulated, firm and rubbery lesions. On immunohistochemistry, they have mesenchymal and epithelial cells, and are positive for both vimentin and epithelial membrane antigen. Histologically, they are classified by the World Health Organization (WHO) as Grade I to III. Grade I (typical) comprise 90% of meningiomas and are fibroblastic, transitional, psammomatous, or meningotheliomatous (angiomatous). Atypical meningiomas (WHO II) show hypercellularity, frequent mitosis, and necrosis. Malignant/anaplastic meningiomas (WHO III) are characterized by brain invasion, rapid recurrence, increased mitosis, and rarely metastasize.[3,91] Characteristic MRI features are extra-axial, durally based lesions involving the anterior skull base which are iso- to hypo-intense on T1-weighted images. These are contrast-enhancing and have characteristic dense calcification on CT scan (Fig. 17.14). Preoperatively, it is important to define adjacent neurovascular structures, especially the anterior cerebral arteries and their branches (Fig. 17.15A). Surgical resection is the primary modality of treatment for symptomatic lesions. These have a good long-term prognosis with a 5-year survival over 90%. However, they may recur even after total removal.[3,91] Over the past decade, extended/expanded endoscopic endonasal skull base approaches have developed and a wide variety of skull base lesions, including meningioma are favorable for such approaches[50-52] (Figs 17.15A to D).

Schwannomas

They frequently involve the head and neck region (25–45% of all cases). Approximately 4% of head and neck lesions involve the nasal and paranasal cavities. Most cases of schwannoma occur between the second and fifth decade of life with equal involvement of males and females of all races. These are found mainly in the nasoethmoid compartment and occur less frequently in the other

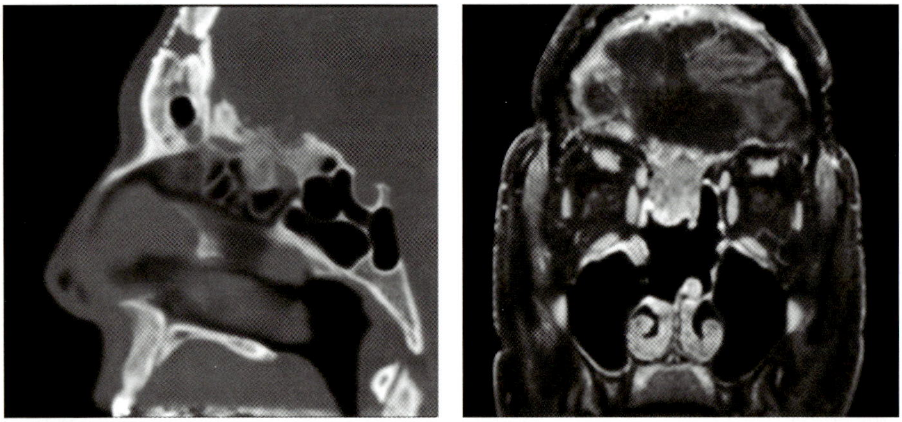

Fig. 17.14: Recurrent low-grade meningioma of the anterior skull base. They have characteristic dense calcification, best seen on CT scan. The iso to hypointense on T1-weighted images and are contrast-enhancing, as seen in this T1 with contrast MR sequence.

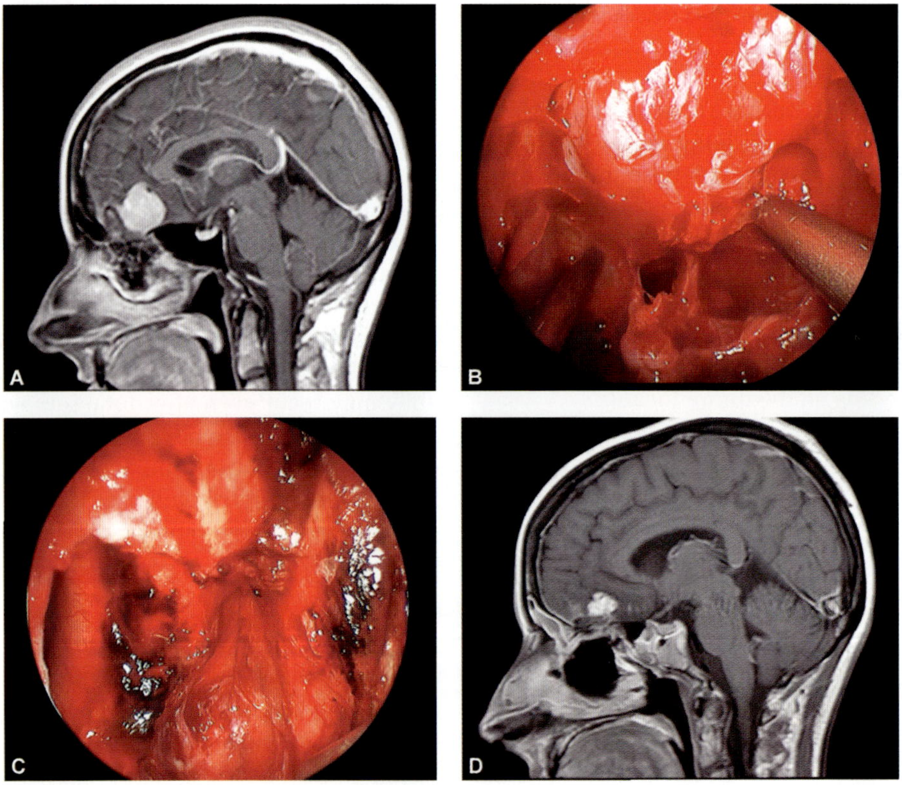

Figs 17.15A to D: Olfactory groove meningioma. (A) Preoperative sagittal T-1 with contrast MR sequence. Note the flow void anterior to the tumor mass from a branch of the anterior cerebral artery; (B) Endoscopic intra-operative appearance of the tumor; (C) The gyrus recti are visualized after tumor resection; (D) T1 with contrast image 3 months postoperatively shows complete removal of tumor. The fat used for skull base reconstruction lights up brightly. The nasoseptal flap used for anterior skull base reconstruction is also nicely healed and enhances with contrast.

sinuses. The tumor appears as well-delineated grossly, but can be un-encapsulated, rubbery yellow-tan mass.[92,93] Histologically, schwannomas are composed of cellular Antoni A areas with Verocay bodies and hypocellular myxoid Antoni B areas. Tumor cells are immunoreactive for S-100 protein. Differential diagnoses for schwannoma include neurofibroma, solitary fibrous tumor, leiomyoma, fibrous histiocytoma, and fibrosarcoma. There is a very low risk of malignant degeneration, increase to 10–15% in those associated with Von Recklinghausen's disease. Radical surgery is the treatment of choice for sinonasal schwannoma.[3] Before the advent of endoscopic surgery, external approaches were used based on the site and size of the lesion.

HAMARTOMATOUS LESIONS

Hamartomatous lesions are tumors composed of persistent rests of cells that, at some point during embryologic development, were a normal part of the local anatomy.[94-96] These are categorized into epithelial, mesenchymal and mixed epithelial mesenchymal types, with respiratory epithelial adenomatoid hamartoma (REAH) being the most common lesions. REAH is an uncommon lesion of the upper aerodigestive tract. It was first described by Wenig and Heffner in 1995 as prominent glandular proliferations lined by ciliated respiratory epithelium originating from the surface epithelium.[97] Inflammation is a common feature and may represent the background in which these lesions develop. REAH is seen most often in adult males as a polypoid mass (Fig. 17.16). It may occur in one or both nasal cavities. REAH is a benign lesion, but recognition of the lesion is important because it can be easily confused grossly and microscopically with other tumors such as inverted papilloma and sinonasal carcinomas.[95] REAHs with mesenchymal elements, cartilage or bone, are labeled chondro-osseous respiratory epithelial adenomatoid hamartomas. A much rarer type of epithelial hamartoma is the seromucinous (glandular) hamartoma. These are polypoid masses with an epithelial proliferation of small glands, acini and tubules growing in clusters, lobules, or haphazardly. Seromucinous hamartomas were first described by Baillie

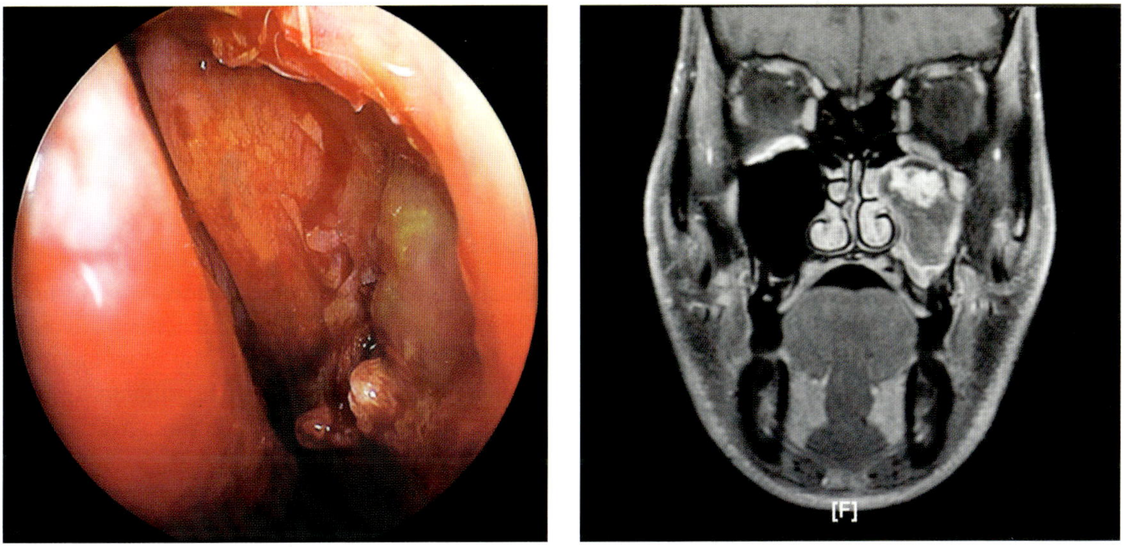

Fig. 17.16: Hamartoma of the left maxillary sinus. This appears to be polypoid on endoscopy. MR with contrast showing a variegated lesion with areas of contrast enhancement and other areas of cystic degeneration. This appears in similar to that of inverted papilloma and sinonasal malignancy.

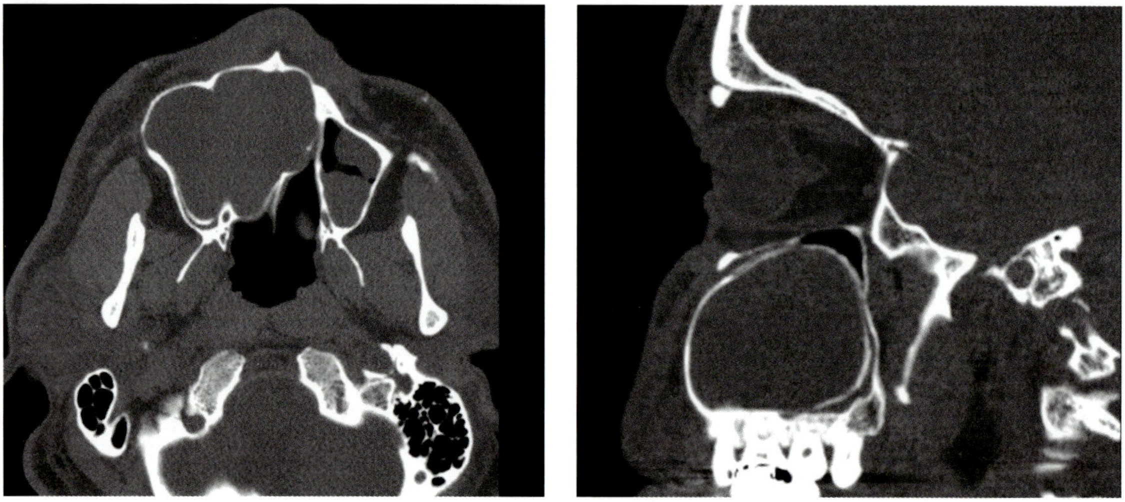

Fig. 17.17: Right maxillary ameloblastoma. Note the rim of the bony cyst pushing against the posterior maxillary wall and occupying the entire maxillary sinus.

and Batsakis[98] with only a few additional cases reported since.[94] These can be misdiagnosed as low-grade adenocarcinomas.[96]

ODONTOGENIC TUMORS

The two hamartomas of odontogenic origin presenting in the sinonasal cavity are ameloblastoma and the calcifying epithelial tumor of Pindborg.[3] Twenty percent of all ameloblastomas arise in the bone of the maxilla. The sinuses themselves get involved after secondary growth into these air-containing spaces (Fig. 17.17).[99] Pindborg's tumors are much rarer and can present clinically in a fashion similar to ameloblastoma.

OTHER TUMORS

Pleomorphic adenoma arising from minor salivary glands is the third most common benign tumor of the sinonasal tract following osteoma and inverted papilloma. It usually affects patients in the fifth decade of life, with no significant gender predominance. The nasal septum most frequently affected, followed by maxillary sinus.[100]

There are many other benign tumors such as leiomyoma, paraganglioma, hemangioma, myoepithelioma, oncocytoma that occur sporadically in the sinonasal area. Odontogenic cysts (Figs 17.18A to D) and inflammatory lesions such as mucoceles, sinonasal polyps, allergic fungal sinusitis (Fig. 17.19), and autoimmune diseases (Sarcoidosis, Wegener's granulomatosis) may be difficult to tell apart from nasal tumors on clinical and radiologic examination. While the clinical and radiographic appearance of these may offer subtle clues to a differential diagnosis, histopathological examination (and occasionally, serologic testing) is key to diagnosis. Individual discussion of these is beyond the scope of this chapter.

CONCLUSIONS

A vast diversity of benign tumors occurs in the nose, although benign sinonasal tumors themselves occur rarely in the population. The most common benign sinonasal tumors include osteoma, inverted papilloma and juvenile angiofibroma. The behavior and spread of individual pathologies is distinct, and dictates treatment. Surgical resection by minimally invasive endoscopic endonasal approaches can offer success rates equivalent or superior to those achieved by external approaches in carefully selected cases. Increased experience with the

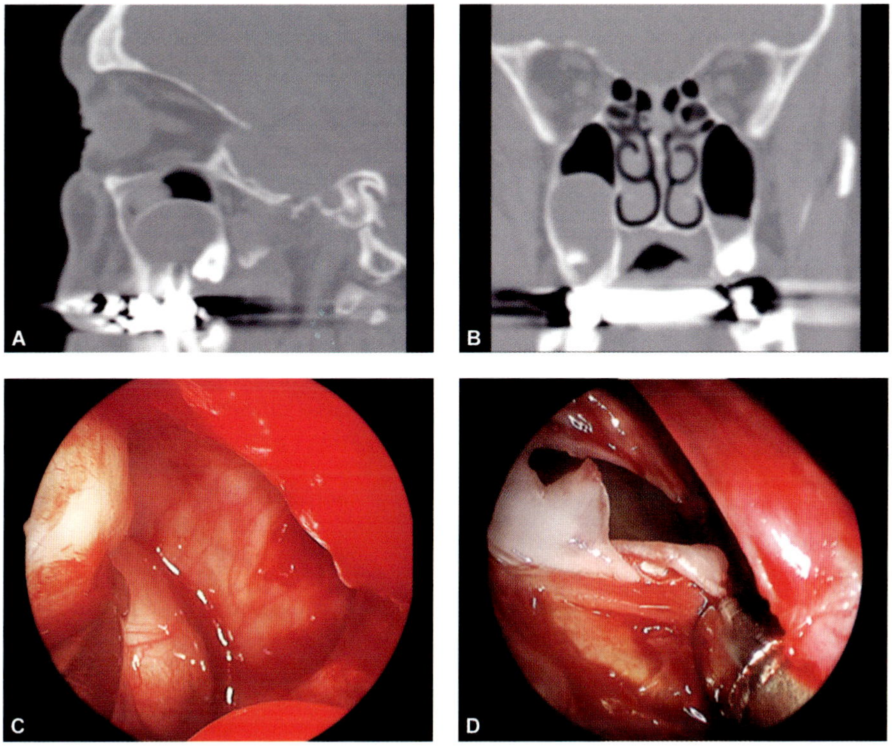

Figs 17.18A to D: Odontogenic keratocyst can be confused with ameloblastoma and other tumors. (A and B) CT showing bony cyst growing around a tooth root expanding into the right maxillary sinus; (C) Cyst is exposed via a right endoscopic medial maxillectomy approach; (D) The bony cyst wall is opened and keratotic fluid-filled cyst is drained, and then will be further marsupialized.

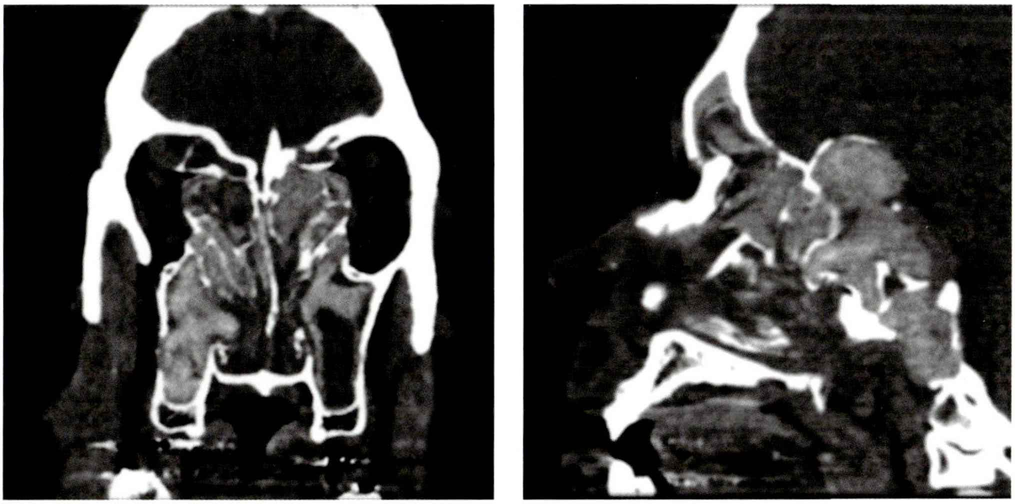

Fig. 17.19: Massive bilateral allergic fungal sinusitis on CT. Note that though there is bony erosion, this is accompanied by remodeling and bowing of the bone (suggesting a slow expansion). Characteristic calcification and differential density in the opacified sinuses is also noted.

endoscopic technique, better understanding of the complex anatomy along with technological innovations in instrumentation and imaging have made the shift in the paradigm from open to endoscopic techniques possible.

REFERENCES

1. Barnes LEJ, Reichart P, Sidransky D, et al. Pathology and genetics of head and neck tumours. 2005;Lyon:ARC Press.
2. Earwaker J. Paranasal sinus osteomas: a review of 46 cases. Skeletal Radiol. 1993;22(6):417-23.
3. Lund VJ, Stammberger H, Nicolai P, et al. European position paper on endoscopic management of tumours of the nose, paranasal sinuses and skull base. Rhinol Suppl. 2010;(22):1-143.
4. Hullar TE, Lustig LR. Paget's disease and fibrous dysplasia. Otolaryngol Clin North Am. 2003;36(4):707-32.
5. Lloyd G, Lund VJ, Howard D, et al. Optimum imaging for sinonasal malignancy. J Laryngol Otol. 2000;114(7):557-62.
6. Fatterpekar GM, Delman BN, Som PM. Imaging the paranasal sinuses: where we are and where we are going. Anat Rec (Hoboken). 2008;291(11):1564-72.
7. Atallah N, Jay MM. Osteomas of the paranasal sinuses. J Laryngol Otol. 1981;95(3):291-304.
8. Smith ME, Calcaterra TC. Frontal sinus osteoma. Ann Otol Rhinol Laryngol. 1989;98(11):896-900.
9. Koivunen P, Löppönen H, Fors AP, et al. The growth rate of osteomas of the paranasal sinuses. Clin Otolaryngol Allied Sci. 1997;22(2):111-4.
10. MacDonald-Jankowski DS. Fibro-osseous lesions of the face and jaws. Clin Radiol. 2004;59(1):11-25.
11. Pacini F, Perri G, Bagnolesi P, et al. McCune-Albright syndrome with gigantism and hyperprolactinemia. J Endocrinol Invest. 1987;10(4):417-20.
12. Pensler JM, Langman CB, Radosevich JA, et al. Sex steroid hormone receptors in normal and dysplastic bone disorders in children. J Bone Miner Res. 1990;5(5):493-8.
13. Lietman SA, Schwindinger WF, Levine MA. Genetic and molecular aspects of McCune-Albright syndrome. Pediatr Endocrinol Rev. 2007;4 Suppl 4:380-5.
14. Fu YS, Perzin KH. Non-epithelial tumors of the nasal cavity, paranasal sinuses, and nasopharynx. A clinicopathologic study. II. Osseous and fibro-osseous lesions, including osteoma, fibrous dysplasia, ossifying fibroma, osteoblastoma, giant cell tumor, and osteosarcoma. Cancer. 1974;33(5):1289-305.
15. Zacharin M, O'Sullivan M. Intravenous pamidronate treatment of polyostotic fibrous dysplasia associated with the McCune Albright syndrome. J Pediatr. 2000;137(3):403-9.
16. Kingdom TT, Delgaudio JM. Endoscopic approach to lesions of the sphenoid sinus, orbital apex, and clivus. Am J Otolaryngol. 2003;24(5):317-22.
17. Wenig BM, Vinh TN, Smirniotopoulos JG, et al. Aggressive psammomatoid ossifying fibromas of the sinonasal region: a clinicopathologic study of a distinct group of fibro-osseous lesions. Cancer. 1995;76(7):1155-65.
18. Khoury NJ, Naffaa LN, Shabb NS, et al. Juvenile ossifying fibroma: CT and MR findings. Eur Radiol. 2002;12 Suppl 3:S109-13.
19. Brodish BN, Morgan CE, Sillers MJ. Endoscopic resection of fibro-osseous lesions of the paranasal sinuses. Am J Rhinol. 1999;13(2):111-6.
20. Howard DJ, Lund VJ, Wei WI. Craniofacial resection for tumors of the nasal cavity and paranasal sinuses: a 25-year experience. Head Neck. 2006;28(10):867-73.
21. Lampertico P, Russell WO, Maccomb WS. Squamous papilloma of upper respiratory epithelium. Arch Pathol. 1963;75:293-302.
22. Skolnik EM, Loewy A, Friedman JE. Inverted papilloma of the nasal cavity. Arch Otolaryngol. 1966;84(1):61-7.
23. Hyams VJ. Papillomas of the nasal cavity and paranasal sinuses. A clinicopathological study of 315 cases. Ann Otol Rhinol Laryngol. 1971;80(2):192-206.
24. Mirza S, Bradley PJ, Acharya A, et al. Sinonasal inverted papillomas: recurrence, and synchronous and metachronous malignancy. J Laryngol Otol. 2007;121(9):857-64.
25. Chiu AG, Jackman AH, Antunes MB, et al. Radiographic and histologic analysis of the bone underlying inverted papillomas. Laryngoscope. 2006;116(9):1617-20.
26. Jeon TY, Kim HJ, Choi JY, et al. 18F-FDG PET/CT findings of sinonasal inverted papilloma with or without coexistent malignancy: comparison with MR imaging findings in eight patients. Neuroradiology. 2009;51(4):265-71.
27. Jeon TY, Kim HJ, Chung SK, et al. Sinonasal inverted papilloma: value of convoluted cerebriform pattern on MR imaging. AJNR Am J Neuroradiol. 2008;29(8):1556-60.

28. Lawson W, Patel ZM. The evolution of management for inverted papilloma: an analysis of 200 cases. Otolaryngol Head Neck Surg. 2009;140(3):330-5.
29. Phillips PP, Gustafson RO, Facer GW. The clinical behavior of inverting papilloma of the nose and paranasal sinuses: report of 112 cases and review of the literature. Laryngoscope. 1990;100(5):463-9.
30. Garavello W. Gaini RM. Histopathology of routine nasal polypectomy specimens: a review of 2,147 cases. Laryngoscope. 2005;115(10):1866-8.
31. Garavello W, Gaini RM. Incidence of inverted papilloma in recurrent nasal polyposis. Laryngoscope. 2006;116(2):221-3.
32. Sham CL, Lee DL, van Hasselt CA, et al. A case-control study of the risk factors associated with sinonasal inverted papilloma. Am J Rhinol Allergy. 2009. [Epub ahead of print].
33. Mansell NJ, Bates GJ. The inverted Schneiderian papilloma: a review and literature report of 43 new cases. Rhinology. 2000;38(3):97-101.
34. Tanvetyanon T, Qin D, Padhya T, et al. Survival outcomes of squamous cell carcinoma arising from sinonasal inverted papilloma: report of 6 cases with systematic review and pooled analysis. Am J Otolaryngol. 2009;30(1):38-43.
35. Lawson W, Schlecht NF, Brandwein-Gensler M. The role of the human papillomavirus in the pathogenesis of Schneiderian inverted papillomas: an analytic overview of the evidence. Head Neck Pathol. 2008;2(2):49-59.
36. Kim JY, Yoon JK, Citardi MJ, et al. The prevalence of human papilloma virus infection in sinonasal inverted papilloma specimens classified by histological grade. Am J Rhinol. 2007;21(6):664-9.
37. Yoon JH, Kim CH, Choi EC. Treatment outcomes of primary and recurrent inverted papilloma: an analysis of 96 cases. J Laryngol Otol. 2002;116(9):699-702.
38. Christensen WN, Smith RR. Schneiderian papillomas: a clinicopathologic study of 67 cases. Hum Pathol. 1986;17(4):393-400.
39. Lawson W, Le Benger J, Som P, et al. Inverted papilloma: an analysis of 87 cases. Laryngoscope. 1989;99(11):1117-24.
40. Cannady SB, Batra PS, Sautter NB, et al. New staging system for sinonasal inverted papilloma in the endoscopic era. Laryngoscope. 2007;117(7):1283-7.
41. Han JK, Smith TL, Loehrl T, et al. An evolution in the management of sinonasal inverting papilloma. Laryngoscope. 2001;111(8):1395-400.
42. Krouse JH. Development of a staging system for inverted papilloma. Laryngoscope. 2000;110(6):965-8.
43. Oikawa K, Furuta Y, Nakamaru Y, et al. Preoperative staging and surgical approaches for sinonasal inverted papilloma. Ann Otol Rhinol Laryngol. 2007;116(9):674-80.
44. Landsberg R, Cavel O, Segev Y, et al. Attachment-oriented endoscopic surgical strategy for sinonasal inverted papilloma. Am J Rhinol. 2008;22(6):629-34.
45. Kamel R, Khaled A, Kandil T. Inverted papilloma: new classification and guidelines for endoscopic surgery. Am J Rhinol. 2005;19(4):358-64.
46. Calcaterra TC, Thompson JW, Paglia DE. Inverting papillomas of the nose and paranasal sinuses. Laryngoscope. 1980;90(1):53-60.
47. Vrabec DP. The inverted Schneiderian papilloma: a 25-year study. Laryngoscope. 1994;104(5 Pt 1):582-605.
48. Bielamowicz S, Calcaterra TC, Watson D. Inverting papilloma of the head and neck: the UCLA update. Otolaryngol Head Neck Surg. 1993;109(1):71-6.
49. Fortes FS, Sennes LU, Carrau RL, et al. Endoscopic anatomy of the pterygopalatine fossa and the transpterygoid approach: development of a surgical instruction model. Laryngoscope. 2008;118(1):44-9.
50. Kassam A, Snyderman CH, Mintz A, et al. Expanded endonasal approach: the rostrocaudal axis. Part II. Posterior clinoids to the foramen magnum. Neurosurg Focus. 2005;19(1):E4.
51. Kassam A, Snyderman CH, Mintz A, et al. Expanded endonasal approach: the rostrocaudal axis. Part I. Crista galli to the sella turcica. Neurosurg Focus. 2005;19(1):E3.
52. Kassam AB, Gardner P, Snyderman C, et al. Expanded endonasal approach: fully endoscopic, completely transnasal approach to the middle third of the clivus, petrous bone, middle cranial fossa, and infratemporal fossa. Neurosurg Focus. 2005;19(1):E6.
53. Prevedello DM, Kassam AB, Snyderman C, et al. Endoscopic cranial base surgery: ready for prime time? Clin Neurosurg. 2007; 54:48-57.
54. Lawson W, Kaufman MR, Biller HF. Treatment outcomes in the management of inverted papilloma: an analysis of 160 cases. Laryngoscope. 2003;113(9):1548-56.

55. Woodworth BA, Bhargave GA, Palmer JN, et al. Clinical outcomes of endoscopic and endoscopic-assisted resection of inverted papillomas: a 15-year experience. Am J Rhinol. 2007;21(5):591-600.
56. Busquets JM, Hwang PH. Endoscopic resection of sinonasal inverted papilloma: a meta-analysis. Otolaryngol Head Neck Surg. 2006;134(3):476-82.
57. Carrillo JF, Albores O, Ramírez-Ortega MC, et al. An audit of nasopharyngeal fibromas. Eur J Surg Oncol. 2007;33(5):655-61.
58. Farag MM, Ghanimah SE, Ragaie A, et al. Hormonal receptors in juvenile nasopharyngeal angiofibroma. Laryngoscope. 1987;97(2):208-11.
59. Coutinho-Camillo CM, Brentani MM, Nagai MA. Genetic alterations in juvenile nasopharyngeal angiofibromas. Head Neck. 2008;30(3):390-400.
60. Brunner C, Urbschat S, Jung V, et al. [Chromosomal alterations in juvenile angiofibromas]. HNO. 2003;51(12):981-5.
61. Schick B, Rippel C, Brunner C, et al. Numerical sex chromosome aberrations in juvenile angiofibromas: genetic evidence for an androgen-dependent tumor? Oncol Rep. 2003;10(5):1251-5.
62. Schick B, Urbschat S. New aspects of pathogenesis of juvenile angiofibroma. Hosp Med. 2004;65(5):269-73.
63. Schick B, Veldung B, Wemmert S, et al. p53 and Her-2/neu in juvenile angiofibromas. Oncol Rep. 2005;13(3):453-7.
64. Schick B, Wemmert S, Bechtel U, et al. Comprehensive genomic analysis identifies MDM2 and AURKA as novel amplified genes in juvenile angiofibromas. Head Neck. 2007;29(5):479-87.
65. Schick B, Wemmert S, Jung V, et al. Genetic heterogeneity of the MYC oncogene in advanced juvenile angiofibromas. Cancer Genet Cytogenet. 2006;164(1):25-31.
66. Beham A, Beham-Schmid C, Regauer S, et al. Nasopharyngeal angiofibroma: true neoplasm or vascular malformation? Adv Anat Pathol. 2000;7(1):36-46.
67. Lloyd G, Howard D, Lund VJ, et al. Imaging for juvenile angiofibroma. J Laryngol Otol. 2000;114(9):727-30.
68. Chandler JR, Goulding R, Moskowitz L, et al. Nasopharyngeal angiofibromas: staging and management. Ann Otol Rhinol Laryngol. 1984;93(4 Pt 1):322-9.
69. Dandekar M, McHugh JB. Sinonasal glomangiopericytoma: case report with emphasis on the differential diagnosis. Arch Pathol Lab Med. 2010;134(10):1444-9.
70. Howard DJ, Lloyd G, Lund V. Recurrence and its avoidance in juvenile angiofibroma. Laryngoscope. 2001;111(9):1509-11.
71. Lloyd G, Howard D, Phelps P, et al. Juvenile angiofibroma: the lessons of 20 years of modern imaging. J Laryngol Otol. 1999;113(2):127-34.
72. Casasco A, Houdart E, Biondi A, et al. Major complications of percutaneous embolization of skull-base tumors. AJNR Am J Neuroradiol. 1999;20(1):179-81.
73. Tranbahuy P, Borsik M, Herman P, et al. Direct intratumoral embolization of juvenile angiofibroma. Am J Otolaryngol. 1994;15(6):429-35.
74. Sessions RB, Bryan RN, Naclerio RM, et al. Radiographic staging of juvenile angiofibroma. Head Neck Surg. 1981;3(4):279-83.
75. Radkowski D, McGill T, Healy GB, et al. Angiofibroma. Changes in staging and treatment. Arch Otolaryngol Head Neck Surg. 1996;122(2):122-9.
76. Andrews JC, Fisch U, Valavanis A, et al. The surgical management of extensive nasopharyngeal angiofibromas with the infratemporal fossa approach. Laryngoscope. 1989;99(4):429-37.
77. Bremer JW, Neel HB 3rd, DeSanto LW, et al. Angiofibroma: treatment trends in 150 patients during 40 years. Laryngoscope. 1986;96(12):1321-9.
78. Antonelli AR, Cappiello J, Di Lorenzo D, et al. Diagnosis, staging, and treatment of juvenile nasopharyngeal angiofibroma (JNA). Laryngoscope. 1987;97(11):1319-25.
79. Onerci M, Ogretmenoglu O, Yucel T. Juvenile nasopharyngeal angiofibroma: a revised staging system. Rhinology. 2006;44(1):39-45.
80. Carrillo JF, Maldonado F, Albores O, et al. Juvenile nasopharyngeal angiofibroma: clinical factors associated with recurrence, and proposal of a staging system. J Surg Oncol. 2008;98(2):75-80.
81. Snyderman CH, Pant H, Carrau RL, et al. A new endoscopic staging system for angiofibromas. Arch Otolaryngol Head Neck Surg. 2010;136(6):588-94.
82. Douglas R, Wormald PJ. Endoscopic surgery for juvenile nasopharyngeal angiofibroma: where are the limits? Curr Opin Otolaryngol Head Neck Surg. 2006;14(1):1-5.
83. Nicolai P, Berlucchi M, Tomenzoli D, et al. Endoscopic surgery for juvenile angiofibroma: when and how. Laryngoscope. 2003;113(5):775-82.
84. Nicolai P, Villaret AB, Farina D, et al. Endoscopic surgery for juvenile angiofibroma: a critical review

of indications after 46 cases. Am J Rhinol Allergy. 2010;24(2):e67-72.

85. Robinson S, Patel N, Wormald PJ. Endoscopic management of benign tumors extending into the infratemporal fossa: a two-surgeon transnasal approach. Laryngoscope. 2005;115(10):1818-22.
86. Khalifa MA, Ragab SM. Endoscopic assisted antral window approach for type III nasopharyngeal angiofibroma with infratemporal fossa extension. Int J Pediatr Otorhinolaryngol. 2008;72(12):1855-60.
87. Hofmann T, Bernal-Sprekelsen M, Koele W, et al. Endoscopic resection of juvenile angiofibromas-long-term results. Rhinology. 2005;43(4):282-9.
88. Lee JT, Chen P, Safa A, et al. The role of radiation in the treatment of advanced juvenile angiofibroma. Laryngoscope. 2002;112(7 Pt 1):1213-20.
89. Goepfert H, Cangir A, Lee YY. Chemotherapy for aggressive juvenile nasopharyngeal angiofibroma. Arch Otolaryngol. 1985;111(5):285-9.
90. Gupta AK, Rajiniganth MG, Gupta AK. Endoscopic approach to juvenile nasopharyngeal angiofibroma: our experience at a tertiary care centre. J Laryngol Otol. 2008;122(11):1185-9.
91. Whittle IR, Smith C, Navoo P, et al. Meningiomas. Lancet. 2004;363(9420):1535-43.
92. Berlucchi M, Piazza C, Blanzuoli L, et al. Schwannoma of the nasal septum: a case report with review of the literature. Eur Arch Otorhinolaryngol. 2000;257(7):402-5.
93. Hillstrom RP, Zarbo RJ, Jacobs JR. Nerve sheath tumors of the paranasal sinuses: electron microscopy and histopathologic diagnosis. Otolaryngol Head Neck Surg. 1990;102(3):257-63.
94. Figures MR, Nayak JV, Gable C, et al. Sinonasal seromucinous hamartomas: clinical features and diagnostic dilemma. Otolaryngol Head Neck Surg. 2010;143(1):165-6.
95. Fitzhugh VA, Mirani N. Respiratory epithelial adenomatoid hamartoma: a review. Head Neck Pathol. 2008;2(3):203-8.
96. Weinreb I, Gnepp DR, Laver NM, et al. Seromucinous hamartomas: a clinicopathological study of a sinonasal glandular lesion lacking myoepithelial cells. Histopathology. 2009;54(2):205-13.
97. Wenig BM, Heffner DK. Respiratory epithelial adenomatoid hamartomas of the sinonasal tract and nasopharynx: a clinicopathologic study of 31 cases. Ann Otol Rhinol Laryngol. 1995;104(8):639-45.
98. Baillie EE, Batsakis JG. Glandular (seromucinous) hamartoma of the nasopharynx. Oral Surg Oral Med Oral Pathol. 1974;38(5):760-2.
99. Schafer DR, Thompson LD, Smith BC, et al. Primary ameloblastoma of the sinonasal tract: a clinicopathologic study of 24 cases. Cancer. 1998;82(4):667-74.
100. Compagno J, Wong RT. Intranasal mixed tumors (pleomorphic adenomas): a clinicopathologic study of 40 cases. Am J Clin Pathol. 1977;68(2):213-8.

18

Malignant Sinonasal Tumors

Vijay R Ramakrishnan, MD; Jeffrey D Suh, MD

INTRODUCTION

Cancers of the nasal cavity and paranasal sinuses are relatively uncommon, representing roughly 3% of head and neck cancers, and less than 1% of all cancers. A number of malignancies can arise from the nose and sinuses. Although presentation may be similar, each type is unique in its pathologic behavior and response to treatment. As such, biopsy proven diagnosis should be sought prior to definitive treatment. During biopsy, representative deep tumor samples should be obtained while leaving natural planes and tumor boundaries undisturbed. Sinonasal malignancies are generally associated with a poor prognosis; this may be due to delays in diagnosis as early tumors can mimic benign diseases such as allergic rhinitis or sinusitis. Frequently, tumors are large on presentation and approach critical neighboring structures of the orbit and skull base, or extend into nearby foramina or pathways of least resistance. The complex anatomy of these areas may lead to incomplete tumor removal or the desire for open approaches to augment surgeon comfort in these potentially dangerous areas.

Evidence for endoscopic surgery of sinonasal malignancy is based mostly on retrospective chart analysis of survival data, disease control, cost-benefit analyses, quality of life and complications. When reviewing available literature, endoscopic resection of malignant tumors appears favorable when compared to open surgery. However, there is a general selection bias in favor of reports on successful surgical outcomes when new techniques are presented. In addition, endoscopic surgery for malignant disease was initially performed for smaller tumors and earlier stage disease, as is appropriate with any technical innovation or paradigm shift. Additional factors such as operative parameters and patient postoperative course may support endoscopic surgical approaches over traditional open approaches in some cases. The majority of these retrospective analyses consist of heterogeneous tumor groups, or small cohorts of specific tumor types with limited follow-up. Due to relative rarity of disease, tumor heterogeneity, and technical differences between surgeons and radiation therapists, it is extremely difficult to come to any definitive conclusions with meta-analyses, and is exceedingly difficult to design prospective comparison studies. Table 18.1 represents a simplified guideline for treating a variety of sinonasal tumors discussed in this chapter. However, we must make decisions for patients-based on all available data, physician experience and hospital resources.

Table 18.1 Management guidelines for select sinonasal malignancies

Tumor type	*Surgery*	*XRT**	*w Chemo*	*Notes*
Squamous cell carcinoma	Yes	Yes	+/-	
Adenocarcinoma	Yes	Yes	?	May consider surgery alone for small, low-grade tumors
Adenoid cystic carcinoma	Yes	Yes	?	
Sinonasal melanoma	Yes	Yes	?	
Esthesioneuroblastoma	Yes	Yes	+/-	Protocols widely vary by institution. Can consider neoadjuvant chemoradiation versus surgery + adjuvant therapy
Sinonasal undifferentiated Carinoma	Yes	Yes	Yes	Surgery followed by chemoradiation or chemoradiation alone for unresectable lesions

*Combination therapy usually indicated for (+) margins, perineural/perivascular invasion, (+) lymph nodes or recurrent tumors. Actual management depends on a variety of factors (stage, margin status, etc.) which must be taken into consideration.

En-bloc versus piecemeal resection does not appear to change prognosis.[1] The necessity of *en-bloc* resection for head and neck tumors has been questioned by the success of techniques such as laryngeal laser microsurgery and Moh's micrographic surgery. However, with malignant sinus tumors, the *en-bloc* principle is ideally followed at the site of tumor origin. Prognostic factors, such as pterygomaxillary, dural or periorbital invasion, negatively impact survival. In both open and endoscopic resection of sinonasal malignancy, there is a trend toward recurrence with advanced stage disease.[2,3] But, the most important prognostic factor is the presence of a positive margin, and therefore this is the ultimate deciding factor in the approach to a given tumor for a given surgical team.

General staging systems for malignant tumors, such as the tumor-node metastasis (TNM) classification, are useful for research purposes and possibly patient counseling, but less so for surgical planning in individual tumor cases. Staging systems, such as the TNM classification, correlate poorly with prognosis and do not determine suitability for an endoscopic approach.[4-6] The World Health Organization (WHO) has categorized sinus cancers by etiology into epithelial, neuroectodermal, soft tissue, bone and cartilage, hematolymphoid, and metastatic subdivisions. In this chapter, we will discuss the presentation, workup and management of each of these tumors in detail.

SQUAMOUS CELL CARCINOMA

As the most common malignancy of the sinonasal tract, squamous cell carcinoma (SCC) represents between 27% and 92% of all sinonasal malignancies.[3,7] There is a 2:1 male:female ratio, with a peak incidence in the 6th decade.[8] There is a known relationship between nickel exposure and delayed SCC development, and a number of other chemical and environmental exposures may be factors, as well.[9] Alcohol and tobacco use are major contributors to SCC of the head and neck, but do not appear to be risk factors in the pathogenesis of sinonasal SCC.[10] Inverted papilloma carries a roughly 10% association with SCC, which may arise within, nearby or subsequent to papilloma development.[11]

The maxillary sinus is the most common site of presentation, followed by the ethmoid sinus. Presenting symptoms are usually nasal obstruction, epistaxis, pain and postobstructive sinusitis. Due to the common nature of early complaints, most SCC on presentation is advanced. Tumors may expand into the orbit, skull base, pterygopalatine and infratemporal fossae, maxillary soft tissues, gingiva and palate. Orbital symptoms of proptosis, diplopia, loss of acuity, and pain with movement may result from pressure on the orbit, frank orbital invasion, or extension into the inferior or superior orbital fissures. Lateral extension into the pterygoid musculature can cause significant trismus (Fig. 18.1). Approximately 10% of all maxillary SCC will have nodal metastasis on presentation; this is notably less for SCC of the other sinuses. The rate of regional metastasis on presentation or regional recurrence is significant for T2 tumors and larger, and portends a sharp decrease in overall survival.[12]

Both computed tomography (CT) and magnetic resonance imaging (MRI) are needed to provide adequate information for sinonasal SCC. CT scan provides detail about bony destruction and invasion which occurs in nearly 80% of SCC, and is used for image guidance during surgery.[13] MRI will help distinguish tumor from mucosal inflammation and secretions, and can help determine spread into surrounding soft tissues of the skin, orbit, pterygopalatine and infratemporal fossae, intracranial cavity and along major nerves. Positron emission tomography (PET) scanning is helpful for metastatic evaluation at diagnosis, and all three modalities may be of use in surveillance. Perineural spread may be detected in up to 22% of sinonasal SCC on pathologic analysis, and is a frequent site of failure to obtain clear surgical margins. 5-year overall survival for SCC drops from 66% to 57% in patients with perineural invasion noted on pathologic analysis.[14]

Pathologically, SCC should be graded as well-, moderate, or poorly-differentiated. Most sinonasal SCC are keratinizing, but can be poorly differentiated or nonkeratinizing. Unusual variants include basaloid, verrucous, papillary, adenosquamous and spindle cell SCC, with varying prognoses. Tumors of the nasal cavity, maxillary and ethmoid sinuses are staged according to the TNM system of the Union Internationale Contre le Cancer (UICC)/ American Joint Cancer Committee (AJCC) (Table 18.2).

There are no randomized trials comparing treatment modalities for sinonasal SCC. Multimodality treatment is recommended for anything beyond a T1 lesion. Surgery with postoperative radiotherapy with or without concurrent chemotherapy is the most commonly recommended treatment plan for sinonasal SCC. Results for radiotherapy alone are very poor; with 5-year survival rates less than 21%.[15] Little data exist for concurrent chemoradiation

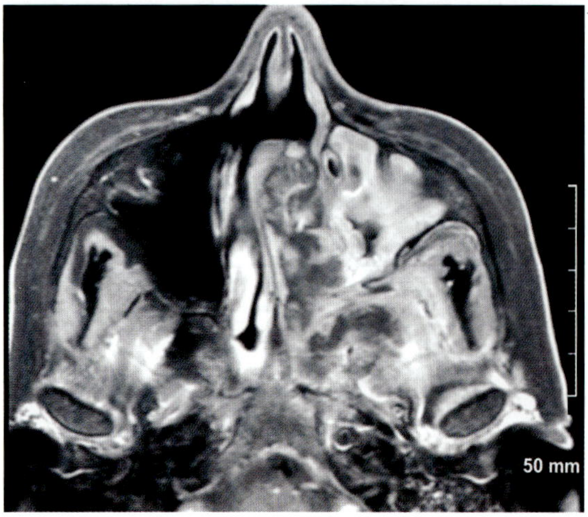

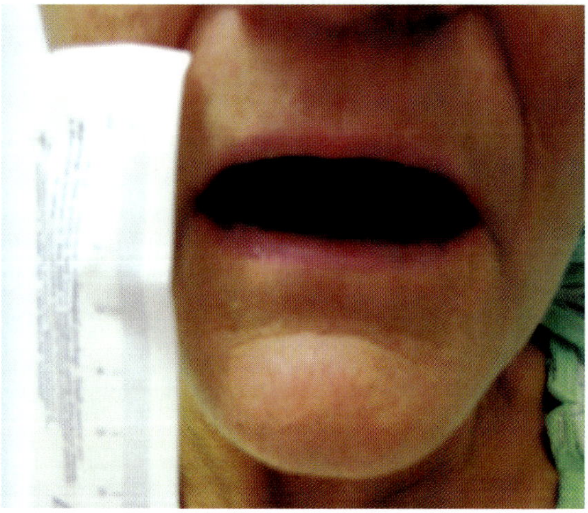

Fig. 18.1: Photograph and axial postcontrast MRI of a patient with SCC arising within an inverted papilloma. Extension into the pterygoid musculature results and infratemporal fossa in this patient has resulted in significant trismus.

Table 18.2 Description of the AJCC staging system for sinonasal tumors

Nasal cavity and ethmoid sinus

- T1—Tumor restricted to one subsite, with or without bony invasion
- T2—Tumor invading two subsites in a single region or involving an adjacent region within the nasoethmoidal complex, with or without bony invasion
- T3—Tumor invades the medial wall or floor of the orbit, maxillary sinus, palate or cribriform plate
- T4a—Tumor involves any of the following: anterior orbital contents, skin of nose or cheek, minimal extension to anterior cranial fossa, pterygoid plates, sphenoid or frontal sinuses
- T4b—Tumor involves any of the following: orbital apex, dura, brain, middle cranial fossa, cranial nerves, other than V2, nasopharynx or clivus

Maxillary sinus

- T1—Tumor limited to the maxillary sinus mucosa without bony destruction
- T2—Tumor causing bone destruction including erosion into the hard palate and/or middle nasal meatus, except extension to posterior maxillary wall and pterygoid plates
- T3—Tumor invades any of the following: bone of the posterior wall of the maxillary sinus, subcutaneous tissues, floor or medial wall of the orbit, pterygoid fossa, ethmoid sinuses
- T4a—Tumor invades anterior orbital contents, skin of cheek, pterygoid plates, infratemporal fossa, cribriform plate, sphenoid or frontal sinuses
- T4b—Tumor invades any of the following: orbital apex, dura, brain, middle cranial fossa, cranial nerves other than V2, nasopharynx or clivus

as definitive therapy. Postoperative radiation or chemoradiation is universally recommended for microscopically positive margins and perineural spread. Neoadjuvant chemotherapy (cisplatin or 5-FU) or chemoradiation may be entertained for large "unresectable" lesions, which may be subsequently resected if significant tumor response is obtained. Metastasis mandates adjuvant chemoradiation, and possibly neck dissection.

The overall survival of maxillary sinus SCC is about 25% T1 tumors are more favorable, and are about 55%.[3] Promising case series of endoscopic resection of SCC have been successfully reported; however, there is insufficient data to recommend endoscopic or endoscopic-assisted surgery over open approaches.[16] Pooled data suggest comparable overall disease-free survival at four years, but there is a selection bias for T1 and T2 tumors to undergo endoscopic treatment.[17] Known prognostic factors for sinonasal SCC include: T stage, N stage, positive margin status, dural or orbital involvement, pterygopalatine and infratemporal spread, skin invasion, unfavorable tumor histology and perineural spread. Ohngren's line, drawn from the medial canthus through the mandibular angle, is a traditional way to describe many of these factors. Tumors extending superiorly and laterally to this line portend a worse prognosis, generally due to disease spread outside of the sinus. The most common cause of treatment failure is local recurrence, which portends an extremely poor prognosis.

Salivary Gland Tumors

Adenocarcinoma

Sinonasal adenocarcinoma accounts for up to 10% of all primary malignant tumors of the nasal cavity and paranasal sinuses, making it the second most common malignancy after SCC. These tumors are associated with a better prognosis than SCC. Sinonasal adenocarcinoma usually presents as a locally aggressive neoplasm, predominating in males aged 40–70 years. The nasal cavity, the maxillary sinus and the ethmoid sinus are the most common sites of origin. Like SCCA, the primary symptoms can range from nasal obstruction, epistaxis and pain to a facial mass with deformation and/or proptosis, depending on the size and tumor location. Two main categories of adenocarcinoma are recognized: (1) intestinal-type adenocarcinoma (ITAC) and (2) Nonintestinal-type adenocarcinoma (non ITAC), which can be further subdivided into low-grade and high-grade.

Intestinal-type adenocarcinoma shares histopathologic features with gastroenterologic adenocarcinomas. Therefore, metastatic adenocarcinomas from the gastrointestinal tract must be excluded by appropriate imaging or endoscopic studies. These tumors occur primarily in men aged 55–60 years. The tumors are common in workers in the hardwood and shoe industries. Exposure to wood dust increases the risk of adenocarcinoma by 900–1000x.[18,19] The time between the first occupational exposure to wood dust and the development of adenocarcinoma of the sinonasal tract averages 40 years.[20] Occupational nasal and paranasal adenocarcinomas most commonly arise in the ethmoid sinus. In contrast, sporadic adenocarcinoma usually affects women and is found in the maxillary sinus.[21] Adenocarcinomas associated with wood dust exposure have a better prognosis than sporadic cases. Immunohistochemical staining for carcinoembryonic antigen (CEA) has been proposed as a method of differentiating metastatic colonic adenocarcinomas from primary ITAC. Tumors that stain strongly positive favor metastatic disease.[22]

Salivary gland adenocarcinoma (non ITAC) has a variety of histologic patterns. Papillary adenocarcinoma is composed of complex papillary fronds, lined by columnar or pseduostratified cells. The cytoplasm is eosinophilic containing mucin. In general, the papillary-tubular types show a better prognosis than intestinal-type adenocarcinoma.[21] Sinonasal non ITAC occurs predominantly in adults, but have been identified over a wide age range 9–80 years. These well-differentiated tumors with predominantly papillary and tubular structures are associated with a better prognosis (5-year survival: 80%) than their poorly differentiated counterparts (5-year survival: 40%). The high-grade, non ITAC are invasive tumors with a predominantly solid growth pattern. These tumors are characterized by marked cellular pleomorphism, high mitotic activity and areas of necrosis.

Treatment is surgical resection and postoperative radiotherapy. Endoscopic approaches have been used for select tumors with good results.[23] High grade adenocarcinoma is locally aggressive with frequent local recurrences in up to 53% of cases. Metastasis to regional lymph nodes occurs infrequently in 8% of cases. Elective neck dissections are not warranted. Distant metastases are also rare. When death occurs, it usually results from uncontrolled local disease or cranial nerve extension.

Adenoid Cystic Carcinoma

Adenoid cystic carcinoma (ACC) is of salivary gland origin and is the second most common salivary gland tumor of the nasal cavity and paranasal sinuses after adenocarcinoma.[24-26] Histologic types include solid, tubular, and cribriform subtypes. ACC is characterized by having an indolent but aggressive clinical course, the presence of early perineural invasion, frequent local recurrence, and a high rate of delayed distant metastasis. The maxillary sinus is the most common site for ACC in the sinuses.[24,25] Presenting symptoms are usually vague and nonspecific, and include nasal obstruction, facial pain and epistaxis, which can delay diagnosis. Clinicians should be aware of more concerning symptoms including V2 numbness, epiphora and diplopia which can be suggestive of a more aggressive process and perineural invasion. ACC is different from SCCs of the head and neck in that cervical lymph node metastases are uncommon.

Surgical resection with postoperative adjuvant radiation therapy is considered to be the optimal therapeutic regimen. The goal is complete tumor resection with negative margins. Perineural involvement may be difficult to clear. However, despite aggressive surgery, there is a high rate of local recurrences and distant metastasis. Thus, the surgeon must balance the value of radical surgery when planning treatment. Lupinnetti et al[25] found that surgery with postoperative radiation provided the best overall and disease—specific survival compared with other treatment modalities. Typically intensity—modulated radiation therapy (IMRT) or neutron-based radiotherapy is given for ACC; however, a recent study from Massachusetts General Hospital using high-dose proton beam radiation showed encouraging short and long-term (5 year 93%, 8 year 82%) local control rates in a group of 23 patients with advanced skull base ACC.[27] Chemotherapy is generally reserved for palliative treatment of metastatic disease or locoregional recurrence for which further surgery or radiation is not possible.

Despite aggressive surgery and postoperative radiotherapy, about 70% of patients will experience a tumor recurrence. Due to the indolent nature of this tumor, long-term follow-up is necessary to convey the outcome of ACC. Patients may present with local recurrence or hematogenous distant metastases more than 10 years after initial treatment. Although radiation therapy is known to decrease local recurrence, its contribution to overall survival is unclear, and it does not appear to affect the rate of distant metastasis. Wiseman et al[26] found that patients who had surgery alone had a higher rate of local recurrence than did those in the surgery plus radiation group; however, this was not statistically significant. The surgery and radiation group also had a higher 10-year survival rate (67 vs 57%; p = 0.49), but this was also not statistically significant.

ESTHESIONEUROBLASTOMA

Esthesioneuroblastoma (ENB) (also known as olfactory neuroblastoma), a malignant neuroendocrine tumor, is one of the many "small blue cell tumors" that may occur in the sinonasal tract. There is a bimodal age distribution (second and third decades and sixth and seventh decades) and slight male predilection. There are no known etiologic factors. Delayed presentation is the norm, as the initial presenting symptoms are generally overlooked (Fig. 18.2). ENB presents similarly to other sinonasal tumors, although epistaxis and hyposmia may be more common. Intracranial extension rarely causes symptoms, except in the most extreme of cases. The tumor is thought to arise from the olfactory basal reserve cell in the nasal roof, and may present due to either intranasal or intracranial growth. Bilateral nasal cavity involvement is frequent, as the superior septum is often

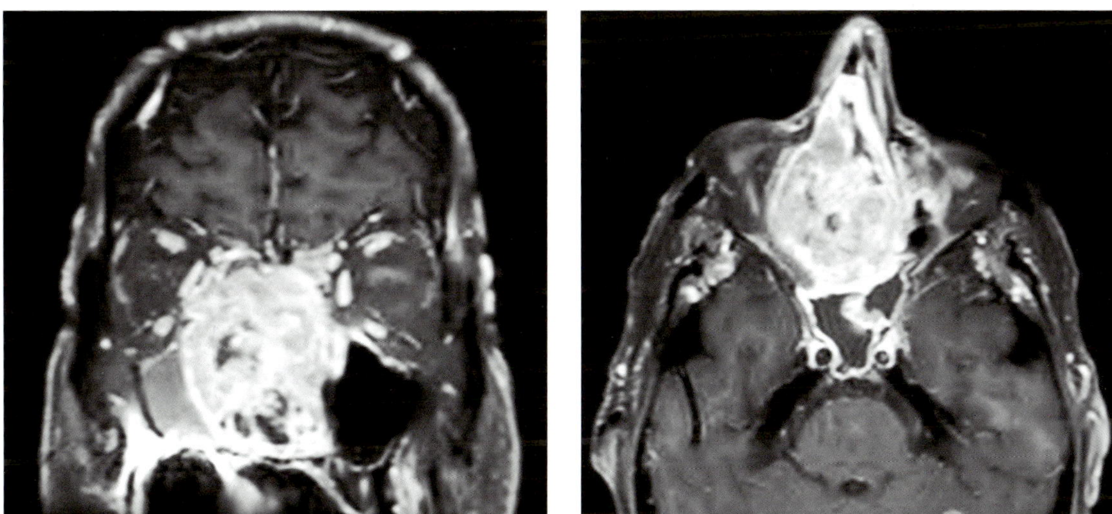

Fig. 18.2: Axial and coronal postcontrast T1-weighted MRI scan. Mild nasal symptoms of obstruction and congestion were ignored for several years, until the patient finally presented with ear fullness.

involved early in the process. The tumor presents as a polypoid mass in the superior nasal vault that is often quite friable and bleeds easily with manipulation. The tumor frequently encroaches upon the orbital periosteum, but it is uncommon for frank orbital invasion to occur.

CT and MRI are mandatory in the initial workup to extent of skull base erosion and degree of local tumor extension. Site of the tumor may suggest ENB, but there are no particular defining characteristics radiologically. Coronal CT scans are helpful to examine the presence and degree of skull base erosion. Occasionally, the tumor will be entirely intranasal and the bony skull base will appear intact. The tumor will enhance with contrast, but MRI assessment of orbital and dural invasion is not entirely reliable. In a review of 15 series, cervical metastasis on presentation occurred in 23.4%, with increasing frequency based on tumor stage.[28] CT or ultrasound of the neck, or PET scan, should be included in the initial metastatic workup. It is highly unusual to have distant metastatic spread on initial presentation, but treatment may fail with distant metastases, usually skeletal or pulmonary.

Histologically, rosette or pseudorosette formation is the hallmark, where clusters of cells palisade around blood vessels. When the tumor is not as well-differentiated, immunohistochemical markers are necessary to distinguish this tumor from other "small, blue-cell" tumors such as lymphoma, melanoma, SNUC, Ewing's sarcoma and primitive neuroectodermal tumors. ENB will stain positive for neuron-specific enolase, chromogranin, synaptophysin and S-100. The Hyams grading system is based on preservation of lobular architecture, mitotic activity, nuclear polymorphism, fibrillary matrix, necrosis and presence of rosettes.[29] This grading system may carry some prognostic value.[30]

The modified Kadish staging system is the most frequently used clinical staging tool, although several others have been proposed (Table 18.3).[31] This type of staging system is beneficial to potentially categorize tumors according to size and spread, but is not entirely prognostic. Spread into adjacent sinuses, or even a small degree of spread intracranially, may no longer portend a poor prognosis, as these tumors can reliably be resected with negative margins.

Table 18.3 Modified Kadish staging for esthesioneuroblastoma

A	Nasal cavity
B	Nasal cavity + paranasal sinus involvement
C	Involvement of orbit, skull base and/or intracranial cavity
D	Metastatic spread

Craniofacial resection with radiation therapy is considered the standard treatment for ENB.[32] Craniofacial resection can be performed from an open approach, endoscopically, or combined. A number of publications have described small series of endoscopically resected ENB patients with excellent early outcomes; longer follow-up and larger cohorts are needed, however.[33-36] Regardless of the approach, the oncologic principles are the same. In the setting of an entirely intranasal tumor, it is controversial whether or not the skull base needs to be removed and the dura and olfactory bulb needs to be biopsied. There are anecdotal reports of intranasal tumors with negative dural biopsies and tumor presence within the olfactory bulb. Radiation and possibly concurrent chemoradiation should be part of the management of this disease. Generally, postoperative radiation is preferred. However, if the tumor is extremely large or considered "unresectable", neoadjuvant chemotherapy or chemoradiation may be administered initially. Neoadjuvant chemotherapy has been shown to significantly reduce tumor burden in two-thirds of patients, and response to chemotherapy is a predictor of long-term survival.[37,38]

Prognosis is generally good with craniofacial resection and postoperative radiotherapy, with 5-year survival ranging 52–89%.[39-41] Brain or orbit involvement, cervical or CNS metastasis and distant metastasis are poor prognostic factors. Local recurrence is common (10–30%), as is regional (15–20%), and delayed distant metastasis (8%).[42]

Local recurrence may be treated with revision surgery or stereotactic radiosurgery. Long-term follow-up is required.

SINONASAL UNDIFFERENTIATED CARCINOMA

Sinonasal undifferentiated carcinoma (SNUC) is an aggressive malignancy on the spectrum of neuroendocrine carcinoma which include ENB and small cell neuroendocrine carcinoma (SNEC). Presentation and workup is similar to other sinonasal malignancies, although SNUC is usually more advanced when discovered. Regional metastasis is common, but distant metastasis or CSF seeding is rare. Pathologically, SNUC is a small, round, blue-cell tumor with an undifferentiated appearance, and may be difficult to diagnose. Immunohistochemical staining may be helpful to exclude certain diagnoses, but the cytologic features used to distinguish between SNUC, SNEC and undifferentiated nasopharyngeal carcinomas are subtle. The management of SNUC is often debated, but relies upon both surgery and radiation. It is unclear whether adjuvant chemotherapy is of any benefit. Our standard treatment is surgery followed by postoperative radiation therapy (which includes the neck) and concomitant single-agent cisplatin chemotherapy, similar to the University of Florida protocol.[43] Initial treatment with concurrent multidrug chemotherapy and radiation, followed by surgery, has shown similar success rates at the University of Virginia. This may be a viable alternative, especially for advanced disease.[44] Nearly one-third of patients present with unresectable disease, and are offered initial radiation therapy. Overall 5-year survival is about 50%.

Sinonasal Melanoma

Epidemiology and Presentation

Primary mucosal malignant melanoma of the nasal cavity, paranasal sinuses and nasopharynx is rare, accounting for between 0.3% and 2% of all malignant melanomas and about 4% of head and neck melanomas. Overall, melanomas account for 3.5–7% of all sinonasal neoplasms.[45,46] Melanoma is a malignancy of ectodermal origin, arising from melanocytes which are found in respiratory mucosa. The most frequent sites of noncutaneous melanoma are the eye (5.3%), melanoma of unknown origin (2.2%) and then mucosal melanoma. Microscopically, sinonasal melanoma (SNMM) is another "small blue cell tumor" with similarities to lymphoma, rhabdomyosarcoma, plasmacytoma, olfactory neuroblastoma and poorly differentiated carcinoma. The most common histological subtypes of sinonasal melanoma include spindle cell, epithelioid and pleomorphic. Immunohistochemical analysis is crucial to differentiated sinonasal melanoma from other small, round blue cell tumors. In one study of 115 cases of SNMM from the Armed Forces Institute of Pathology, nearly all stained with vimentin (97.1%), S-100 protein (91%), HMB-45 (75.9%), Tyrosinase (77.7%) and Melan A (64.8%).[47] Representative histology is illustrated in Figures 18.3A to F.

The mean age of presentation of sinonasal melanoma is 65 years, with a range of 50–80 years. There is a slight male predominance. Risk factors for mucosal melanoma are unknown, although there are links to a variety of occupational exposures, including formaldehyde. Within the nasal cavity, the lateral nasal wall and the inferior turbinate are the most common sites. Within the sinuses, the most common site of origin is the maxillary sinus, followed by the ethmoid and sphenoid sinuses. However, most sinonasal melanomas present with advance disease, making it difficult to ascertain the exact origin. Ganly et al reported that 50% of patients with skull base melanomas had tumors infiltrating the cribriform plate, 34% had periorbital invasion and 17% had dural invasion.[48]

Staging

In contrast to cutaneous melanomas, there is not a widely accepted classification and staging system and evidence-based treatment concept specifically focused on SNMM. Ballantyne described

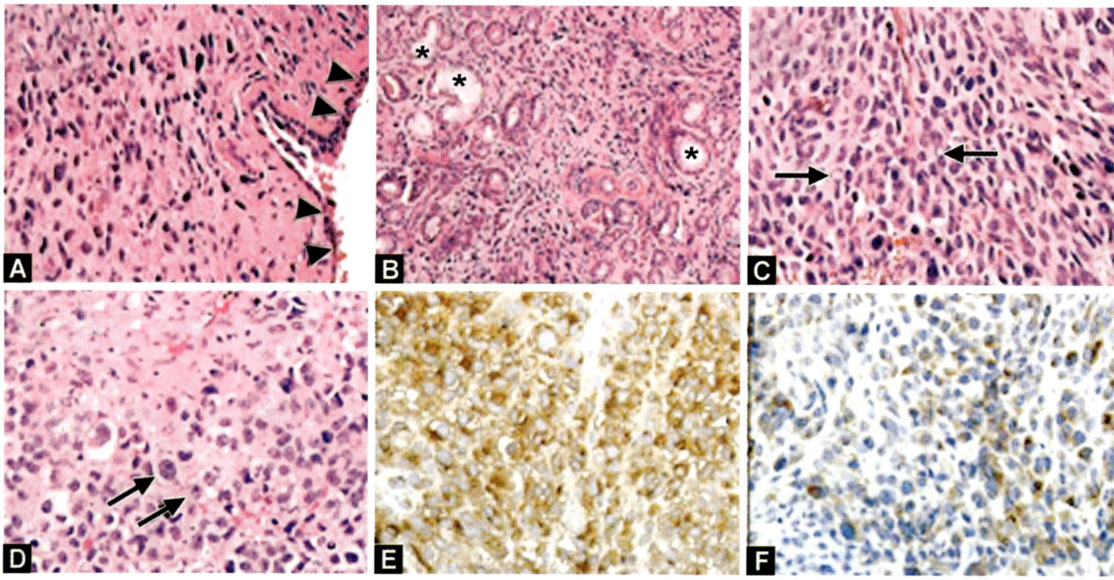

Figs 18.3A to F: Mucosal malignant melanoma. (A) Partially denuded respiratory epithelium (arrowheads) with underlying malignant spindle cells exhibiting marked cytologic atypia [H and E stain; original magnification, 400X]; (B) These cells infiltrate deep into the submucosa and surround the seromucous glands (asterisks) [H and E stain; original magnification, 200X]; (C) Scattered malignant cells demonstrate intranuclear inclusions (arrows) [H and E stain; original magnification, 400X]; (D) In some areas, the malignant cells appear epithelioid with prominent macronucleoli (arrows); (E) HMB45; (F) MART1 immunostains exhibit strong, diffuse, cytoplasmic positivity within malignant cells [original magnification, 400X].

a simplified staging system for head and neck mucosal melanomas in 1970, which continues to be the most widely utilized.[49] This system classifies tumors in the following three stages: stage I for localized lesions; stage II for cervical lymph node metastasis and stage III for distant metastasis. The advantages of this system are its simplicity and the fact that it can be used for oral and mucosal primaries. Unfortunately, since the vast majority of patients present with local disease only (stage I), the prognostic value of this staging system is relatively limited, and it appears that the current AJCC sinonasal staging system to be useful.[50,51]

Specific clinical and histological features have been suggested to be of prognostic significance. Thompson et al found that age over 60 years, those who developed recurrences, presented with obstructive symptoms, had tumors located in the nasopharynx, an undifferentiated histology, and greater than 10 mitotic figures per 10 HPFs were each more likely to experience a worse clinical outcome.[47] SNMM also has a lower frequency of lymph node metastasis than oral cavity melanoma. Roth found that tumor size did not correlate with survival rate, and that distant metastasis occurred in both small and large sinonasal melanomas.[45] Melanoma of the sinonasal mucosa often demonstrates deep invasion, necrosis and vascular invasion. These characteristics have been found to be predictors of reduced survival. Perineural invasion, while occurring more frequently in ACC and SCC, can also occur with sinonasal melanoma.

Treatment

The standard treatment of sinonasal melanoma continues to be surgical. There is also growing evidence to support an improvement in locoregional control with postoperative adjuvant radiation. However, there is no evidence of improved overall survival with adjuvant radiotherapy.[51] Data from the treatment of cutaneous melanoma suggests that therapy, like chemotherapy and/or immunotherapy, can be considered for patients with distant metastasis. Since neck lymph nodes are rarely encountered in cases of sinonasal melanoma, neck dissection should be reserved for those with clinically or radiologically positive neck disease.

Outcomes

The 5-year overall survival ranges from 20% to 35% among different series. Recently, Lund et al. reported a 28% and 20% 5-year and 10-year overall survival rate respectively, with a 21-month median survival.[52] A large cohort study by AFIP showed that there was no statistical difference in survival between patients managed by surgery alone, surgery with chemotherapy, surgery with radiotherapy, or surgery with combined therapy. After a mean follow-up of almost 14 years, 35% of the patients in the study were alive or died without evidence of disease. Ganly et al. demonstrated a threefold increase in overall and disease-free survival following adjuvant conventional radiation therapy.[48] The risk of recurrence was 4x higher in patients not receiving radiotherapy. Despite aggressive treatment, 37% of patients will ultimately fail at distant sites, more than 2/3 of whom will also develop local or regional disease. The most common sites of distant metastases are the lung and brain (33% and 14% respectively). The medial survival period from the time of detection of distant metastases to death is 7.1 months.[50]

Sarcoma

Sarcomas are rare and diverse malignancies, despite their common mesenchymal origin. Head and neck sarcomas represent less than 1% of all head and neck malignancies. However, 14–30% of sarcomas occur in the paranasal sinuses.[53-55] Presentation and diagnosis are similar to other sinonasal tumors. Tissue diagnosis generally requires at least a core biopsy, as fine needle aspirate may not be sufficient to make the diagnosis. Imaging modalities used are similar to other sinonasal tumors, as well. Particular attention is paid to local tumor extension and assessment of metastatic disease.

Chondrosarcomas

They are divided into three grades (well-, intermediate and poorly differentiated) based on pathologic features of cellularity, mitotic activity, nuclear size and atypia. Classic chondrosarcoma of the head and neck affects the maxilla, nasal septum, clivus or spheno-petrous junction. Locally aggressive and destructive behavior is typical. A rare subtype, e.g. mesenchymal chondrosarcoma, has the potential for both locally aggressive behavior and metastasis. Complete surgical excision is the primary management of this disease. Incompletely excised tumors, or intermediate- and high-grade tumors, require postoperative radiation therapy. Chondrosarcoma is known as a relatively radioresistant tumor, as doses of greater than 60 Gy are needed for local control. If tumor is at the skull base, significant side-effects result from such doses. Proton beam therapy has been successful in these scenarios.[56] Overall 5-year survival for chondrosarcoma is 56–87%, depending on grade, and is poorer with the mesenchymal subtype.[57]

Osteosarcoma

It is characterized by the production of osteoid. Osteosarcoma of the paranasal sinuses is different from that of long bones in that the affected population is 10–15 years older, with mean age ranges between 26 and 40 years.[58] Radiation exposure, bone dysplasias, rare genetic syndromes and genetic mutations (retinoblastoma gene) are predisposing factors (Fig. 18.4). A number of histologic variants exist, but do not affect prognosis. Treatment includes surgical excision followed by adjuvant chemotherapy for elimination of micrometastatic disease. In a multi-institutional study, patients with osteosarcoma of the extremities treated surgically followed by adjuvant chemotherapy had a statistically higher 6- year event free survival (61% vs 11%) than those not receiving chemotherapy.[59] However, chemotherapy has not been shown to

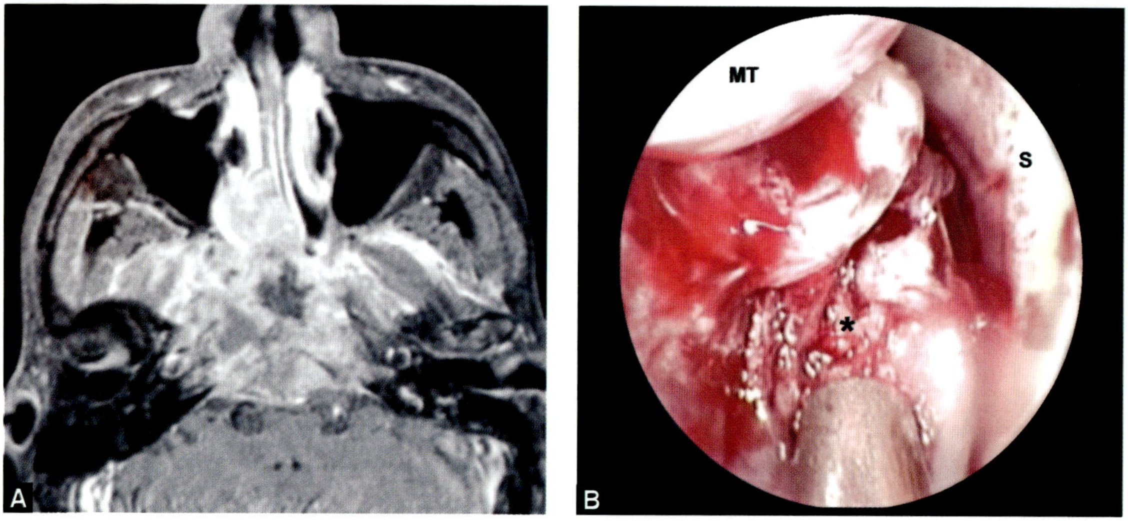

Figs 18.4A and B: Postcontrast coronal MRI scan (A) and endoscopic photograph during biopsy (B) of a patient who underwent radiation therapy for nasopharyngeal carcinoma nearly 10 years prior to presentation with headache, nasal obstruction and 6th nerve palsy. He was found to have a locally aggressive osteosarcoma.

improve survival in head and neck osteosarcoma without obvious metastatic disease. Radiation therapy is recommended when margins are close or cannot be obtained. Overall 5 and 10-year survival of head and neck osteosarcoma is 63% and 55% respectively.[60]

Hemangiopericytoma

This is a tumor derived from pericytes surrounding capillaries (pericytes of Zimmerman). These cells are thought to be immature smooth muscle cells of mesenchymal origin, and tumors can have an aggressive clinical course. Aggressive surgery and postoperative radiation are crucial to achieving local control. 5-year local control was 84% with gross total resection versus 38% for subtotal resections.[61] Increased tumor volume (> 25 ml) is associated with lower control rates.[62] With postoperative radiation, 5-year overall survival was 100%, and 10-year overall survival was 64%.[63]

Summary

Surgical management of sarcomas requires wide excision; however, this is frequently not possible at the skull base given the abundance of critical neurovascular structures. Adjuvant radiation is essential for all but the smallest low-grade tumors, as adequate margins are rarely obtained secondary to tumor location. Local control of head and neck sarcomas increases from 52% with surgery alone to 90% with the addition of postoperative radiation.[64] We prefer to use radiation postoperatively in these patients; however, some centers advocate preoperative radiation. Proton beam radiation may be of use at the skull base, as the favorable physical properties of decreased scatter and rapid dose drop-off allow maximal tumoricidal effect with decreased collateral damage. Currently, only a few centers have access to this type of therapy. The efficacy of chemotherapy for varying sarcomas has been established through the management of metastatic disease. Anthracyclines, ifosfamide and combination chemotherapy may be appropriate in certain situations. Particular histologic subtypes appear to be more responsive to certain agents. No known chemotherapeutic regimen has demonstrated value in the management of chondrosarcoma, stressing the need for surgery and radiation with this tumor. Local recurrence is the main concern, ranging from 22% in low-grade histologic lesions to 48% in high-grade tumors.

Overall 5-year survival ranges from 45% to 68% in general for skull base sarcoma.[53-55] Low-grade tumors, such as well-differentiated chondrosarcoma, carry a much better prognosis.

NASOPHARYNGEAL CARCINOMA

Nasopharyngeal carcinoma (NPC) is a tumor arising from the epithelial cells that cover the surface of the nasopharynx. Its incidence is relatively high in Southeast Asia, North Africa and part of the Mediterranean basin where about 80 cases per 100,000 of population are reported. A clear etiology for nasopharyngeal carcinoma is still lacking. In general, NPC is thought to be the result of both genetic susceptibility and environmental factors such as carcinogens and infection with Epstein-Barr virus (EBV). Possible environmental or cultural factors that may be associated with NPC include the ingestion of Cantonese-style salted fish and preserved foods that contain carcinogenic nitrosamines, especially during childhood.[65] The WHO recognizes three different histologic subtypes: (1) SCCA; (2) nonkeratinizing carcinoma and (3) undifferentiated carcinoma.[66] The NPC is observed predominantly in males, with a male-to-female ratio of 3:1.[65,67] The AJCC staging for NPC is shown in Table 18.4.

Nasopharyngeal carcinoma is highly radiosensitive, and radiotherapy is the mainstay treatment, achieving a 5-year overall survival of 90% and 84% for early stage disease. However, the vast majority of patients with NPC presents with advanced disease. The timing and addition of chemotherapy in advanced NPC is controversial, and review of the literature is complicated by different chemotherapy regimens, radiation types and doses, and overall heterogeneity of clinical trials.[67,68] The addition of chemotherapy appears to be most beneficial when given concurrently with radiotherapy. Surgery plays relatively a limited role in the initial management of NPC; however, it can be an important treatment option for patients who experience recurrence after definitive radiation or chemoradiation therapy. Isolated recurrence in the cervical lymph nodes without evidence of distant metastasis or local disease can be addressed with surgery. Treatment of the primary site is usually an option when the residual or recurrent tumor is of limited size and localized in the nasopharynx.

Table 18.4 Staging for nasopharyngeal carcinoma

Primary tumor (T)

- T1—Tumor confined to the nasopharynx
- T2—Tumor extends to soft tissues:
  - T2a—Tumor extends to the oropharynx and/or nasal cavity without parapharyngeal extension*
  - T2b—Any tumor with parapharyngeal extension*
- T3—Tumor invades bony structures and/or paranasal sinuses
- T4—Tumor with intracranial extension and/or involvement of cranial nerves, infratemporal fossa, hypopharynx, orbit or masticator space

Regional lymph nodes (N)

NX—Regional lymph nodes cannot be assessed
N0—No regional lymph node metastasis
N1—Unilateral metastasis in lymph node(s), not more than 6 cm in greatest dimension, above the supraclavicular fossa
N2—Bilateral metastasis in lymph node(s), not more than 6 cm in greatest dimension, above the supraclavicular fossa
N3—Metastasis in a lymph node(s) larger than 6 cm and/or to supraclavicular fossa:
N3a—Larger than 6 cm
N3b—Extension to the supraclavicular fossa

* Parapharyngeal extension denotes posterolateral infiltration of tumor beyond the pharyngobasilar fascia

The prognostic factors for patients with NPC include tumor stage (i.e. skull base invasion, cranial nerve involvement, parapharyngeal infiltration), histologic subtype, age and the sex of the patient, and the type and technique of radiotherapy. Survival rates are generally better in females than in males.

The 5-year overall survival rate is 85–95% for stage I NPC and 70–80% for stage II NPC treated with radiation alone. For stages III and IV NPC treated with radiation alone, the 5-year overall survival rate ranges from 24% to 80%, with better results generally occurring in patients from Southeast Asia.[65-69] Current research is exploring the use of epidermal growth factor receptor monoclonal antibodies and immunotherapy to EBV antigens in the treatment of NPC.

Treatment of local recurrences of NPC is usually managed with a second course of external radiotherapy, usually at a higher dose than the initial course. However, reirradiation can have significant side-effects. Other options for recurrent NPC include brachytherapy or salvage surgery. Endoscopic approaches are most applicable when the tumor is small and localized to the posterior or superior wall of the nasopharynx, but not extending to the fossa of Rosenmüller. Fee et al[70] described approaching the nasopharynx via a transpalatal, transmaxillary and transcervical approach. Wei et al[71] first described the anterolateral approach to the nasopharynx in 1991. This approach exposes the entire nasopharynx and the paranasopharyngeal space to allow an oncological surgical resection of the nasopharynx and Eustachian tube *en bloc* while identifying and preserving the internal carotid artery.

Lymphoma/Plasmacytoma

Non-Hodgkin's lymphoma (NHL) represents 5% of head and neck malignancies, and may involve the sinonasal tract. NHL is more common in the immunosuppressed, those with known systemic disease, and the Asian population. It is more common in the elderly male demographic, but can present in females and children. Endoscopically, lymphoma typically appears as a submucosal mass without overlying ulceration. Pathologically, most are diffused large cell B-lymphomas, although nearly any subtype can be found. Sclerotic or osteoblastic features may be seen on CT scan. On MRI, lesions are isointense on T1, variable on T2 and heterogeneously enhance with gadolinium. Disease stage may be more prognostic than histologic subtype; staging is performed according to the Ann Arbor system (Table 18.5). The International Pronostic Index (IPI) is another clinical tool used to predict the prognosis of patients with aggressive NHL. (Table 18.6) The IPI predicts the risk of disease recurrence and overall survival by taking into

Table 18.5 Ann Arbor staging system

- Stage 1—Limited to one lymph node group above or below the diaphragm or extranodal disease that has not spread to other organs or lymph nodes
- Stage 2—Limited to two lymph node groups on the same side of the diaphragm or limited to one extranodal organ and has spread to one or more lymph node groups on the same side of the diaphragm
- Stage 3—NHL is in two lymph node groups, with/without partial involvement of an extranodal organ or site above and below the diaphragm
- Stage 4—NHL is extensive in one organ or site, with/without NHL in distant lymph nodes

Additional designations

- A—Absent (no) symptoms
- B—Presence of any of the following B symptoms: fever, night sweats, weight loss of >10% within the last 6 months, pruritis
- E—Involvement of a single extranodal site that directly adjoins or is next to the known nodal group
- X—Presence of "bulky" disease, that is, a nodal mass whose greatest dimension is > 10 cm in size, and/or a widening of the mediastinum by more than one-third

Table 18.6 International prognostic index for non-Hodgkin's lymphoma

- Age over 60 years
- Late-stage disease (stages 3 and 4)
- More than one extranodal site
- High LDH
- Poor general health

International prognostic index scoring (score 1 point for each)

Risk	*IPI score*	*Complete response rate (%)*	*Relapse-free 5-year survival (%)*	*Overall 5-year survival (%)*
Low	0–1	87	70	73
Low/intermediate	2	67	50	51
High/intermediate	3	55	49	43
High	>4	44	40	26

account factors such as age, stage of disease, general health, number of extranodal sites, and the presence of elevated lactate dehydrogenase. The role of surgery in lymphoma is for diagnosis. Combination chemotherapy and radiation is typically used for therapy, although in some cases radiation alone may suffice. Concurrent chemotherapy has been shown to decrease the rates of local and distant recurrence. T-cell lymphomas, including angiocentric lymphoma, are more commonly found in Asian populations. Five-year overall survival for all types is 50%, but varies based on subtype and stage.[72]

Plasma cell neoplasms are classified as either multiple myeloma or plasmacytoma. Extramedullary plasmacytomas arise from the plasma cells in the submucosa of the aerodigestive tract. The nasal cavity and sinuses are common sites for these rare tumors. They present as a solitary sinonasal lesion, with a 4:1 male:female preponderance, and usually in the fifth to sixth decade.[73] Nonspecific sinonasal symptoms are typically found on presentation. CT often shows local bone destruction. Pathologic diagnosis requires a deep biopsy, as the tumor is submucosal and the overlying thickened mucosa will show chronic inflammation only.[74] Workup should include serum or urine protein electrophoresis, complete blood count (CBC), chemistry panel, bone marrow biopsy and possibly plain film X-rays of the skull and extremities. Treatment consists of surgery if the lesion can be completed resected; otherwise, radiation or a combination of the two modalities are used for larger tumors. Overall 10-year disease specific survival is 50–89%.[75] In a large review, 22% of patients experienced recurrence after treatment, and 15% of patients went on to develop multiple myeloma.[74] Chemotherapy may be considered for multifocal disease, which carries a poor prognosis. Lifelong surveillance is mandatory.

Metastasis

Metastasis must be considered in the differential diagnosis of sinonasal masses. While rare, metastases from tumors of the kidney, lung, thyroid and breast have been reported in the literature.[76] Other unusual primary sites for metastatic sinus tumors include the uterus, colon and prostate.[77-78] In a review of the available literature, Prescher and Brors[76] found that the maxillary sinus was the most commonly affected site of metastasis, followed by the sphenoid, ethmoid and frontal sinus. Symptoms and imaging results are not specific and usually are similar to primary neoplasms of the affected region. There is little literature on the frequency of metastasis to the paranasal sinuses. In a study looking at skull base metastasis, Laigle-Donadey et al[79] found that the overall median survival with skull base metastasis is 31 months. Metastatic breast cancer carried the best prognosis (60 months), while lung and colon cancers had the worst (2.5 months and 1.5 months respectively). In general, the metastases are treated with radiotherapy, but in some cases, a small or single focus of metastatic disease in the sinuses can be removed at the time of biopsy to improve symptoms or quality of life.

CONCLUSION

Despite advances of imaging and endoscopy, sinonasal malignancies remain a challenge to diagnose and treat. Advanced tumors are usually associated with poor prognosis, often due to late diagnosis, difficult surgical anatomy limiting complete tumor removal and a lack of large scale studies evaluating adjuvant therapies due to the rarity of these tumors. Treatment of paranasal sinus malignancies should therefore be tailored to the individual tumors, taking into consideration the nature of the tumor including its size and extent, the patient's comorbidities, and the available literature on the surgical and non-surgical treatment modalities.

REFERENCES

1. Wellman BJ, Traynelis BC, McCulloch TM, et al. Midline anterior craniofacial approach for malignancy: results of en bloc versus piecemeal resections. Skull Base Surgery. 1999;9(1):41-6.
2. Har-El G, Casiano RR. Endoscopic management of anterior skull base tumors. Otolaryngol Clin N Am. 2005;38(1):133-44.
3. Bhattacharyya N. Factors predicting survival for cancer of the ethmoid sinus. Am J Rhinol. 2002; 16(5):281-6.
4. Bogaerts S, Vander P, Nuyts S, et al. Results of endoscopic resection followed by radiotherapy for primarily diagnoses adenocarcinomas of the paranasal sinuses. Head and Neck. 2008;30(6):728-36.
5. Cantu G, Solero CL, Miceli R, et al. Which classification for ethmoid malignant tumors involving the anterior skull base? Head and Neck. 2005;27(3):224-31.
6. Lee CH, Hur DG, Roh HJ, et al. Survival rates of sinonasal squamous cell carcinoma with the new AJCC staging system. Arch Otololaryngol Head Neck Surg. 2007;133(2):131-4.
7. Magnani C, Ciambelloti E, Salvi U, et al. The incidence of tumors of the nasal cavity and the paranasal sinuses in the district of Biella, 1970-1986. Acta Otorhinolaryngologica Italica. 1989;9(5):511-9.
8. McKay SP, Shibuya TY, Armstrong WB, et al. Cell carcinoma of the paranasal sinuses and skull base. Am J Otolaryngol. 2007;28(5):294-301.
9. Pedersen E, Hogetveit AC, Andersen A. Cancer of respiratory organs among workers at a nickel refinery in Norway. Intl J Cancer. 1973;12(1):32-41.
10. Jackson RT, Fitz-Hugh GS, Constable WC. Malignant neoplasms of the nasal cavities and paranasal sinuses: a retrospective study. Laryngoscope. 1977;87(5 Pt 1):726-36.
11. von Buchwald C, Bradley PJ. Risks of malignancy in inverted papilloma of the nose and paranasal sinuses. Curr Op Otolaryngol Head Neck Surgery. 2007;15(2):95-8.
12. Cantu G, Bimbi G, Micelli R, et al. Lymph node metastasis in malignant tumors of the paranasal sinuses: prognostic value and treatment. Arch Oto HNS. 2008;134(2):173-9.
13. Yousem DM. Imaging in sinus disease. In: Kennedy DW, Bolger WE, Zinreich SJ, (Eds). Diseases of the Sinuses: Diagnosis and Management. London: BC Decker; 2001. pp. 129-48.
14. Gil Z, Carson DL, Gupta A, et al. Patterns and incidence of neural invasion in patients with cancer of the paranasal sinuses. Arch Oto HNS. 2009;135(2):173-9.
15. Guntinas-Lichias O, Kreppel MP, Stuetzer H, et al. Single modality and multimodality treatment of nasal and paranasal sinuses cancer: a single institution experience of 229 patients. Eur J Surg Oncol. 2007;33:222-8.
16. Shipchandler TZ, Batra PS, Citardi MJ, et al. Outcomes for endoscopic resection of sinonasal squamous cell carcinoma. Laryngoscope. 2005;115(11):1983-7.
17. Lund VJ, Stammberger H, Nicolai P, et al. European position paper on endoscopic management of tumours of the nose, paranasal sinuses, and skull base. Rhinology Suppl. 2010;1(22):1-143.
18. Luce D, Gerin M, Leclerc A, et al. Sinonasal cancer and occupational exposure to formaldehyde and other substances. Int J Cancer. 1993;53(2):224-31.
19. Wills JH. Nasal carcinoma in woodworkers: a review. J Occup Med. 1982;24(7):526-30.
20. Nylander LA, Demart JM. Carcinogenic effects of wood dust: review and discussion. Am J Ind Med. 1993;24:619-47.
21. Abecasis J, Viana G, Pissarra C, et al. Adenocarcinomas of the nasal cavity and paranasal sinuses: a clinicopathological and immunohistochemical study of 14 cases. Histopathology. 2004;45(3):254-9.

22. McKinney CD, Mills SE, Franquemont DW. Sinonasal intestinal-type adenocarcinoma: Immunohistochemical profile and comparison with colonic adenocarcinoma. Mod Pathol. 1995;8:421-6.
23. Van Gerven L, Jorissen M, Nuyts S, et al. Long-term follow-up of 44 patients with adenocarcinoma of the nasal cavity and sinuses primarily treated with endoscopic resection followed by radiotherapy. Head Neck. 2010 Oct 21 [Epub ahead of print].
24. Rhee CS, Won TB, Lee CH, et al. Adenoid cystic carcinoma of the sinonasal tract: treatment results. Laryngoscope. 2006;116(6):982-6.
25. Lupinnetti AD, Roberts DB, Williams MD, et al. Sinonasal adenoid cystic carcinoma: the MD Anderson cancer center experience. Cancer. 2007;110(12):2726-31.
26. Wiseman SM, Popat SR, Rigual NR, et al. Adenoid cystic carcinoma of the paranasal sinuses or nasal cavity: a 40-year review of 35 cases. Ear Nose Throat J. 2002;81(8):510-4, 516-7.
27. Pommier P, Liebsch NJ, Deschler DG, et al. Proton beam radiation therapy for skull base adenoid cystic carcinoma. Arch Otolaryngol Head Neck Surg. 2006;132(11):1242-9.
28. Rinaldo A, Ferlito A, Shaha AR, et al. Esthesioneuroblastoma and cervical lymph node metastases: clinical and therapeutic implications. Acta Otolaryngol. 2002;122:125-221.
29. Hyams VJ. Olfactory neuroblastoma. In: Hyams V, Batsakis J, Michaels L (Eds). Tumours of the Upper Aerodigestive Tract and Ear. Washington DC: Armed Forces Institute of Pathology; 1988. pp. 240-8.
30. Miyamoto R, Gleich LL, Biddinger PW, et al. Esthesioneuroblastoma and sinonasal undifferentiated carcinoma: impact of histological grading and clinical staging on survival and prognosis. Laryngoscope. 2000;110(8):1262-5.
31. Kadish S, Goodman M, Wang C. Olfactory neuroblastoma: a clinical analysis of 17 cases. Cancer. 1976;37:1571-6.
32. Dulguerov P, Abdelkarim SA, Calcaterra TC. Esthesioneuroblastoma: a meta-analysis and review. Lancet Oncol. 2001;2:683-8.
33. Lund VJ. Endoscopic resection of malignant tumours of the nose and sinuses. Am J Rhinol. 2007;21:89-94.
34. Walch C, Stammberger H, Anderhuber W, et al. The minimally invasive approach to olfactory neuroblastoma: combined endoscopic and sterotactic treatment. Laryngoscope. 2000;110:635-40.
35. Casiano RR, Numa WA, Falquez AM. Endoscopic resection of esthesioneuroblastoma. Am J Rhinol. 2001;15:271-9.
36. Batra PS, Citardi MJ, Worley S, et al. Resection of anterior skull base tumors: comparison of combined traditional and endoscopic techniques. Am J Rhinol. 2005;19:521-8.
37. Polin RS, Sheehan JP, Chenelle AG, et al. The role of preoperative adjuvant treatment in the management of esthesioneuroblastoma: the University of Virginia experience. Neurosurgery. 1998;42(5):1029-37.
38. Sheehan JM, Sheehan JP, Jane JA Sr., et al. Chemotherapy for esthesioneuroblastoma. Neurosurg Clin N Am. 2000;11(4):693-701.
39. Dulgeurov P, Calcaterra T. Esthesioneuroblastoma: the UCLA experience 1970-1990. Laryngoscope. 1992;102(8):843-9.
40. Lund VJ, Howard D, Wei W, et al. Olfactory neuroblastoma. Laryngoscope. 2003;113:502-7.
41. Diaz E, Johnigan R, Pero C, et al. Olfactory neuroblastoma. The 22 year experience and one comprehensive cancer center. Head Neck. 2005;27:138-49.
42. Dulgeurov P, Allal AS, Calcaterra C. Esthesioneuroblastoma: a meta-analysis and review. Lancet Oncol. 2001;2(11):683-90.
43. Tanzler ED, Morris CG, Orlando CA, et al. Management of sinonasal undifferentiated carcinoma. Head Neck. 2008;30(5):595-9.
44. Musy PY, Reibel JF, Levine PA. Sinonasal undifferentiated carcinoma: the search for a better outcome. Laryngoscope. 2002;112:1450-5.
45. Roth TN, Gengler C, Huber GF, et al. Outcome of sinonasal melanoma: clinical experience and review of the literature. Head Neck. 2010;32(10):1385-92.
46. Conley JJ, Ackerman AB. Melanoma of the Head and Neck, 1st edition. New York: Georg Thieme Verlag; 1990. pp. 154-78.
47. Thompson LD, Wieneke JA, Miettinen M. Sinonasal tract and nasopharyngeal melanomas: a clinicopathologic study of 115 cases with a proposed staging system. Am J Surg Pathol. 2003;27:594-611.
48. Ganly I, Patel SG, Singh B, et al. Craniofacial resection for malignant melanoma of the skull base: report of an international collaborative study. Arch Otolaryngol Head Neck Surg. 2006;132(1):73-8.
49. Ballantyne AJ. Malignant melanoma of the skin of the head and neck. An analysis of 405 cases. Am J Surg. 1970;120:425-31.

50. Patel SG, Prasad ML, Escrig M, et al. Primary mucosal malignant melanoma of the head and neck. Head Neck. 2002;24:247-57.
51. Moreno MA, Roberts DB, Kupferman ME, et al. Mucosal melanoma of the nose and paranasal sinuses, a contemporary experience from the M. D. Anderson Cancer Center. Cancer. 2010;116(9):2215-23.
52. Lund VJ, Howard DJ, Harding L, et al. Management options and survival in malignant melanoma of the sinonasal mucosa. Laryngoscope. 1999;109(2 Pt 1):208-11.
53. Weber RS, Benjamin RS, Peters LJ, et al. Soft tissue sarcomas of the head and neck in adolescents and adults. Am J Surg. 1986;152:386-92.
54. Freedman AM, Reiman HM, Woods JE. Soft tissue sarcomas of the head and neck. Am J Surg. 1989;158:367-72.
55. Farhood AI, Hajdu SI, Shiu MH, et al. Soft tissue sarcomas of the head and neck in adults. Am J Surg. 1990;160:365-9.
56. Nguyen QN, Chang EL. Emerging role of proton beam radiation therapy for chordoma and chondrosarcoma of the skull base. Curr Oncology Reports. 2008;10(4):338-43.
57. Howard DJ, Lund VJ, Wei WI. Craniofacial resection for tumors of the nasal cavity and paranasal sinuses: a 17 year experience. Head Neck. 1998; 20(2):97-105.
58. Ha PK, Eisels DW, Frassica FJ, et al. Osteosarcoma of the head and neck: a review of the Johns Hopkins experience. Laryngoscope. 1999;109(6):964-9.
59. Link MP, Goorin AM, Horowitz M, et al. Adjuvant chemotherapy of high-grade osteosarcoma of the extremity. Updated results of the multi-institutional osteosarcoma study. Clin Ortho Rel Res. 1991; 270:8-14.
60. Guadagnolo BA, Zagars GK, Raymond K, et al. Osteosarcoma of the jaw/craniofacial region: outcomes after multimodality treatment. Cancer. 2009;115(14):3262-70.
61. Soyeur S, Chang EL, Selek U, et al. Intracranial meningeal hemangiopericytoma: the role of radiotherapy. Report of 29 cases and review of the literature. Cancer. 2004;100:1491-7.
62. Gelderblom H, Hogendoorn PC, Djikstra SD, et al. The clinical approach towards chondrosarcoma. Oncologist. 2008;13(3):320-9.
63. Combs S, Thilmann C, Debus J, et al. Precision radiotherapy for hemangiopericytomas of the central nervous system. Cancer. 2005;104:2457-65.
64. Tran LM, Mark R, Meier R, et al. Sarcomas of the head and neck: prognostic factors and treatment strategies. Cancer. 1992;70:169-77.
65. Yu MC, Yuan JM. Epidemiology of nasopharyngeal carcinoma. Semin Cancer Biol. 2002;12(6):421-9.
66. Caponigro F, Longo F, Ionna F, et al. Treatment approaches to nasopharyngeal carcinoma: a review. Anticancer Drugs. 2010;21(5):471-7.
67. Chan AT. Nasopharyngeal carcinoma. Ann Oncol. 2010;21(Suppl 7):vii308-12.
68. Al-Sarraf M. Treatment of locally advanced head and neck cancer: historical and critical review. Cancer Control. 2002;9(5):387-99.
69. Kwong DL, Nicholls J, Wei WI, et al. The time course of histologic remission after treatment of patients with nasopharyngeal carcinoma. Cancer. 1999;85(7):1446-53.
70. Fee WE Jr, Moir MS, Choi EC, et al. Nasopharyngectomy for recurrent nasopharyngeal cancer: a 2 to 17-year follow-up. Arch Otolaryngol Head Neck Surg. 2002;128:280-4.
71. Wei WI, Lam KH, Sham JS. New approach to the nasopharynx: the maxillary swing approach. Head Neck. 1991;13:200-7.
72. Longsdon M, Ha C, Kavadi V, et al. Lymphoma of the nasal cavity and paranasal sinuses. Improved outcome and altered prognostic factors with combined modality therapy. Cancer. 1997;80:477-88.
73. Kayrouz T, Jose B, Chu Am, et al. Solitary plasmacytoma. J Surg Oncol. 1983;24:46-8.
74. Alexious C, Kau RJ, Dietzfelbinger H, et al. Extramedullary plasmacytoma: tumor occurrence and therapeutic concepts. Cancer. 1999;85:2305-14.
75. Shreif J, Covonas P, Mastonikolis N, et al. Extramedullary plasmacytomas of the nasal cavity. Otolaryngol Head Neck Surg. 2001;124:119-20.
76. Prescher A, Brors D. Metastases to the paranasal sinuses: case report and review of the literature. Laryngorhinootologie. 2001;80(10):583-94.
77. McClatchey KD, Lloyd RV, Schaldenbrand JD. Metastatic carcinoma to the sphenoid sinus. Case report and review of the literature. Arch Otorhinolaryngol. 1985;241(3):219-24.
78. Mickel RA, Zimmerman MC. The sphenoid sinus—a site for metastasis. Otolaryngol Head Neck Surg. 1990;102(6):709-16.
79. Laigle-Donadey F, Taillibert S, Martin-Duverneuil N, et al. Skull-base metastases. J Neurooncol. 2005;75(1):63-9.

Index

Page numbers followed by *f* refer to figures and *t* refer to tables.

T

U

V

W

Z